Emergency Department Resuscitation

Editors

SUSAN R. WILCOX
MICHAEL E. WINTERS

EMERGENCY MEDICINE
CLINICS OF NORTH AMERICA

www.emed.theclinics.com

Consulting Editor
AMAL MATTU

November 2020 • Volume 38 • Number 4

ELSEVIER

1600 John F. Kennedy Boulevard • Suite 1800 • Philadelphia, Pennsylvania, 19103-2899

http://www.theclinics.com

EMERGENCY MEDICINE CLINICS OF NORTH AMERICA Volume 38, Number 4
November 2020 ISSN 0733-8627, ISBN-13: 978-0-323-76107-9

Editor: John Vassallo
Developmental Editor: Casey Potter

Emergency Medicine Clinics of North America (ISSN 0733-8627) is published quarterly by Elsevier Inc., 360 Park Avenue South, New York, NY, 10010-1710. Months of issue are February, May, August, and November. Business and Editorial Offices: 1600 John F. Kennedy Boulevard, Suite 1800, Philadelphia, PA 19103-2899. Customer Service Office: 6277 Sea Harbor Drive, Orlando, FL 32887-4800. Periodicals postage paid at New York, NY, and additional mailing offices. Subscription prices are $100.00 per year (US students), $352.00 per year (US individuals), $716.00 per year (US institutions), $220.00 per year (international students), $462.00 per year (international individuals), $882.00 per year (international institutions), $100.00 per year (Canadian students), $411.00 per year (Canadian individuals), and $882.00 per year (Canadian institutions). International air speed delivery is included in all *Clinics'* subscription prices. All prices are subject to change without notice. POSTMASTER: Send address changes to *Emergency Medicine Clinics of North America*, Elsevier Periodicals Customer Service, 11830 Westline Industrial Drive, St. Louis, MO 63146. Customer Service (orders, claims, online, change of address): Elsevier Periodicals **Customer Service, 11830 Westline Industrial Drive, St. Louis, MO 63146. Tel: 1-800-654-2452 (U.S. and Canada); 314-453-7041 (outside U.S. and Canada). Fax: 314-453-5170. E-mail: journalscustomerservice-usa@elsevier.com (for print support); journalsonlinesupport-usa@elsevier.com (for online support)**.

Reprints. For copies of 100 or more of articles in this publication, please contact the Commercial Reprints Department, Elsevier Inc., 360 Park Avenue South, New York, NY 10010-1710. Tel.: 212-633-3874; Fax: 212-633-3820; E-mail: reprints@elsevier.com.

Emergency Medicine Clinics of North America is covered in *MEDLINE/PubMed (Index Medicus), Current Contents/Clinical Medicine, EMBASE/Excerpta Medica, BIOSIS, SciSearch, CINAHL, ISI/BIOMED,* and *Research Alert*.

Contributors

CONSULTING EDITOR

AMAL MATTU, MD
Professor and Vice Chair of Academic Affairs, Department of Emergency Medicine, University of Maryland School of Medicine, Baltimore, Maryland, USA

EDITORS

SUSAN R. WILCOX, MD
Chief, Division of Critical Care, Department of Emergency Medicine, Massachusetts General Hospital, Boston, Massachusetts, USA

MICHAEL E. WINTERS, MD
Professor of Emergency Medicine and Medicine, Vice Chair for Clinical and Administrative Affairs, Department of Emergency Medicine, University of Maryland School of Medicine, Baltimore, Maryland, USA

AUTHORS

JENELLE H. BADULAK, MD
Division of Pulmonary, Critical Care and Sleep Medicine, Department of Emergency Medicine, Acting Assistant Professor, University of Washington, Harborview Medical Center, Seattle, Washington, USA

NICOLE BENZONI, MD, MPHS
Department of Emergency Medicine, Indiana University, Indianapolis, Indiana, USA

KATRINA D'AMORE, DO, MPH
Core Faculty, Department of Emergency Medicine, Good Samaritan Hospital Medical Center, West Islip, New York, USA

TIMOTHY ELLENDER, MD
Department of Emergency Medicine, Indiana University, Indianapolis, Indiana, USA

JONATHAN ELMER, MD, MSc
Assistant Professor, Departments of Emergency Medicine, Critical Care Medicine, and Neurology, University of Pittsburgh, Pittsburgh, Pennsylvania, USA

MICHAEL S. FARRELL, MD, MS
Clinical Fellow, Department of Surgery, University of California, San Francisco, San Francisco, California, USA

SAMUEL FRANCIS, MD
Division of Emergency Medicine, Department of Surgery, Duke University Hospital, Durham, North Carolina, USA

DAVID GORDON, MD
Fellow, Department of Medicine, University of Maryland Medical Center, Baltimore, Maryland, USA

SARA H. GRAY, MD, FRCPC, MPH
Emergency Medicine and Critical Care, St. Michael's Hospital, Associate Professor, University of Toronto, Toronto, Ontario, Canada

DANIEL HAASE, MD
Assistant Professor of Emergency Medicine and Critical Care, Department of Emergency Medicine, University of Maryland School of Medicine, Baltimore, Maryland, USA

CHRISTOPHER HICKS, MD, MEd, FRCPC
Emergency Physician, Trauma Team Leader, St Michael's Hospital, Toronto, Ontario, Canada

ALETA S. HONG, MD
Clinical Instructor, Department of Internal Medicine, University of Maryland School of Medicine, Baltimore, Maryland, USA

CINDY H. HSU, MD, PhD
Assistant Professor, Departments of Emergency Medicine, and Surgery, Michigan Center for Integrative Research in Critical Care, University of Michigan Medical School, Ann Arbor, Michigan, USA

KAMI M. HU, MD, FAAEM
Assistant Professor, Departments of Emergency Medicine and Internal Medicine, University of Maryland School of Medicine, Baltimore, Maryland, USA

CHRISTOPHER KABRHEL, MD, MPH
Department of Emergency Medicine, Center for Vascular Emergencies, Massachusetts General Hospital, Boston, Massachusetts, USA

WOON CHO KIM, MD, MPH
Clinical Fellow, Department of Surgery, University of California, San Francisco, San Francisco, California, USA

VIVIAN LAM, MD, MPH
Resident Physician, Department of Emergency Medicine, University of Michigan Medical School, Ann Arbor, Michigan, USA

MICHAEL J. LAURIA, MD, NRP, FP-C
Department of Emergency Medicine, University of New Mexico School of Medicine, Albuquerque, New Mexico, USA

SARA MANNING, MD
Assistant Professor, Department of Emergency Medicine, University of Maryland School of Medicine, Baltimore, Maryland, USA

NATHAN W. MICK, MD, FACEP
Vice Chair, Department of Emergency Medicine, Division Director, Pediatric Emergency Medicine, Maine Medical Center, Portland, Maine, USA; Associate Professor, Tufts University School of Medicine, Boston, Massachusetts, USA

JESSICA MONAS, MD
Senior Associate Consultant, Assistant Professor, Department of Emergency Medicine, Mayo Clinic Alix School of Medicine, Mayo Clinic Hospital, Phoenix, Arizona, USA

ZACHARY SHINAR, MD
Attending Physician, Department of Emergency Medicine, Sharp Memorial Hospital, San Diego, California, USA

AARON SKOLNIK, MD
Senior Associate Consultant, Department of Critical Care Medicine, Assistant Professor, Department of Emergency Medicine, Mayo Clinic Alix School of Medicine, Mayo Clinic Hospital, Phoenix, Arizona, USA

RORY SPIEGEL, MD
Attending Emergency Medicine, Georgetown University Hospital, Washington Hospital Center, Faculty Critical Care, Washington, DC, USA

DEBORAH M. STEIN, MD, MPH
Vice Chair of Trauma and Critical Care Surgery, Department of Surgery, University of California, San Francisco, Professor and Chief of Surgery, Zuckerberg San Francisco General Hospital, San Francisco, California, USA

ALEXIS STEINBERG, MD
Assistant Professor, Departments of Neurology and Critical Care Medicine, University of Pittsburgh, Pittsburgh, Pennsylvania, USA

ANAND SWAMINATHAN, MD, MPH
Assistant Professor of Emergency Medicine, St. Joseph's University Medical Center, Paterson, New Jersey, USA

WILLIAM TEETER, MD, MS
Assistant Professor of Emergency Medicine and Critical Care, Department of Emergency Medicine, University of Maryland School of Medicine, Baltimore, Maryland, USA

RACHEL J. WILLIAMS, MD
Assistant Professor, Tufts University School of Medicine, Boston, Massachusetts, USA; Pediatric Emergency Medicine, Maine Medical Center, Portland, Maine, USA

DAVID P. YAMANE, MD
Assistant Professor, Departments of Emergency Medicine, Anesthesia and Critical Care Medicine, George Washington University, Washington, DC, USA

Contents

Excellent resuscitation requires technical skills and knowledge, but also the right mindset. Expert practitioners must master their internal affective state, and create the environment that leads to optimal team performance. Leaders in resuscitation should use structured approaches to prepare for resuscitation, and psychological skills to enhance their performance including mental rehearsal, positive self-talk, explicit communication strategies, and situational awareness skills. Postevent recovery is equally important. Providers should have explicit plans for recovery after traumatic cases, including developing resilience and self-compassion. Experts in resuscitation can improve their performance (and that of their team) by consciously incorporating psychological skills into their armamentarium.

There are approximately 350,000 out-of-hospital cardiac arrests and 200,000 in-hospital cardiac arrests annually in the United States, with survival rates of approximately 5% to 10% and 24%, respectively. The critical factors that have an impact on cardiac arrest survival include prompt recognition and activation of prehospital care, early cardiopulmonary resuscitation, and rapid defibrillation. Advanced life support protocols are continually refined to optimize intracardiac arrest management and improve survival with favorable neurologic outcome. This article focuses on current treatment recommendations for adult nontraumatic cardiac arrest, with emphasis on the latest evidence and controversies regarding intracardiac arrest management.

Patients resuscitated from cardiac arrest require complex management. An organized approach to early postarrest care can improve patient outcomes. Priorities include completing a focused diagnostic work-up to identify and reverse the inciting cause of arrest, stabilizing cardiorespiratory instability to prevent rearrest, minimizing secondary brain injury,

This article examines, using an organ-systems based approach, rapid diagnosis, resuscitation, and critical care management of the crashing poisoned patient in the emergency department. The topics discussed in this article include seizures and status epilepticus, respiratory failure, cardiovascular collapse and mechanical circulatory support, antidotes and drug-specific therapies, acute liver failure, and extracorporeal toxin removal.

The obesity pandemic now affects hundreds of millions of people worldwide. As obesity rates continue to increase, emergency physicians are called on with increasing frequency to resuscitate obese patients. This article discusses important anatomic, physiologic, and practical challenges imposed by obesity on resuscitative care. Impacts on hemodynamic monitoring, airway and ventilator management, and pharmacologic therapy are discussed. Finally, several important clinical scenarios (trauma, cardiac arrest, and sepsis), in which alterations to standard treatments may benefit obese patients, are highlighted.

Massive gastrointestinal hemorrhage is a life-threatening condition that can result from numerous causes and requires skilled resuscitation to decrease patient morbidity and mortality. Successful resuscitation begins with placement of large-bore intravenous or intraosseous access; early blood product administration; and early consultation with a gastroenterologist, interventional radiologist, and/or surgeon. Activate a massive transfusion protocol when initial red blood cell transfusion does not restore effective perfusion or the patient's shock index is greater than 1.0. Promptly reverse coagulopathies secondary to oral anticoagulant or antiplatelet use. Use thromboelastography or rotational thromboelastometry to guide further transfusions. Secure a definitive airway and minimize aspiration.

Evaluating and treating traumatic cardiac arrest remains a challenge to the emergency medicine provider. Guidelines have established criteria for patients who can benefit from treatment and resuscitation versus those who will likely not survive. Patient factors that predict survival are penetrating injury, signs of life with emergency medical services or on arrival to the Emergency Department, short length of prehospital cardiopulmonary resuscitation, cardiac motion on ultrasound, pediatric patients, and those with reversible causes including pericardial tamponade and tension pneumothorax. Newer technologies such as resuscitative endovascular balloon occlusion of the aorta, selective aortic arch perfusion, and extracorporeal membrane oxygenation may improve outcomes, but remain primarily investigational.

Care of the critically ill pregnant patient is anxiety-provoking for those unprepared, as the emergency physician must consider not only the welfare of the immediate patient, but of the fetus as well. Familiarity with the physiologic changes of pregnancy and how they affect clinical presentation and management is key. Although some medications may be safer in pregnancy than others, stabilizing the pregnant patient is paramount. Emergency physicians should target pregnancy-specific oxygen and ventilation goals and hemodynamics and should be prepared to perform a perimortem cesarean section, should the mother lose pulses, to increase chances for maternal and fetal survival.

The geriatric population is growing and is the largest utilizer of emergency and critical care services; the emergency clinician should be comfortable in the management of the acutely ill geriatric patient. There are important physiologic changes in geriatric patients, which alters their clinical presentation and management. Age alone should not determine the prognosis for elderly patients. Premorbid functional status, frailty, and severity of illness should be considered carefully for the geriatric population. Emergency clinicians should have honest conversations about goals of care based not only a patient's clinical presentation but also the patient's values.

Emergency physicians must be prepared to rapidly diagnose and resuscitate patients with pulmonary embolism (PE). Certain aspects of PE resuscitation run counter to typical approaches. A specific understanding of the pathophysiology of PE is required to avoid cardiovascular collapse potentially associated with excessive intravenous fluids and positive pressure ventilation. Once PE is diagnosed, rapid risk stratification should be performed and treatment guided by patient risk class. Although anticoagulation remains the mainstay of PE treatment, emergency physicians also must understand the indications and contraindications for thrombolysis and should be aware of new therapies and models of care that may improve outcomes.

 Video content accompanies this article at http://www.emed. theclinics.com.

Extracorporeal membrane oxygenation (ECMO) is a mechanical way to provide oxygenation, ventilation, and perfusion to patients with severe cardiopulmonary failure. Extracorporeal cardiopulmonary resuscitation (ECPR) describes the use of ECMO during cardiac arrest. ECPR requires an organized approach to resuscitation, cannula insertion, and pump initiation. Selecting the right patients for ECPR is an important aspect of successful programs. A solid understanding of the components of the ECMO circuit is critical to troubleshooting problems. Current evidence suggests a substantial benefit of ECPR compared with traditional CPR for refractory cardiac arrest but is limited by lack of randomized trials to date.

EMERGENCY MEDICINE
CLINICS OF NORTH AMERICA

SERIES OF RELATED INTEREST

Orthopedic Clinics
https://www.orthopedic.theclinics.com/

THE CLINICS ARE NOW AVAILABLE ONLINE!
Access your subscription at:
www.theclinics.com

Erratum

In the May 2019 issue, in the article, "Postdelivery Emergencies" (Volume 37, number 2, pages 287-300), by Natasha Wheaton, Aws Al-Abdullah, and Tyler Haertlein, please note the following changes:

- On page 288: The sentence, "It occurs when the uterus does not contract after the third stage of labor (delivery of the baby)" should be changed to: "It occurs when the uterus does not adequately contract after delivery of the baby, during the third stage of labor."
- On page 290, Figure 1 should be replaced with the following figure:

California Maternal Quality Care Collaborative Four Stages of Postpartum Hemorrhage	
Stage 0	Normal postpartum bleeding
Stage 1	Cumulative blood loss >500 mL via Vaginal Birth (>1000 mL via Cesarean Section) OR- Vital Signs>15% change or HR ≥110, BP ≤85/45, O2 sat <95% OR- Increased bleeding during recovery or postpartum
Stage 2	Continued Bleeding or Vital Sign instability, and 1000–1500mL cumulative blood loss
Stage 3	Cumulative Blood Loss >1500 ml, >2 units pRBCs given, Vital Sign instability, or suspicion for Disseminated Intravascular Coagulopathy

- On page 292, in Box 2: The correct carboprost dose is 250 μg, not 0.25 μg as stated in the article.

Emerg Med Clin N Am 38 (2020) xiii
https://doi.org/10.1016/j.emc.2020.06.016
0733-8627/20/© 2020 Elsevier Inc. All rights reserved.

Foreword

Resuscitation

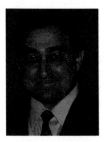

Amal Mattu, MD
Consulting Editor

During the early years in the creation of emergency medicine as its own specialty, questions continually arose about why emergency medicine should be a separate specialty. What is unique about emergency medicine that warrants its own standing as a specialty? After all, every other specialty involves emergencies, so why should there be a specialty focused just on emergencies? If a patient has a heart attack, the cardiologist can manage the emergency; if a patient has profuse hematemesis, the gastroenterologist can manage the emergency; if a patient is the victim of a gunshot wound to the abdomen, a surgeon can manage the emergency, and so on.

With time, however, physicians in other specialties realized that they were not well prepared to manage the *undifferentiated* emergency. For example, which specialist should be called if a patient presents in shock with a decreased level of consciousness and no obvious precipitating cause? In addition, they realized that none of the individual specialties were trained to manage patients with multisystem crises. For example, when a patient presents with sepsis leading to diabetic ketoacidosis, respiratory failure, and disseminated intravascular coagulopathy, does that patient need the infectious disease specialist, the endocrinologist, the anesthesiologist, or the hematologist? The answer eventually became clear: the patient needs a "multisystem undifferentiated resuscitationist." In other words, the patient needs the specialist that we now know of today as an "emergency physician."

Emergency medicine as a specialty developed from this need of physicians that were comprehensively trained in resuscitation. The primary goal of our specialty is to resuscitate and stabilize; diagnosis and definitive treatment are secondary goals, and in fact, are often not even accomplished during the emergency department stay. Resuscitation, however, is the sine qua non of our work. Consequently, we emergency physicians must be 100% committed to maintaining the most up-to-date knowledge of resuscitation at all times.

Emerg Med Clin N Am 38 (2020) xv–xvi
https://doi.org/10.1016/j.emc.2020.08.001
0733-8627/20/© 2020 Published by Elsevier Inc.

With this commitment in mind, I suggest to you that this issue of *Emergency Medicine Clinics of North America* should be considered must-reading for anyone who considers himself or herself an emergency physician. Trainees, advanced practice providers, and emergency medical services personnel should take note as well. Guest editors, Dr Susan Wilcox and Dr Michael Winters, both accomplished authors and educators in emergency resuscitation, have assembled an outstanding group of authors to teach us about the latest advances in resuscitation. The first article is a particularly interesting one that allows us to get inside the minds of expert resuscitationists. Subsequent articles focus on the bread-and-butter of resuscitation—cardiac arrest and postarrest care. Articles address the management of various causes of shock, including sepsis, trauma, overdose, and gastrointestinal bleeding. The authors have also addressed special populations, including resuscitation of pediatric patients, elder patients, obese patients, and pregnant patients. The final 2 articles address the critically ill patient with a pulmonary embolus and the use of extracorporeal membrane oxygenation in the emergency department.

Resuscitation is the foundation of our specialty. Drs Wilcox, Winters, and their excellent group of authors have significantly contributed to this foundation. Knowledge and practice of the concepts that are discussed in this issue are certain to save lives. Kudos to the guest editors and authors for providing us with this valuable addition to our specialty.

Amal Mattu, MD
Department of Emergency Medicine
University of Maryland School of Medicine
110 South Paca Street
6th Floor, Suite 200
Baltimore, MD 21201, USA

E-mail address:
amattu@som.umaryland.edu

Preface

Resuscitation in Emergency Medicine: Now More Important than Ever

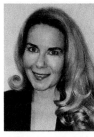
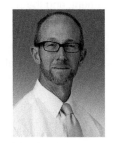

Susan R. Wilcox, MD   Michael E. Winters, MD
Editors

Resuscitation has long been a cornerstone of emergency medicine. Whether it is caring for the patient with cardiac arrest, acute respiratory distress, multisystem trauma, or undifferentiated shock, the emergency physician must be an expert at resuscitation. For many critically ill patients, it is the crucial initial hours of illness, when the patient is in the emergency department (ED), when lives can be saved. With our collective goal of saving lives, we have focused this issue of *Emergency Medicine Clinics of North America* on the resuscitation of our sickest ED patients. This issue begins with an outstanding article on how to best prepare yourself, and your team, for a successful resuscitation. The remaining articles provide critical resuscitation pearls on important topics that include cardiac arrest, post–cardiac arrest care, fluid resuscitation, sepsis, emergency transfusions, toxicologic emergencies, gastrointestinal hemorrhage, the crashing pregnant patient, and the initiation of extracorporeal membrane oxygenation in the ED. Written by experts in emergency medicine resuscitation, the articles in this issue provide the latest, evidence-based approaches to commonly encountered critical conditions. Quite simply, we feel this issue will help the emergency physician save lives!

As we completed the publication of this issue, we witnessed the unfolding of one of the greatest public health challenges and tragedies of the last century: the COVID-19 pandemic. Since this pandemic hit, starting in late February of 2020, Emergency Medicine has taken a strong leadership role within the health care system. Emergency physicians have not only provided outstanding clinical care in their EDs but also provided operational expertise as leaders within organizations locally, regionally, and nationally. Emergency physicians have been offering clinical innovations, authoring research papers, and leading national conversations around resuscitation of

Emerg Med Clin N Am 38 (2020) xvii–xviii
https://doi.org/10.1016/j.emc.2020.07.001
0733-8627/20/© 2020 Published by Elsevier Inc.   **emed.theclinics.com**

patients with COVID-19. This public health emergency has led to a deluge of critically ill patients in many EDs, with emergency clinicians now being called upon to resuscitate and manage critically ill patients at a much higher volume and for even longer periods of time than baseline.

Importantly, the articles in this issue were written and edited prior to this pandemic. However, increased experience with caring for patients with COVID-19 has shown us that the fundamentals of resuscitation and critical care still apply. As such, the approaches outlined in these articles provide an excellent foundation for taking care of all critically ill and injured patients in the ED, with COVID-19 or otherwise. For example, articles on fluid resuscitation, sepsis management, and the crashing obese patient are applicable to patients with COVID-19.

As we as a specialty look to move beyond this pandemic, returning to caring for our broad ED population is essential. As our patients return to the ED for customary care, it is essential that we as a specialty provide the most up-to-date evidence-based approaches. For the emergency physician, expertise in resuscitation may be more important now than ever.

Susan R. Wilcox, MD
Zero Emerson Place, Suite 3B
Boston, MA 02114, USA

Michael E. Winters, MD
2103 Huntington Terrace
Mt. Airy, MD 21771, USA

E-mail addresses:
Swilcox1@partners.org (S.R. Wilcox)
mwinters@som.umaryland.edu (M.E. Winters)

The Mindset of the Resuscitationist

Sara H. Gray, MD, FRCPC, MPH[a],*, Michael J. Lauria, MD, NRP, FP-C[b],
Christopher Hicks, MD, MEd, FRCPC[a]

KEYWORDS

• Resuscitation • Performance • Psychology • Resilience • Communication

KEY POINTS

• Expert resuscitation requires much more than just technical skill and knowledge: we must also understand and master our internal affective state and analyze the interplay between self and team.
• The Zero Point Survey provides a structured approach to self, team, and environmental preparation that should occur before the primary survey commences.
• Mental rehearsal and positive self-talk can realign subjective appraisal of a stressful event and facilitate performance. Specific techniques to improve communication and situation awareness help multimember teams to stay on task during dynamic events.
• Recovery is as important as preparation: reflection, self-compassion, and self-care can build resilience and prevent burnout.

INTRODUCTION

Developing strategies to optimize performance during crisis is an essential component of resuscitation. It is possible to practice for excellence, even under acutely stressful conditions. This article reviews strategies for optimizing performance before crisis arrives, during resuscitation, and for recovery after difficult cases, so that one can effectively return to work.

CASE SCENARIO

You are working your typical Saturday evening shift when you get a telephone call from a paramedic. A gunman has opened fire at a local concert where there are thousands of people in the audience. It is not clear how many people have been injured and there is chaos at the scene. You are the closest hospital. Patients will be arriving in 10 minutes. Are you prepared?

[a] St Michael's Hospital, Emergency Department Administration, 30 Bond Street, Toronto, ON M5B 1W8, Canada; [b] Department of Emergency Medicine, University of New Mexico School of Medicine, Albuquerque, NM, USA
* Corresponding author.
E-mail address: sara.gray@unityhealth.to
Twitter: @EmICUcanada (S.H.G.)

Emerg Med Clin N Am 38 (2020) 739–753
https://doi.org/10.1016/j.emc.2020.06.002
emed.theclinics.com
0733-8627/20/© 2020 Elsevier Inc. All rights reserved.

BEFORE THE CRISIS OCCURS

In an organized resuscitation, the primary survey should be preceded by a series of steps to ensure self, team, and environmental preparation. Ideally, effective teams start preparing to resuscitate before patients arrive.

The Zero Point Survey (ZPS) is a consensus-derived framework for organizing pre-primary survey discussions around self, team, and environmental preparation.[1] The ZPS is designed to create shared mental models, facilitate adaptive team coordination by direct team-based discussion and preparation before patient arrival, and is updated periodically once the resuscitation commences. The STEP-UP mnemonic is used to recall the elements of the ZPS (**Fig. 1**). Before patient arrival, team members are prompted to examine their own sense of psychological preparedness via I'M SAFE (illness, medication, stress, alcohol, fatigue, eating/elimination), followed by a focused examination of shared team roles, anticipated early priorities, and an environmental scan for equipment safety and logistics.

A preprimary survey accomplishes several key tasks relevant to coordination during chaotic and dynamic clinical events:

1. *Establishing clear and flexible shared mental models.* A mental model is a cognitive representation of current and anticipated features of an event or situation.[2,3] A mental model becomes shared when that same cognitive representation is mutually understood and acknowledged among team members.[4] Shared mental models

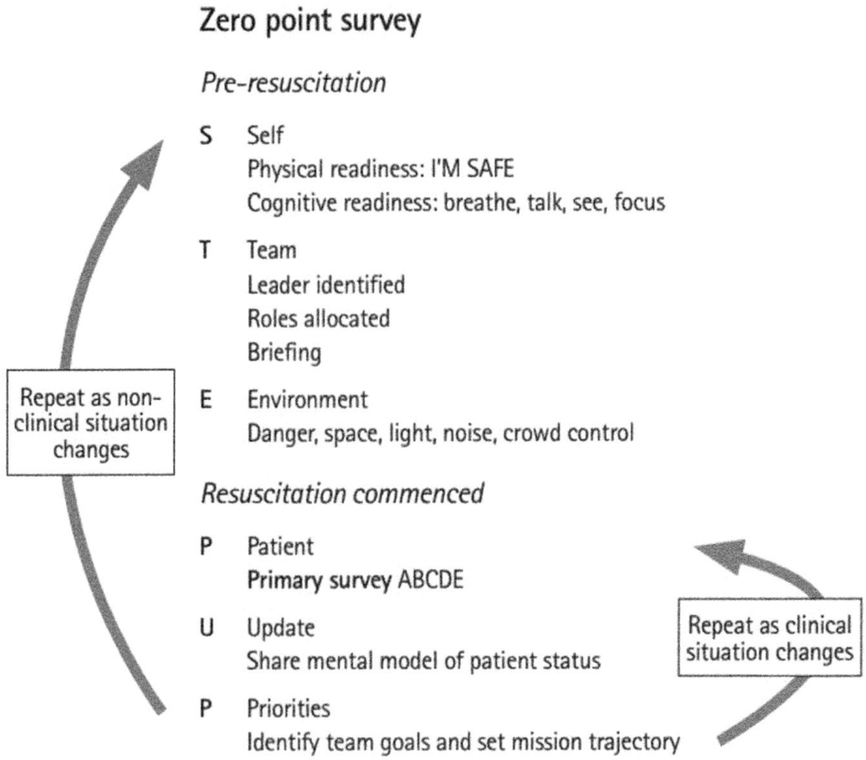

Zero point survey

Pre-resuscitation

S   Self
     Physical readiness: I'M SAFE
     Cognitive readiness: breathe, talk, see, focus

T   Team
     Leader identified
     Roles allocated
     Briefing

E   Environment
     Danger, space, light, noise, crowd control

Repeat as non-clinical situation changes

Resuscitation commenced

P   Patient
     Primary survey ABCDE

U   Update
     Share mental model of patient status

Repeat as clinical situation changes

P   Priorities
     Identify team goals and set mission trajectory

Fig. 1. Zero Point Survey and the STEP-UP mnemonic.

allow team members of varied backgrounds and clinical experience to create a common understanding of teamwork and task work relevant to the situation at hand.[5] As a dynamic event progresses, the mental model needs to be periodically updated to incorporate new data and changing priorities.[6] A structured preprimary survey can help to clarify elements of an ambiguous clinical event, allow for team input and challenge-response queries, and allow the team leaders to establish early goals and priorities.

2. *Creating a shared sense of psychological safety.* To function cohesively under stressful, time-pressured conditions, team members need to be reassured that they have the permission to ask questions, admit mistakes, or challenge the team leader. The key to facilitating positive social interactions within teams is establishing a sufficient sense of psychological safety: that is, that the team environment is safe for interpersonal risk-taking.[7] Psychological safety is correlated with improved safety behaviors, such as error reporting, and promotes knowledge and power sharing, cogeneration, and team learning.[7] Structured briefings can help create psychological safety by clarifying what is known, and by extension what remains unknown about a clinical scenario and provide an avenue for team members to ask questions and request clarification ahead of engaging in the hands-on work of the primary survey.

3. *Conducting a methodical environmental and safety scan.* The resuscitation environment is hazardous for providers, and in many situations team hazards are accepted as an unavoidable or unnoticed element of resuscitation practice. It is our contention that the clinical environment should not be unsafe for patient or provider, and a simple focused environmental and equipment scan can help identify and mitigate latent safety hazards before they can inflict harm.[8] This may include: the provision of adequate lighting, positioning and spacing of procedure trays and carts in relation to the provider, positioning the stretcher centrally to ensure 360° patient access, unencumbering monitoring wires and sterile equipment, and appointing a logistics and safety officer to monitor and mitigate emerging hazards as the case progresses.

CASE SCENARIO

You have divided into teams, prebriefed, and assigned roles. You have selected rooms and thoughtfully arranged your equipment. The first patients arrive: a woman with a gunshot to her leg, and man with multiple gunshots to his torso. The paramedics describe the scene as chaotic and overwhelming. They say "countless" more patients are coming. You fear your resources will be overwhelmed, and your anxiety levels are rising. You want to focus on the patient in front of you but you feel distracted by thoughts of the impending disaster.

DURING THE RESUSCITATION

Once the resuscitation is commenced, an ABCDE primary survey is undertaken and periodic updates are provided to ensure accurate and flexible shared mental models and set priorities dynamically. The STEP-UP process can be repeated throughout the resuscitation based on evolving clinical and nonclinical demands.

Strategies to Facilitate the Zero Point Survey During Resuscitation

1. *Use short, structured prebriefings.* In the authors resuscitation practice, we use four simple questions in a challenge-response format:
   i. What do *we know*, based on limited prehospital notification?

    ii. What will *we do* based on what we know (Plan A)?

    iii. What will *we change* based on changing information or failure of Plan A (Plan B)?

    iv. What are *the roles* for all team members?

2. *Perform tactical pauses and 10-for-10 snap briefs.* As the resuscitation progresses, the mental model needs to be updated in an equally concise fashion. A tactical pause refers to a deliberate break in case action to summarize, reflect, and set priorities for next stages in care. During a tactical pause all nonessential clinical activity stops and all team members listen, reflect, and are asked to respond as needed. The 10-for-10 snap briefs involve 10-second updates provided by the team leader every 10 minutes, and include a brief recap of the case, clinical events happening now, anticipated next steps and priorities, and role allocation or clarification.

Psychological Skills to Manage Stress and Improve Performance

Psychological skills are discrete, trained interventions that leverage higher level thought processes and innate physiology to mitigate the sequelae of the human stress response.[9] These skills incorporate everything from breathing and relaxation techniques to cognitive restructuring interventions (the process of identifying and stopping negative or irrational thoughts).[10] They have been adapted to a host of different domains and shown benefit: musicians, business executives, and military personnel.[11–15] Psychological skills are used before and during resuscitation to optimize stress levels and performance.

    Recently, the US military has specifically explored the applications of teaching psychological skills to medical personnel with the intention of improving their ability to provide emergency medical care under the most stressful of circumstances.[16,17] Outside the military, civilians have also demonstrated the benefit of developing these skills as it pertains to specific surgical procedures[18] or trauma resuscitation.[19] There are a handful of skills, in particular, that may be most helpful in emergency care.

1. *Controlled breathing.* There is a strong relationship between respiration and emotion.[20–22] Breathing techniques have been shown to increase an individual's ability to regulate emotion: decreasing anxiety, hyperarousal, and attention selectivity.[23] When a slow, deep, controlled respiratory cycle is used there are significant, measurable decreases in heart rate.[20,24] Perhaps the most practical method for using this in resuscitation is to use what many performance psychology experts refer to as "square breathing" or "box breathing."[25–27] Inhale deeply for approximately 4 seconds, engaging your diaphragm and attempting to pull the breath down into your abdomen. Hold the breath for 4 seconds. Then, exhale slowly over the course of 4 seconds and hold the lungs empty for 4 seconds.

2. *Positive self-talk.* An individual's internal monologue is critical when it comes to how one assesses and responds to the challenges one is presented with.[28,29] Self-talk is used to enhance one's perception of the situation, which psychologists refer to as "cognitive reframing," and increases the likelihood of successful task completion.[30–32] Psychologists have identified several types of self-talk that are helpful, two of which seem to be most helpful in emergency medical situations: instructional and motivational. Instructional self-talk entails walking yourself through the discrete steps or technical maneuvers of a procedure; for example, when placing a thoracostomy tube saying "now advance over the rib and into the pleural cavity." Motivational self-talk, however, is affirmative statements that bolster confidence, such as "I can do this."[33–36]

3. *Visualization or mental practice.* Visualizing is a specific technique that acts as a mental video of what successful execution should look like. Evidence suggests that just thinking through the steps of a task activates the same neural architecture needed to actually perform it.[37,38] Over the years, there has been significant data from athletics demonstrating the performance benefit of mental practice, also referred to as the use of "mental imagery."[39–42] However, it was not until recently that mental practice has been used to enhance performance of specific surgical skills,[43,44] cardiac arrest resuscitation,[45] or trauma resuscitation.[46] Some authors have even characterized the most effective way to implement the use of mental imagery: imagine the physical nature of the ask, the environment the task will be carried out in, the timing of critical steps, and the perspective of the person performing the task.[47,48]

4. *Trigger or cue words.* Using a trigger word can drive attention control. Cognitive science experts often explain attention, the concentration of mental effort on sensory inputs or executive processes, using the metaphor of a spotlight.[49,50] Selective attention on important resuscitation technical skills, such as laryngoscopy, is important and requires a clinician to keep their mental spotlight fixed for a period of time. Any internal or external stimulus that distracts attention can result in failure to accomplish a task or induce errors.[51–55] Attention, however, can be consciously controlled.[9] Specifically, in the presence of distractions a trigger or cue word, such as "focus" or "concentrate," can be used to turn selective attention to a specific task.[56,57]

Communication

Effective communication is essential to successful teamwork, particularly in stressful and dynamic situations. Failure of communication has been cited as a primary contributor to mishaps and accidents in several high-risk industries[58,59] including clinical medicine.[60,61] Therefore, in resuscitation, it is important to understand what constitutes good communication.

1. *Use clear and direct language.* First and foremost, the structure of our communication is critical. During emergency situations when time pressure exists and the cognitive load on individual participants is high, being explicit is important. It is best to avoid mitigating language (vague or noncommittal).[62] In combat aviation, language is structured such that the most important information comes first, follow by information that augments the most critical content. The mantra used in these circumstances is "directive, descriptive, informative." An example during the resuscitation of a critically ill patient might be, "John, please place a right humoral intraosseous access immediately [directive]. We have no other vascular access after several attempts [descriptive] and need to administer medications emergently [informative]." In the civilian world experts in communication and crew resource management refer to the "C's of Communication"; two important characteristics being *clear* and *concise* communication.[63,64]

2. *Use standard terminology.* Standardizing language is also important. In general, team performance is more efficient when standardized terminology is used.[65,66] When people hear expected or predictable words or phrases they seem to be able to coordinate activities and perform critical tasks more effectively. This seems to hold true when validated team performance tools are used to compare the work of teams that use a standardized vernacular with teams that communicate in nonstandardized ways. It is also important to acknowledge that standardized communication does not mean inflexible or rigid communication. Some

authors have suggested that using standard phraseology is important, but when faced with an uncertain, time-sensitive situation more flexible communication is effective.[67]

3. *Time your communication effectively.* Knowing when to communicate is equally imperative. At times, team members are so focused on activities or busy completing other critical tasks, they may not be prepared to receive a message. Actually, under high-cognitive workload conditions, decreased (or limited) team communication correlated with better team performance.[68] Anticipating that a team member may need a key piece of information relayed is paramount. Studies demonstrate that an important characteristic of high-functioning teams is that members anticipate the needs of others and communicate important information before it is requested.[69]

4. *Use closed-loop communication.* One challenge when it comes to communication is ensuring that certain information is heard, acknowledged, and processed by those that may be in charge. Therefore, closed-loop communication is important. This means that instructions between team members are reinforced by verbal feedback.[70,71] The important aspect of this behavior is that information is provided to the message originator with positive confirmation that a task is complete.

5. *Use graded assertiveness.* At times, even though a message is received the communication may not be met with appropriate action. Problems with cognitive overload or challenge with authority gradients have been found to cause communication breakdown and untoward results.[59,72,73] As a result in many high-risk occupations, not only are team members taught to speak up, but they are also taught how to used increased grades of assertiveness to bring important information to light. One common method is using the four-step PACE communication method.[74] In this graded communication approach, one starts by asking a probing question, then escalates to an alert, followed by challenging statement, and ultimately and emergency warning if the concern is still not acknowledged.

6. *Align your body language with your words.* In addition to the actual words that are spoken, the body language that accompanies words is critical. Nonverbal communication is the deliberate or unintentional signaling of emotional state without words. In certain situations authors have suggested that in face-to-face communication most communication (up to 55%) is nonverbal.[75] Facial expressions, body posture, hand gestures, and eye movements are all critical accompaniments to the words we use.[76] For these reasons, it is important that body language also be directly aligned with verbal communication so that the verbal message is reinforced as opposed to contradicted.

7. *Facilitate psychological safety and encourage team input.* During a stressful event, team members are markedly responsive to verbal and nonverbal cues. Social contagion describes the process by which team members adopt the attitudes and behaviors of others around them. By viewing teams as tightly coupled social networks, psychological safety can spread outward, based on the phrasing and posture of the team leader, a process termed "contagion by cohesion."[77] To that end, specific phrases can help to establish psychological safety by expressing, where appropriate, optimism, uncertainty, or the need for team input. Some examples include:

- I'm glad I'm here, with you, to do our best.
- What am I missing/What are we missing?
- I really need your help and input with the following …

CASE SCENARIO

In the end, 50 patients arrived in your emergency department from the concert. You stayed at work hours late before you finally go home. Once there, you feel exhausted, but you cannot sleep. Your mind keeps returning to the images from the disaster. Six weeks later, you still are not sleeping. You are having flashbacks. You are irritable at work. You are wondering if you will ever recover.

AFTER THE CRISIS HAS ENDED

To enter a resuscitation fully prepared, with the optimized mindset, it is essential to have healed from previous difficult cases. Working as a first responder or in the emergency department is a challenging, high-stress workplace. Over time, these environments take a psychological toll on front-line health care providers.

This is evidenced by high rates of burnout. Burnout is characterized by emotional depletion, cynicism, and a low sense of personal accomplishment.[78] Burnout has garnered significant media attention lately, in addition to scientific investigations, which cite alarming rates of burnout among doctors. Emergency medicine physicians show the highest burnout rates among all specialties assessed.[79] Burnout is also highly prevalent in nurses, with 33% of in-hospital nurses showing burnout in a 2001 study.[80] Physician assistants' burnout rates are in the initial phases of investigation, but early reports suggest that their burnout rates may also be elevated.[81] This is not merely personally relevant; burnout has been associated with worsened patient outcomes across doctors, nurses, and medical students.[82] Burnout and stress also impact the ability to perform stressful procedures, and to resuscitate effectively **(Fig. 2)**.[83]

Suicide rates for health care providers are similarly terrifying. In the United States, one physician commits suicide every day, and the rate of physician suicide (28–40 per 100,000) is more than double the rate in the general population (12.3 per 100,000).[84] For resident physicians, suicide is the second leading cause of death after malignancy.[85] Nurses are impacted similarly, with higher rates of nurse suicide than gender-matched control subjects.[86]

When providers experience exhaustion, fatigue, and burnout, they may struggle to optimize their resuscitation performance. Accordingly, embracing strategies for wellness and resilience become essential components of effective resuscitation.

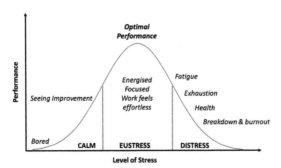

Fig. 2. Performance efficacy varies with stress level. (*Data from* Yerkes RM, Dodson JD (1908). "The relation of strength of stimulus to rapidity of habit-formation". Journal of Comparative Neurology and Psychology. 18 (5): 459–482. https://doi.org/10.1002/cne. 920180503.)

Strategies for Recovery from Your Last Case

1. *Do not stay silent.* One common strategy includes developing a supportive network for discussing difficult cases and sharing reactions and emotions. Providers may talk to colleagues, friends, or family. In recent commentary, these confidants have been termed "failure friends"; people selected for empathy, kindness, and listening skills.[87] Good social support is strongly associated with lower rates of burnout.[88–90]

2. *Practice self-compassion.* Practicing self-compassion is associated with healing after trauma. Self-compassion includes three main components: self-kindness, common humanity, and mindfulness.[91] Self-kindness includes the ability to treat ourselves kindly, even after failure. Common humanity is the concept that we are not alone and isolated, that other people have experienced similar emotions and reactions. Lastly, mindfulness allows us to hold emotions in a balanced perspective, rather than overidentifying with them.[91] Mindfulness can provide the difference between "it was all my fault" and "I played a small role in a large series of mishaps that led to an unfortunate outcome." Readers who want to assess their own level of self-compassion can pursue a validated quiz at www.selfcompassion.org. It can also be valuable to simply listen to your own inner voice during moments of difficulty or stress, and to assess whether your inner voice is kind and supportive, or critical and judgmental. Self-compassion is a crucial component of recovering after a difficult case, and is also associated with lower rates of burnout, lower stress, and increased ability to provide compassionate care to patients.[92] Physicians who are higher in self-compassion are more engaged in work, less exhausted, and more satisfied with their work lives.[93] Medical students who are higher in self-compassion have lower rates of burnout and maladaptive perfectionism,[94] which raises the possibility of future interventions based on training and practice in self-compassion. Compassion fatigue is an important concept that can arise after secondary traumatic stress.[95] Health care providers may benefit from targeted strategies to reduce compassion fatigue including debriefing with colleagues, exercise, spiritual practices, and spending time with family.[96]

3. *Build resilience.* Resilience is the ability with bounce back after hardship or to maintain competency during prolonged stress.[97–99] Resilience is comprised of a combination of factors:
   - Internal (eg, genetics, optimism, self-regulation)[98,99]
   - External (eg, social supports, workplace characteristics, experience of trauma)[98]
   - Skill-based (eg, finding meaning, problem-solving, practicing mindfulness)[97,100]
   It is vital to recognize the skill-based nature of resilience. Health care providers can develop strategies for building their own personal resilience, based on their individual needs and strengths.[100] Different authors highlight the wide variety of available interventions, which are summarized in **Table 1**.[83,101–104]

Health care providers who choose to build their resilience can focus on developing the factors most relevant to them. It should also be noted that many strategies can be developed at the level of the workplace or organization, which can significantly impact the wellbeing of the workforce. The concept of professional coaching is gaining increasing traction in health care after a recent pilot study demonstrating that coaching reduced burnout and increased quality of life among a cohort of physicians.[105] One proposed mechanism is that professional coaching reduces burnout by increasing the client's sense of control.[101] This can increase efficacy and self-determination, which have been associated

Table 1
Strategies to increase resilience and reduce burnout

Personal Strategies	Workplace Strategies
Focus on optimism and gratitude	Develop supportive management
Keep a sense of humor	Encourage supportive professional
Stay adaptable	relationships
Pursue a healthy lifestyle (nutrition,	Decrease workload/hours
sleep, exercise)	Increase participation in decision-making
Spend time in mindfulness, prayer, or self-	Develop supportive team culture and
reflection	mentorship
Reduce stress where possible	Change evaluation of work goals
Spend time with supportive family and	Engage in professional coaching
friends	
Engage in hobbies	
Schedule time for self-care	
Choose work you are passionate about	

Data from Refs.[83,101–104]

with decreased rates of burnout.[106,107] Coaching is an option that either workplaces or individuals can pursue.

4. *Get professional help when you need it* After traumatic events, health care providers can develop post-traumatic stress symptoms or disorder. Many treatment options are available with documented evidence for efficacy.[108] Providers with ongoing symptoms should be encouraged to consider professional help and to reach out for support. Efforts to reduce stigma around this issue are vital. Encouraging a colleague to seek help can save a life. Providers in crisis in the United States can reach out to the National Suicide Prevention Lifeline at https://suicidepreventionlifeline.org/ or call their 24/7 toll-free confidential number at 1-800-273-8255. In Canada, providers can get support from Crisis Services Canada at https://www.crisisservicescanada.ca/en/ or call their 24/7 confidential number at 1-833-456-4566.

CASE RESOLUTION

You talk to friends and colleagues about the disaster, and work to increase your resilience through exercise, nutrition, and a new mindfulness practice. Despite these valuable efforts, you remain traumatized by the disaster and feel your work is being impacted. With the support of your colleagues, you see a therapist who assists you in your recovery. In the end you regain your previous passion and motivation for work, and help your hospital design more robust protocols for mass casualty events.

SUMMARY

Preparing for ideal resuscitation performance starts before the patients arrive, and extends long after they leave the emergency department. Maintaining a knowledge base and technical skills are important, but optimizing ones psychological skillset is also vital. Experts in resuscitation use preplanned approaches to resuscitation, discrete communication skills, psychological skills to manage stress and optimize performance, and resilience and self-compassion skills to recover after challenging cases. These skills are learned, honed and improved with time and attention.

Our job is not easy. We often feel challenged. But preparation for optimal resuscitation is worth the effort.

DISCLOSURE

The authors have nothing to disclose.

REFERENCES

1. Reid C, Brindley P, Hicks C, et al. Zero Point Survey: a multidisciplinary idea to STEP UP resuscitation effectiveness. Clin Exp Emerg Med 2018;5(3):139–43.
2. Wilson MH, Habig K, Wright C, et al. Pre-hospital emergency medicine. Lancet 2015;386(10012):2526–34.
3. Endsley M. Toward a theory of situation awareness in dynamic systems. Hum Factors 1995;37:32–64.
4. Shrestha L, Prince C, Baker D, et al. Understanding situation awareness: concepts, methods, training. Hum Tech Interact Complex Sys 1995;7:45–83. Available at: https://www.air.org/resource/understanding-situational-awareness-concepts-methods-and-training. Accessed July 15 2020.
5. Lim B-C, Klein KJ. Team mental models and team performance: a field study of the effects of team mental model similarity and accuracy. J Organiz Behav 2006; 27(4):403–18.
6. Gaba D, Howard S, Small S. Situation awareness in anesthesiology. Hum Factors 1995;37:20–31.
7. Edmonson A. Psychological safety and learning behavior in work teams. Admin Sci Q 1999;44(2):350–83.
8. Hicks C, Petrosoniak A. The human factor: optimizing trauma team performance in dynamic clinical environments. Emerg Med Clin North Am 2018;36(1):1–17.
9. Weinberg R, Gould D. Foundations of sport and exercise psychology 6th edition with web study guide. 6th edition. Champaign (IL): Human Kinetics; 2014.
10. Greenspan MJ, Feltz DL. Psychological interventions with athletes in competitive situations: a review. Sports Psychol 1989;3(3):219–36.
11. Osborne MS, Greene DJ, Immel DT. Managing performance anxiety and improving mental skills in conservatoire students through performance psychology training: a pilot study. Psychol Well Being 2014;4(1):1–17.
12. Fred Luthans, James BAvey, Jaime LPatera. Experimental Analysis of a Web-Based Training Intervention to Develop Positive Psychological Capital. AMLE 2008;7:209–21. https://doi.org/10.5465/amle.2008.32712618.
13. Luthans BC, Luthans KW, Avey JB. Building the leaders of tomorrow the development of academic psychological capital. J Leadersh Organ Stud 2014;21(2): 191–9.
14. Janelle C, Hatfield B. Visual attention and brain processes that underlie expert performance: implications for sport and military psychology. Mil Psychol 2008; 20(1):39.
15. Saunders T, Driskell JE, Johnston JH, et al. The effect of stress inoculation training on anxiety and performance. J Occup Health Psychol 1996;1(2): 170–86.
16. Herzog TP, Deuster PA. Performance psychology as a key component of human performance optimization. J Spec Oper Med 2014;14(4):99–105.
17. Deuster PA, Schoomaker E. Mindfulness: a fundamental skill for performance sustainment and enhancement. J Spec Oper Med 2015;15(1):93–9.

18. Immenroth M, Bürger T, Brenner J, et al. Mental training in surgical education. Ann Surg 2007;245(3):385–91.
19. Lorello GR, Hicks CM, Ahmed SA, et al. Mental practice: a simple tool to enhance team-based trauma resuscitation. Can J Emerg Med 2015;(suppl 1):1–7.
20. Arch JJ, Craske MG. Mechanisms of mindfulness: emotion regulation following a focused breathing induction. Behav Res Ther 2006;44(12):1849–58.
21. Philippot P, Chapelle G, Blairy S. Respiratory feedback in the generation of emotion. Cogn Emot 2002;16:605–27.
22. Boiten FA, Frijda NH, Wientjes CJ. Emotions and respiratory patterns: review and critical analysis. Int J Psychophysiol 1994;17(2):103–28.
23. Seppälä EM, Nitschke BJ, Tudorascu DL, et al. Breathing-based meditation decreases posttraumatic stress disorder symptoms in U.S. military veterans: a randomized controlled longitudinal study. J Trauma Stress 2014;27(4):397–405.
24. Openshaw P. Breathing and control of heart rate. BMJ 1978;2(6153):1663–4.
25. Whitelock KA, Asken MJ. Code calm on the streets: mental toughness skills for prehospital emergency personnel. Mechanicsburg (PA): Sunbury Press; 2012.
26. Grossman D. On combat: the psychology and physiology of deadly conflict in war and in peace. Mascoutah, IL: PPCT Research Publications; 2008.
27. Siddle BK. Sharpening the warrior's edge. Millstadt, IL: PPCT Management Systems; 1995.
28. Hardy L, Jones G, Gould D. Understanding psychological preparation for sport: theory and practice of elite performers. Chichester (NY): Wiley; 1996.
29. Bunker L, Williams JM, Zinsser N. Cognitive techniques for improving performance and self-confidence. In: Williams JM, Krane V, editors. Applied sport psychology: personal growth to peak performance. 7th edition. New York: McGraw Hill; 2015. p. 274–303.
30. Hatzigeorgiadis ZN. Investigating the functions of self-talk: the effects of motivational self-talk on self-efficacy and performance in young tennis players. Sport Psychol 2008;22:458–71.
31. Hatzigeorgiadis A, Zourbanos N, Goltsios C, et al. Self-talk and sports performance a meta-analysis. Perspect Psychol Sci 2011;6(4):348–56.
32. Tod D, Hardy J, Oliver E. Effects of self-talk: a systematic review. J Sport Exerc Psychol 2011;33(5):666.
33. Hatzigeorgiadis A, Theodorakis Y, Zourbanos N. Self-talk in the swimming pool: the effects of self-talk on thought content and performance on water-polo tasks. J Appl Sport Psychol 2004;16(2):138–50.
34. Hatzigeorgiadis A, Zourbanos N, Theodorakis Y. The moderating effects of self-talk content on self-talk functions. J Appl Sport Psychol 2007;19(2):240–51.
35. Perkos S, Theodorakis Y, Chroni S. Enhancing performance and skill acquisition in novice basketball players with instructional self-talk. Sport Psychol 2002;16(4):368–83.
36. Mikes J, Meyer R. Basketball fundamentals: a complete mental training guide. Champaign (Ill): Human Kinetics Publishers; 1991.
37. Weisinger H, Pawliw-Fry JP. Performing under pressure: the science of doing your best when it matters most. New York: Crown Business; 2015.
38. Olsson CJ, Jonsson B, Nyberg L. Learning by doing and learning by thinking: an fMRI study of combining motor and mental training. Front Hum Neurosci 2008;8(2):5.
39. Richardson A. Mental imagery. London: Routledge & Kegan Paul; 1969.

40. Martin KA, Moritz SE, Hall CR. Imagery use in sport: a literature review and applied model. Sport Psychol 1999;13(3):245–68.

41. Weinberg R. Does imagery work? Effects on performance and mental skills. Journal of Imagery Research in Sport and Physical Activity 2008;3(1), Article 1. https://doi.org/10.2202/1932-0191.1025.

42. Feltz DL, Landers DM. The effects of mental practice on motor skill learning and performance: a meta- analysis. J Sport Psychol 1983;5(1):25–57.

43. Hall JC. Imagery practice and the development of surgical skills. Am J Surg 2002;184(5):465–70.

44. Arora S, Aggarwal R, Sirimanna P, et al. Mental practice enhances surgical technical skills: a randomized controlled study. Ann Surg 2011;253(2):265–70.

45. Institute of Medicine. Hospital-based emergency care: at the breaking point. Washington, DC: National Academy of Sciences, National Academics Press; 2007.

46. Lorello GR, Hicks CM, Ahmed SA, et al. Mental practice: a simple tool to enhance team-based trauma resuscitation. Can J Emerg Med 2016;18(2): 136–42.

47. Smith D, Wright C, Allsopp A, et al. It's all in the mind: PETTLEP-based imagery and sports performance. J Appl Sport Psychol 2007;19(1):80–92.

48. Holmes PS, Collins DJ. The PETTLEP approach to motor imagery: a functional equivalence model for sport psychologists. J Appl Sport Psychol 2001;13(1): 60–83.

49. Moran AP. Attention, concentration and thought management. In: Brewer BW, editor. Sport Psychol. Hoboken (NJ): Wiley-Blackwell; 2009. p. 18–29.

50. Perry C. Concentration: focus under pressure. In: Murphy S, editor. The sport psychology handbook. Champaign (IL): Human Kinetics; 2005. p. 113–25.

51. Wegner DM, Giuliano T. Arousal-induced attention to self. J Pers Soc Psychol 1980;38(5):719–26.

52. Lazarus RS, Folkman S. Stress, appraisal, and coping. New York: Springer; 1984.

53. Bell JJ, Hardy J. Effects of attentional focus on skilled performance in golf. J Appl Sport Psychol 2009;21(2):163–77.

54. Wulf G. Attentional focus and motor learning: a review of 15 years. Int Rev Sport Exerc Psychol 2013;6(1):77–104.

55. Crichton M, O'Connor P, Flin R. Safety at the sharp end: a guide to non-technical skills. Burlington (VT): Ashgate Publishing, Ltd.; 2008.

56. Gucciardi DF, Dimmock JA. Choking under pressure in sensorimotor skills: conscious processing or depleted attentional resources? Psychol Sport Exerc 2008;9(1):45–59.

57. Lam WK, Maxwell JP, Masters R. Analogy learning and the performance of motor skills under pressure. Psychol Sport Exerc 2009;31(3):337–57.

58. HSE. The contamination of the beach incident at British Nuclear Fuels Limited, Sellafield, November 1983. London: HMSO; 1983.

59. NTSB. Air Florida Inc. Boeing 737-222, N62AF, collision with 14th street bridge near Washington national airport, Washington, DC January 13, 1982. (NTSB report number AAR-82/08). Washington, DC: National Transportation Safety Board; 1982.

60. JCAHO. Sentinel event alert, issue No. 30. Oak Brook (IL): Joint Commission for the Accreditation of Healthcare Organizations; 2004.

61. JCAHO. Medication errors related to potentially dangerous abbreviations. Sentinel event alert, Issue No. 23. Oak Brook (IL): Joint Commission for the Accreditation of Healthcare Organizations; 2001.
62. Gladwell M. The ethnic theory of plane crashes. In: Gladwell M, Patel VI, editors. Outliers. New York: Crown Publishers; 2008. p. 177–223.
63. Brindley PG. Patient safety and acute care medicine: lessons for the future, insights from the past. Crit Care 2010;14(2):217–22.
64. Nethercott D, Shelly M. Critical Care. In: Cyna AM, ANdrew MI, Suyin GM, et al, editors. Handbook of communications in aneasthesia and critical care: A practical guide to exploring the art. Oxford (United Kingdom): Oxford University Press; 2010. p. 126–42.
65. Kanki BG, Lozito S, Foushee HC. Communication indices of crew coordination. Aviat Space Environ Med 1989;60:56–60.
66. Kanki BG, Smith GM. Training aviation communication skills. In: Salas E, Bowers CA, Edens E, editors. Improving teamwork in organizations. Mahwah (NJ): Lawrence Erlbaum; 2001. p. 95–127.
67. Tushman M. Special boundary roles in the innovation process. Admin Sci Q 1977;22:587–606.
68. Orasanu JM. Decision-making in the cockpit. In: Wiener EL, Kanki BG, Helmreich RL, editors. Cockpit resource management. San Diego (CA): Academic Press; 1993. p. 137–72.
69. Volpe CE, Cannon-Bowers JA, Salas E. The impact of cross-training on team functioning: an empirical investigation. Hum Factors 1996;38:87–100.
70. Gaba DM, Fish KJ, Howard SK. Crisis management in anesthesiology. New York: Churchill Livingstone; 1994.
71. Gaba DM. Dynamic decision-making in anesthesiology: cognitive models and training approaches. In: Evans DA, Patel VI, editors. Advanced models of cognition for medical training and practice. Berlin: Springer-Verlag; 1992. p. 123–47.
72. Jentsch F, Smith-Jentsch K. Assertiveness and team performance: more than "just say no". In: Salas E, Bowers C, Edens E, editors. Improving teamwork in organizations. Mahwah (NJ): Lawrence Erlbaum; 2001. p. 73–94.
73. Foushee HC, Helmreich R. Group interaction and flightcrew performance. In: Wiener E, Nagel E, editors. Human factors in aviation. San Diego (CA): Academic Press; 1988. p. 189–227.
74. Besco RO. To intervene or not to intervene? The copilots "catch 22": developing flight crew survival skills through the use of "P.A. C.E.". 1994. Available at: http://www.crm-devel.org/resources/paper/PACE.PDF. Accessed Nov 19, 2019.
75. Mehrabian A, Ferris. Inference of attitudes from nonverbal communication in two channels. J Consult Psychol 1967;31:248–52.
76. Malandro L, Barker L, Barker D. Nonverbal communication. 2nd edition. Reading (MA): Addison-Wesley; 1989.
77. SOARES, André Escórcio; PEREIRA LOPES, Miguel. Social networks and psychological safety: A model of contagion. Journal of Industrial Engineering and Management, [S.l.], v. 7, n. 5, p. 995-1012, oct. 2014. ISSN 2013-0953. Available at: https://www.jiem.org/index.php/jiem/article/view/1115 Accessed: July 15, 2020. http://dx.doi.org/10.3926/jiem.1115.
78. Patel RS, Bachu R, Adikey A, et al. Factors related to physician burnout and its consequences: a review. Behav Sci (Basel) 2018;8(11):98.
79. Shanafelt TD, West CP, Sinsky C, et al. Changes in burnout and satisfaction with work-life integration in physicians and the general US working population between 2011 and 2017. Mayo Clin Proc 2019;94(9):1681–94.

80. McHugh MD, Kutney-Lee A, Cimiotti JP, et al. Nurses' widespread job dissatisfaction, burnout, and frustration with health benefits signal problems for patient care. Health Aff (Millwood) 2011;30(2):202–10.

81. Benson MA, Peterson T, Salazar L, et al. Burnout in rural physician assistants: an initial study. J Physician Assist Educ 2016;27(2):81–3.

82. Reith TP. Burnout in United States healthcare professionals: a narrative review. Cureus 2018;10(12):e3681.

83. American Psychiatric Association. APA Wellbeing Ambassador Toolkit: physician burnout and depression: challenges and opportunities. 2018. Available at: https://www.psychiatry.org/psychiatrists/practice/well-being-and-burnout/well-being-resources. Accessed November 15, 2019.

84. Doctors suicide rate highest of any profession. WebMD. Available at: https://www.webmd.com/mental-health/news/20180508/doctors-suicide-rate-highest-of-any-profession#1. Accessed October 4 2019.

85. Yaghmour NA, Brigham TP, Richter T, et al. Causes of death of residents in ACGME-accredited programs 2000 through 2014: implications for the learning environment. Acad Med 2017;92:976–83.

86. Davidson JE, Proudfoot J, Lee K, et al. Nurse suicide in the Unites States: analysis of the Center for Disease Control 2014 National Violent Death Reporting System dataset. Arch Psychiatr Nurs 2019. https://doi.org/10.1016/j.apnu.2019.04.006.

87. Fail better with a failure friend. Feminem. Available at: https://feminem.org/2017/12/05/fail-better-failure-friend/. Accessed November 25 2019.

88. Ma H, Qiao H, Qu H, et al. Role stress, social support and occupational burnout among physicians in China: a path analysis approach. Int Health 2020. https://doi.org/10.1093/inthealth/ihz054. ihz054.

89. Kim B, Jee S, Lee J, et al. Relationships between social support and student burnout: a meta-analytic approach. Stress Health 2018;34:127–34. https://doi.org/10.1002/smi.2771.

90. Velando-Soriano A, Ortega-Campos E, Gómez-Urquiza JL, et al. Impact of social support in preventing burnout syndrome in nurses: a systematic review. Jpn J Nurs Sci 2020. https://doi.org/10.1111/jjns.12269.

91. Neff K. Self-compassion: an alternative conceptualization of a healthy attitude toward oneself. Self Identity 2003;2:85–101.

92. Kemper K, McClafferty H, Wilson P, et al, on behalf of the Pediatric Resident Burnout-Resilience Study Consortium. Do mindfulness and self-compassion predict burnout in pediatric residents? Acad Med 2019;94(6):876–84.

93. Babenko O, Mosewich AD, Lee A, et al. Association of physicians' self-compassion with work engagement, exhaustion, and professional life satisfaction. Med Sci 2019;7:29.

94. Jarrett A. Risk factors, self-compassion, and burnout in medical students: examining relationships through path analysis. [dissertation] ETD collection for University of Nebraska – Lincoln. 2018. AAI10842490. Available at: https://digitalcommons.unl.edu/dissertations/AAI10842490. Accessed November 15, 2019.

95. Cocker F, Joss N. Compassion fatigue among healthcare, emergency and community service workers: a systematic review. Int J Environ Res Public Health 2016;13(6):618.

96. Killian KD. Helping till it hurts? a multimethod study of compassion fatigue, burnout, and self-care in clinicians working with trauma survivors. Traumatology 2008;14(2):32–44.

97. Werner E. Protective Factors and Individual Resilience. In: Zigler (Author) E, Shonkoff J, Meisels S, editors. Handbook of Early Childhood Intervention. Cambridge: Cambridge University Press; 2000. p. 115–32. https://doi.org/10.1017/CBO9780511529320.008.

98. Southwick SM, Bonanno GA, Masten AS, et al. Resilience definitions, theory, and challenges: interdisciplinary perspectives. Eur J Psychotraumatol 2014;5. https://doi.org/10.3402/ejpt.v5.25338.

99. Back AL, Steinhauser KE, Kamal AF, et al. Building resilience for palliative care clinicians: an approach to burnout prevention based on individual skills and workplace factors. J Pain Symptom Manage 2016;52(2):284–91.

100. Jackson R, Watkin C. The resilience inventory: seven essential skills for overcoming life's obstacles and determining happiness. Selection & Development Review 2004;20(6):13–7. Availabe at: https://da7648.approby.com/m/84223279b0001e87.pdf. Accessed July 15, 2020.

101. Patel RS, Sekhri S, Bhimanadham N, et al. A review on strategies to manage physician burnout. Cureus 2019;11(6):e4805.

102. Swetz KM, Harrington SE, Matsuyama RK, et al. Strategies for avoiding burnout in hospice and palliative medicine: peer advice for physicians on achieving longevity and fulfillment. J Palliat Med 2009;12(9):1–5.

103. Lee FJ, Stewart M, Brown JB. Stress, burnout, and strategies for reducing them. What's the situation among Canadian family physicians? Can Fam Physician 2008;54:234–5.e1-5.

104. Matheson C, Robertson HD, Elliott AM, et al. Resilience of primary healthcare professionals working in challenging environments: a focus group study. Br J Gen Pract 2016. https://doi.org/10.3399/bjgp16X685285.

105. Dyrbye LN, Shanafelt TD, Gill PR, et al. Effect of a professional coaching intervention on the well-being and distress of physicians: a pilot randomized clinical trial. JAMA Intern Med 2019;179(10):1406–14.

106. McIntyre TC. The relationship between locus of control and teacher burnout. Br J Educ Psychol 1984;54:235–8.

107. Schmitz N, Neumann W, Oppermann R. Stress, burnout and locus of control in German nurses. Int J Nurs Stud 2000;37(2):95–9.

108. Posttraumatic stress disorder prevention and treatment guidelines, International Society for Traumatic Stress Studies. Available at: https://istss.org/get attachment/Treating-Trauma/New-ISTSS-Prevention-and-Treatment-Guidelines/ISTSS_PreventionTreatmentGuidelines_FNL-March-19-2019.pdf.aspx. Accessed November 15, 2019.

Updates in Cardiac Arrest Resuscitation

Vivian Lam, MD, MPH[a], Cindy H. Hsu, MD, PhD[b,c],*

KEYWORDS

- Cardiac arrest • Cardiopulmonary resuscitation • Airway management
- Vasopressor • Epinephrine • Antiarrhythmic medication • Hypothermia
- Defibrillation

KEY POINTS

- High-quality chest compressions remain a key priority for cardiac arrest management. Mechanical cardiopulmonary resuscitation (CPR) devices may be useful in situations where manual CPR cannot be performed optimally.
- Supraglottic airway is a reasonable alternative to endotracheal intubation in systems with low success rate for endotracheal intubation.
- Epinephrine improves the rate of return of spontaneous circulation, survival to hospital admission, and survival to hospital discharge after cardiac arrest. Its effect on long-term survival and neurologic outcome, however, remains inconclusive.
- Amiodarone or lidocaine may be considered for shock-refractory ventricular fibrillation or pulseless ventricular tachycardia.
- Physiologic monitoring of end-tidal CO_2 and arterial diastolic pressure during cardiac arrest may help guide resuscitative efforts.

INTRODUCTION

There are approximately 350,000 out-of-hospital cardiac arrests (OHCAs)[1] and 200,000 in-hospital cardiac arrests (IHCAs)[2] annually in the United States, with survival rates of approximately 5% to 10%[1] for OHCAs and 24% for IHCAs.[3] The critical factors that have an impact on cardiac arrest survival include prompt recognition and activation of prehospital care, early cardiopulmonary resuscitation (CPR), and rapid

[a] Department of Emergency Medicine, University of Michigan Medical School, 1500 East Medical Center Drive, B1-380 Taubman Center, SPC 5305, Ann Arbor, MI 48109-5305, USA; [b] Department of Emergency Medicine, Michigan Center for Integrative Research in Critical Care, University of Michigan Medical School, NCRC B026-309N, 2800 Plymouth Road, Ann Arbor, MI 48109-2800, USA; [c] Department of Surgery, Michigan Center for Integrative Research in Critical Care, University of Michigan Medical School, NCRC B026-309N, 2800 Plymouth Road, Ann Arbor, MI 48109-2800, USA
* Corresponding author. NCRC B026-309N, 2800 Plymouth Road, Ann Arbor, MI 48109-2800.
E-mail address: hcindy@med.umich.edu
Twitter: @CHsu1012 (C.H.H.)

Emerg Med Clin N Am 38 (2020) 755–769
https://doi.org/10.1016/j.emc.2020.06.003
0733-8627/20/© 2020 Elsevier Inc. All rights reserved.

emed.theclinics.com

defibrillation. Despite recent advances in the evidence for many aspects of intra-arrest management, some controversies persist. They include airway management, mechanical CPR, route of drug administration, role of vasopressors and antiarrhythmic medications, hemodynamic-directed resuscitation, intracardiac arrest hypothermia, double sequential external defibrillation (DSED), and point-of-care echocardiography. **Fig. 1** prioritizes the critical actions based on the timing of interventions and their strength of evidence. **Table 1** summarizes the most updated International Liaison Committee on Resuscitation (ILCOR) and American Heart Association (AHA) treatment recommendations on topics discussed in this article. The AHA provides a Web-based living document of its most recent guidelines at its CPR and emergency cardiovascular care guidelines Web site (https://eccguidelines.heart.org/circulation/cpr-ecc-guidelines/).

AIRWAY MANAGEMENT DURING CARDIAC ARREST

Airway management is an integral component of cardiac arrest management. Previous observational data suggest that endotracheal intubation is superior to supraglottic airway in adult OHCA.[4] Other observational data, however, demonstrate an association between bag-valve mask ventilation and increased rate of neurologically favorable survival compared with endotracheal intubation.[5,6] A potential confounder between the association of advanced airway management and poor outcomes is that patients with longer duration of cardiac arrest are more likely to require advanced

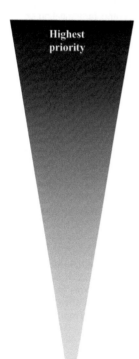

Initiate and maintain high-quality chest compressions. Consider using a mechanical CPR device if manual CPR cannot be performed optimally.

Achieve early defibrillation for shockable rhythm.

Use bag-valve mask or establish advanced airway. A supraglottic airway may be used in settings with low rate of success for endotracheal intubation.

Monitor waveform capnography with goal end-tidal CO_2 >20 mm Hg.

Obtain IV access for drug administration. IO access can be used as alternative if IV access cannot be obtained.

Administer epinephrine as soon as feasible for nonshockable rhythm and after unsuccessful defibrillation attempts for shockable rhythm.

Consider amiodarone or lidocaine administration for shock-refractory ventricular fibrillation or pulseless ventricular tachycardia.

Establish an arterial line for hemodynamic-guided resuscitation with goal arterial diastolic pressure >30–35 mm Hg.

Perform point-of-care echocardiography only if it does not delay other resuscitative efforts.

Fig. 1. Prioritization of critical actions during cardiac arrest.

Table 1
Most updated treatment recommendations for cardiac arrest resuscitation[a,b]

Topic	Most Updated Treatment Recommendations
Airway management[11,12]	2019 ILCOR ALS CoSTR The authors suggest using bag-mask valve or an advanced airway strategy during CPR for adult cardiac arrest in any setting (weak recommendation, low to moderate certainty of evidence). If an advanced airway is used, the authors suggest • Supraglottic airway for adults with OHCA in settings with a low tracheal intubation success rate (weak recommendation, low certainty of evidence) • Supraglottic airway or tracheal intubation for adults with OHCA in settings with a high tracheal intubation success rate (weak recommendation, very low certainty of evidence) • Supraglottic airway or tracheal intubation for adults with IHCA (weak recommendation, very low certainty of evidence)
Mechanical CPR[21]	2015 ILCOR ALS CoSTR The authors suggest against the routine use of automated mechanical chest compression devices to replace manual chest compressions (weak recommendation, moderate certainty of evidence). The authors suggest that automated mechanical chest compression devices are a reasonable alternative to high-quality manual chest compressions in situations where sustained high-quality manual chest compressions are impractical or compromise provider safety (weak recommendation, low certainty of evidence).
IV vs IO[24]	2020 draft ILCOR ALS CoSTR The authors suggest IV access compared with IO access as the first attempt for drug administration during adult cardiac arrest (weak recommendation, very low certainty of evidence). If attempts at IV access are unsuccessful or IV access is not feasible, we suggest IO access as a route for drug administration during adult cardiac arrest (weak recommendation, very low certainty of evidence).
Vasopressors[12,29]	2019 ILCOR ALS CoSTR The authors recommend administration of epinephrine during CPR (strong recommendation, low to moderate certainty of evidence). For nonshockable rhythms, the authors recommend administration of epinephrine as soon as feasible during CPR (strong recommendation, very low certainty of evidence). For shockable rhythms, the authors suggest administration of epinephrine after initial defibrillation attempts are unsuccessful during CPR (weak recommendation, very low certainty of evidence). The authors suggest against the administration of vasopressin in place of epinephrine during CPR (weak recommendation, very low certainty of evidence). The suggest against the addition of vasopressin to epinephrine during CPR (weak recommendation, low certainty of evidence).

(continued on next page)

Table 1
(*continued*)

Topic	Most Updated Treatment Recommendations
Antiarrhythmic medications[22,42]	**2018 ILCOR ALS CoSTR** The authors suggest the use of amiodarone or lidocaine in adults with shock-refractory ventricular fibrillation/pulseless ventricular tachycardia (weak recommendation, low certainty of evidence). The authors suggest against the routine use of magnesium in adults with shock-refractory ventricular fibrillation/pulseless ventricular tachycardia (weak recommendation, very low certainty of evidence).
Hemodynamics-guided resuscitation[21,25,46]	**2015 ILCOR ALS CoSTR** The authors recommend against using $ETCO_2$ cutoff values alone as a mortality predictor or on the decision to stop a resuscitation attempt (strong recommendation, low certainty of evidence). The authors suggest that an $ETCO_2$ greater than or equal to 10 mm Hg measured after tracheal intubation or after 20 minutes of resuscitation, may be a predictor of ROSC (weak recommendation, low certainty of evidence). The authors suggest that an $ETCO_2$ greater than or equal to 10 mm Hg measured after tracheal intubation, or an $ETCO_2$ greater than or equal to 20 mm Hg measured after 20 minutes of resuscitation may be a predictor of survival to discharge (weak recommendation, moderate certainty of evidence). **2015 AHA ACLS guidelines updates** Although no clinical study has examined whether titrating resuscitative efforts to physiologic parameters during CPR improves outcome, it may be reasonable to use physiologic parameters (quantitative waveform capnography, arterial relaxation diastolic pressure, arterial pressure monitoring, and central venous oxygen saturation) when feasible to monitor and optimize CPR quality, guide vasopressor therapy, and detect ROSC (class IIb, LOE C-EO).
Prehospital/intracardiac arrest hypothermia[21]	**2015 ILCOR ALS CoSTR** The authors recommend against routine use of prehospital cooling with rapid infusion of large volumes of cold IV fluid immediately after ROSC (strong recommendation, moderate certainty of evidence).
DSED[62,67]	**2020 draft ILCOR ALS CoSTR** The authors suggest against routine use of dual (or double) sequential defibrillation strategy in comparison to a standard defibrillation strategy for cardiac arrest with a shockable rhythm (weak recommendation, very low certainty of evidence).

(*continued on next page*)

Table 1 *(continued)*	
Topic	**Most Updated Treatment Recommendations**
Point-of-care echocardiography[21,72]	2015 ILCOR ALS CoSTR The authors suggest that if cardiac ultrasound can be performed without interfering with standard ACLS protocol, it may be considered as an additional diagnostic tool to identify potentially reversible causes (weak recommendation, very low certainty of evidence). 2020 Draft ILCOR ALS CoSTR The authors suggest against using point-of-care echocardiography for prognostication during CPR (weak recommendation, very low certainty of evidence).

Abbreviations: ACLS, advanced cardiovascular life support; ALS, advanced life support; ETCO$_2$, end-tidal CO$_2$.; LOE C-EO, Level of Evidence C-Expert Opinion.

 [a] The next ILCOR ALS CoSTR will be published in October 2020.

 [b] ILCOR used the Grading of Recommendations Assessment, Development and Evaluation (www.gradeworkinggroup.org) approach to systematic reviews and guideline development, whereas the AHA used the ILCOR reviews as well as the AHA definition of classes of recommendation and levels of evidence for its 2015 guidelines update. (https://eccguidelines.heart.org/circulation/cpr-ecc-guidelines/).

airway management.[7] Variable prehospital systems also can lead to differences in training, intubation success rates, and complications.

Three randomized controlled trials comparing advanced airway strategies for OHCA were published in 2018. The AIRWAYS-2 trial compared the i-gel supraglottic airway (Intersurgical Ltd, Berkshire, UK) to endotracheal intubation by prehospital providers.[8] No significant difference was found for neurologic outcome at hospital discharge or day 30 in patients randomized to supraglottic airway compared with endotracheal intubation. Among patients who underwent advanced airway management, those who received a supraglottic airway had better outcome. The paramedics randomized to the endotracheal intubation group, however, were less likely to use advanced airway management overall, introducing bias. In a separate study, outcomes of laryngeal tube were compared with endotracheal intubation, and outcomes were improved in the laryngeal tube group.[9] A third trial compared outcomes of bag-valve mask ventilation to endotracheal intubation and did not find any difference.[10]

The most recent systematic review and 2019 Consensus on Science with Treatment Recommendations (CoSTR) stated that the heterogeneity of the aforementioned airway studies limits the ability to perform meaningful meta-analysis or generalize their findings.[11,12] Perhaps most notably, endotracheal intubation success rates were highly variable among studies.[8–10] In situations where likelihood of successful endotracheal intubation is low, a supraglottic airway is recommended as a reasonable alternative. In settings where successful endotracheal intubation rate is high, supraglottic airway or endotracheal intubation is recommended.[11,12] The threshold for high versus low success rates, however, remains ill defined.

MECHANICAL CARDIOPULMONARY RESUSCITATION

High-quality chest compressions are defined as compressions at a depth of 5 cm to 6 cm and a rate of 100 per minute to 120 per minute, allowing full chest recoil between compressions and minimization of interruptions.[13,14] Barriers to achieving optimal CPR include provider fatigue, patient anatomy, transport, and environmental factors.[15,16] Mechanical CPR devices, including the Thumper (Michigan Instruments, Grand Rapids, MI, USA), LUCAS (Physio-Control, Lund, Sweden), and AutoPulse (Zoll Medical, Chelmsford, MA, USA), are designed to improve the quality of CPR and simplify cardiac arrest management in situations where manual CPR cannot be performed optimally. Although the ability to standardize the rate and depth of compressions and eliminate the need to swap providers may increase compression fraction, device deployment also may cause potential delays in cardiac arrest care.

Several studies have compared the outcomes between manual CPR and mechanical CPR for OHCA. Three trials found no significant difference in survival of OHCA patients who received mechanical or manual CPR.[17–19] A 2015 meta-analysis found no difference between manual and mechanical CPR, and there have been inconsistent results regarding survival with good neurologic outcome between the 2 groups.[20] In 2015, ILCOR made a weak recommendation against the routine use of mechanical CPR devices in clinical practice, but they may be considered in circumstances where the delivery of high-quality manual chest compressions may be impractical or dangerous to rescuers.[21]

INTRAVENOUS VERSUS INTRAOSSEOUS DRUG ADMINISTRATION DURING CARDIAC ARREST

Current advanced life support guidelines recommend the administration of epinephrine[12] and antiarrhythmics[22] during cardiac arrest. The most optimal route of drug administration during cardiac arrest, however, remains unclear. Intravenous (IV) access requires additional skill and may be difficult to obtain during cardiac arrest. As such, intraosseous (IO) access may be a reasonable alternative. A recent observational study found that IO access was associated with faster drug delivery in OHCAs.[23]

The outcome differences between IO and IV access in adult OHCAs have been compared in observational studies with varied protocols. Pooled analysis[24] from 3 observational studies showed worse outcomes with the use of IO access compared with IV access for of return of spontaneous circulation (ROSC) and survival to hospital discharge. Given current available data showing that outcomes might be better with IV access during cardiac arrest, the current ILCOR recommendation[14,21,24,25] is that IV access should be attempted first and that IO access is a reasonable alternative if IV access cannot be obtained. It remains unclear whether the effectiveness of drug administration during cardiac arrest is dependent on the type of drug, its dose, or the anatomic location of access.

ROLE OF VASOPRESSORS
Epinephrine

The use of epinephrine is widely accepted in cardiac arrest management; however, its implementation into guidelines was based mainly on animal studies. The α-adrenergic effect of epinephrine increases aortic diastolic pressure, therefore increasing the coronary perfusion pressure (CPP) and likelihood of ROSC. It has, however, the potential to increase dysrhythmias, increase myocardial demand, and decrease cerebral microcirculation in animal studies.[26] Concerns regarding the association of epinephrine with worse neurologic outcome were based largely on older cohort studies that were highly susceptible to uncontrolled confounders and selection bias.[7,27]

The PARAMEDIC2 trial is the largest randomized study on epinephrine for OHCA to date.[28] The epinephrine group had significantly higher ROSC compared with placebo (36.3% vs 11.7%, respectively), but severe neurologic impairment was more common in the epinephrine group than the placebo group (31.0% vs 17.8%, respectively, at hospital discharge). Similar results for survival and survival with favorable neurologic outcome also were found at 3 months. There were several limitations to this study. The median time to epinephrine administration was relatively long at 21 minutes, and the neurologic outcome at 3 months was limited by very low overall survival rate (3.2% in epinephrine vs 2.3% in placebo) and loss to follow-up. As such, the study was underpowered to detect a difference in survival and survival with favorable neurologic outcome between the groups.[29]

A systematic review[29] found robust associations between epinephrine and improved short-term outcomes of ROSC and survival to hospital admission compared to placebo. Epinephrine also was associated with improved survival to hospital discharge and 30-day survival. No difference was found in 30-day neurologic outcome, and only the PARAMEDIC2 trial reported long-term outcomes of 3-month survival and neurologic outcome.[28]

Meta-analysis[29] based on initial rhythm reveals that for nonshockable rhythms, there is an association between epinephrine and more robust increase in ROSC and survival to hospital discharge. This is in contrast to shockable rhythms, where these associations with epinephrine are less robust or absent.[28] The differential effect of epinephrine based on initial rhythm could be explained by the availability of other therapies, leading to later epinephrine administration for shockable rhythms.[30–32]

Based on available evidence and the recent systematic review,[29] ILCOR recommended administration of epinephrine as soon as feasible during CPR for nonshockable rhythms and after initial defibrillation attempts are unsuccessful during CPR for shockable rhythm. Further study is needed to clarify the effects of epinephrine on long-term survival and neurologic outcomes, its use in different etiologies of cardiac arrest, and the optimal dose, timing, and route of drug administration.

Vasopressin

Studies comparing vasopressin to epinephrine have found no significant difference in any outcomes regardless of the initial presenting rhythm.[33–35] There also has been no difference in outcome between vasopressin plus epinephrine compared with epinephrine alone.[36–38] Therefore, ILCOR recommended against the administration of vasopressin, either in place of epinephrine or in addition to epinephrine, during CPR.[12]

ROLE OF ANTIARRHYTHMIC MEDICATIONS
Amiodarone Versus Lidocaine

There may be a role for antiarrhythmic medications in ventricular fibrillation and pulseless ventricular tachycardia if defibrillations fail to achieve ROSC. Amiodarone and lidocaine have been studied for this purpose. Two trials[39,40] found that giving amiodarone in refractory cardiac arrest was associated with higher survival to hospital admission compared with placebo and lidocaine. A third randomized trial (ROC-ALPS) compared the effects of amiodarone, lidocaine, and placebo on OHCA with shock-refractory ventricular fibrillation or pulseless ventricular tachycardia.[41] Treatment with amiodarone or lidocaine did not result in a higher rate of survival or favorable neurologic outcome at hospital discharge. Both medications were associated, however, with a higher rate of survival to hospital discharge among witnessed OHCA patients, suggesting that earlier recognition and time to treatment may have an impact on drug efficacy.

A recent systematic review did not find any difference between amiodarone and placebo for ROSC or survival and favorable neurologic outcome at hospital discharge.[42] It also showed no difference between amiodarone and lidocaine for these outcomes. Therefore, the 2018 ILCOR CoSTR suggested the consideration of amiodarone or lidocaine for ventricular fibrillation or pulseless ventricular tachycardia that is unresponsive to defibrillation.[22] Outstanding questions include differences in the effectiveness of antiarrhythmic medications in specific populations, by route and timing of drug administration, and their interactions with other drugs.

Magnesium

Meta-analysis of multiple randomized controlled studies showed no difference between magnesium and placebo for ROSC, survival to hospital discharge, or survival with favorable neurologic outcome at hospital discharge.[42] Thus, ILCOR recommended against the routine use of magnesium in shock-refractory ventricular fibrillation and pulseless ventricular tachycardia.[22]

HEMODYNAMIC-DIRECTED RESUSCITATION
End-Tidal CO_2

End-tidal CO_2 monitoring is a physiologic parameter that has potential utility during cardiac arrest management. During the low-flow state of CPR, when ventilation is held constant, changes in end-tidal CO_2 correlate with changes in cardiac output as pulmonary blood flow primarily determines end-tidal CO_2.[25] Multiple observational studies have found an association between end-tidal CO_2 below 10 mm Hg after 20 minutes of CPR and very poor chances of ROSC or survival in intubated cardiac arrest patients.[43–45] One study found end-tidal CO_2 greater than 20 mm Hg to be associated with greater survival,[43] but, in general, there has been inadequate evidence to determine a clear numerical goal for end-tidal CO_2. Based on current evidence, end-tidal CO_2 of less than 10 mm Hg after 20 minutes of CPR may have utility in predicting poor likelihood of ROSC. A goal end-tidal CO_2 of 20 mm Hg may be reasonable, but it is unclear if even higher end-tidal CO_2 is beneficial.[21,46]

Coronary Perfusion Pressure/Diastolic Blood Pressure

CPP, or the difference between mid-diastolic aortic pressure and mid-diastolic right atrial pressure, is the primary driving force for myocardial blood flow.[47] In a swine cardiac arrest study, chest compression depth was titrated to maintain systolic blood pressure of 90 mm Hg, and vasopressors were titrated to maintain CPP above 20 mm Hg. This protocol was associated with improvement in sustained ROSC and 4-hour survival compared with standard care by AHA guidelines.[48] Given the difficulty in calculating CPP in the clinical setting, arterial diastolic pressure has been proposed as a proxy, with a goal arterial diastolic pressure of 30 mm Hg to 35 mm Hg to approximate CPP of 20 mm Hg to 25 mm Hg, assuming a right atrial pressure of 10 mm Hg to 15 mm Hg. In humans, maximal CPP has been associated with ROSC, although data are limited to pediatric IHCA patients.[49,50]

In hemodynamic-directed resuscitation, continuous monitoring of hemodynamic variables is used to guide chest compressions and vasopressor therapy. Further study is needed to prospectively evaluate arterial diastolic pressure guidance for resuscitation in adult cardiac arrest patients. Specific knowledge gaps include end-tidal CO_2 and arterial diastolic pressure thresholds that are associated with high-quality CPR and improved outcomes for adult cardiac arrest.

PREHOSPITAL AND INTRACARDIAC ARREST HYPOTHERMIA

Hypothermic targeted temperature management is recommended as a neuroprotective strategy for post–cardiac arrest patients.[21,51] It initially was studied for OHCA patients with shockable rhythm in 2 landmark studies,[52,53] then recently showed to also improve the survival with favorable neurologic outcome for cardiac arrest patients with nonshockable presenting rhythms.[54] In addition, multiple animal studies have found protective effects from achieving intracardiac arrest hypothermia[55,56] and hypothermia within 4 hours of ROSC.[57] Previous trials, however, using cold fluid boluses during cardiac arrest, have found associations with significant adverse effects, including pulmonary edema and rearrest.[58] Some of these adverse effects are postulated to be related to the method of hypothermia. As such, the 2015 ILCOR guidelines recommended against routine prehospital hypothermia using IV fluid bolus.[21]

Other studies have examined the feasibility and efficacy of alternative cooling devices without loading intravascular volume. A randomized controlled trial (PRINCE)[59] demonstrated that a transnasal evaporative device resulted in lower temperature at hospital arrival and faster time to targeted temperature but was underpowered to detect outcome differences. A larger trial of prehospital transnasal hypothermia for OHCA (PRINCESS)[60] found that transnasal cooling again was associated with faster time to targeted temperature but without differences in sustained ROSC, survival to hospital admission, survival at 90 days, or survival with good neurologic outcome at 90 days. Propensity-matched subgroup analysis of the PRINCESS trial[61] showed that for patients with initial shockable rhythm, the transnasal hypothermia group had more favorable neurologic outcome. Further prospective studies are necessary to investigate the role of transnasal cooling in different etiologies of cardiac arrest.

DOUBLE SEQUENTIAL EXTERNAL DEFIBRILLATION FOR REFRACTORY VENTRICULAR FIBRILLATION

Shock-refractory ventricular fibrillation generally is defined as persistent ventricular defibrillation after CPR and 3 or more defibrillations. DSED generally describes the use of 2 defibrillators with anterior-anterior and anterior-posterior pad positions to deliver 2 shocks in rapid sequence, although there is no standardized approach.[62] It has been presented as a potential alternate intervention for shock-refractory ventricular fibrillation.[63–66]

A systematic review attempted to compare DSED with standard defibrillation and identified only observational studies.[67] No change in survival to discharge, ROSC, or event survival was found. An updated systematic review[62] considers additional observational data with similar reservations. Therefore, DSED currently is not recommended by ILCOR.[62] The DOSE-VF study is ongoing to compare the feasibility and the effects of standard defibrillation, DSED, and vector change defibrillation on ROSC for prehospital shock-refractory ventricular fibrillation cardiac arrest.

UTILITY OF POINT-OF-CARE ECHOCARDIOGRAPHY DURING CARDIAC ARREST

Point-of-care echocardiography has become an important adjunct for cardiac arrest management because point-of-care ultrasound utilization has increased in the emergency department. Transthoracic echocardiography potentially can provide more direct information on cardiac activity and the etiology of cardiac arrest, especially for pulseless electrical activity or asystole with reversible causes. Thus far, the evidence regarding point-of-care echocardiography in cardiac arrest has come from small observational studies.[68–70]

There currently is no standard definition for cardiac activity and standstill on ultrasound. Prior studies have defined cardiac activity as any myocardial movement/ventricular wall movement, excluding isolated valve movement or movement of blood in the chambers,[71] but this definition has not been used consistently across studies. Although cardiac standstill on transthoracic echocardiography is strongly associated with the lack of ROSC and nonsurvival, there remains a small percentage of patients with cardiac standstill who go on to attain ROSC and subsequent survival. As such, ILCOR suggested against using point-of-care echocardiography for prognostication during CPR.[72]

There are multiple barriers for the incorporation of point-of-care echocardiography during cardiac arrest management. An alternative solution is the utilization of transesophageal echocardiography, which may minimize interruptions in chest compressions, bypass difficulty in obtaining cardiac windows, and guide effective compressions in real time. A single-center, prospective cohort study examined the feasibility and impact of resuscitative transesophageal echocardiography in the emergency department for OHCA. The study demonstrated that tranesophageal echocardiography was safe and feasible and guided therapeutic interventions.[73] Further study is necessary to evaluate the impact of this relatively resource-intensive intervention on cardiac arrest outcome.

SUMMARY

Cardiac arrest resuscitation remains one of the most challenging and dynamic topics for emergency medicine and critical care. Patient heterogeneity, variabilities in prehospital systems, and complex physiology often generate uncertainties in intracardiac arrest management. In OHCA, when the likelihood of successful endotracheal intubation is low, a supraglottic airway is recommended. When endotracheal intubation success rates are high, supraglottic airway or endotracheal intubation is recommended. The routine use of mechanical CPR devices is not recommended, but they may be considered in circumstances where the delivery of high-quality manual chest compressions may be limited. IO access is a reasonable alternative if IV access cannot be obtained. Epinephrine is recommended as soon as feasible during CPR for nonshockable rhythms and after initial unsuccessful defibrillation for shockable rhythms. Further study is needed to clarify the effects of epinephrine on long-term survival and neurologic outcomes. Amiodarone or lidocaine can be considered for ventricular fibrillation or pulseless ventricular tachycardia unresponsive to defibrillation. Hemodynamic monitoring has been associated with improved outcomes in some studies, but precise targets are unclear. DSED, intracardiac arrest hypothermia, and point-of-care echocardiography have inadequate evidence of improved outcomes to make strong recommendations.

DISCLOSURE

The authors have nothing to disclose.

REFERENCES

1. Daya MR, Schmicker RH, May S, et al. Current Burden of Cardiac Arrest in the United States: Report from the Resuscitation Outcomes Consortium. Paper commissioned by the Committee on the treatment of cardiac arrest: current status and future directions. 2015. Available at: http://www.nationalacademies.org/hmd/~/media/Files/Report%20Files/2015/ROC.pdf. Accessed January 5, 2020.

2. Merchant RM, Yang L, Becker LB, et al. Incidence of treated cardiac arrest in hospitalized patients in the United States. Crit Care Med 2011;39(11):2401–6.

3. Chan P. Public Health Burden of In-Hospital Cardiac Arrest. Paper commissioned by the Institute of Medicine Committee on Treatment of Cardiac Arrest: Current Status and Future Directions. Available at: http://www.nationalacademies.org/

hmd/~/media/Files/Report%20Files/2015/GWTG.pdf. Accessed January 5, 2020.

4. Wang HE, Szydlo D, Stouffer JA, et al. Endotracheal intubation versus supraglottic airway insertion in out-of-hospital cardiac arrest. Resuscitation 2012;83(9): 1061–6.

5. Fouche PF, Simpson PM, Bendall J, et al. Airways in Out-of-hospital Cardiac Arrest: Systematic Review and Meta-analysis. Prehosp Emerg Care 2014;18(2): 244–56.

6. Hasegawa K, Hiraide A, Chang Y, et al. Association of prehospital advanced airway management with neurologic outcome and survival in patients with out-of-hospital cardiac arrest. JAMA 2013;309(3):257–66.

7. Andersen LW, Grossestreuer AV, Donnino MW. "Resuscitation time bias"—A unique challenge for observational cardiac arrest research. Resuscitation 2018; 125:79–82.

8. Benger JR, Kirby K, Black S, et al. Effect of a strategy of a supraglottic airway device vs tracheal intubation during out-of-hospital cardiac arrest on functional outcome the AIRWAYS-2 randomized clinical trial. JAMA 2018;320(8):779–91.

9. Wang HE, Schmicker RH, Daya MR, et al. Effect of a strategy of initial laryngeal tube insertion vs endotracheal intubation on 72-hour survival in adults with out-of-hospital cardiac arrest a randomized clinical trial. JAMA 2018;320(8):769–78.

10. Jabre P, Penaloza A, Pinero D, et al. Effect of bag-mask ventilation vs endotracheal intubation during cardiopulmonary resuscitation on neurological outcome after out-of-hospital cardiorespiratory arrest a randomized clinical trial. JAMA 2018;319(8):779–87.

11. Granfeldt A, Avis SR, Nicholson TC, et al. Advanced airway management during adult cardiac arrest: A systematic review. Resuscitation 2019;139:133–43.

12. Soar J, et al. 2019 international consensus on cardiopulmonary resuscitation and emergency cardiovascular care science with treatment recommendations. Circulation 2019;140:e826–80.

13. Kleinman Monica E, Brennan Erin E, Goldberger Zachary D, et al. Part 5: adult basic life support and cardiopulmonary resuscitation quality. Circulation 2015; 132(18_suppl_2):S414–35.

14. Perkins GD, Handley AJ, Koster RW, et al. European resuscitation council guidelines for resuscitation 2015. Resuscitation 2015;95:81–99.

15. Tomlinson AE, Nysaether J, Kramer-Johansen J, et al. Compression force–depth relationship during out-of-hospital cardiopulmonary resuscitation. Resuscitation 2007;72(3):364–70.

16. Perkins GD, Kocierz L, Smith SCL, et al. Compression feedback devices over estimate chest compression depth when performed on a bed. Resuscitation 2009; 80(1):79–82.

17. Perkins GD, Lall R, Quinn T, et al. Mechanical versus manual chest compression for out-of-hospital cardiac arrest (PARAMEDIC): A pragmatic, cluster randomised controlled trial. Lancet 2015;385(9972):947–55.

18. Wik L, Olsen J-A, Persse D, et al. Clinical Paper Manual vs. integrated automatic load-distributing band CPR with equal survival after out of hospital cardiac arrest. The randomized CIRC trial. Resuscitation 2014;85:741–8.

19. Rubertsson S, Lindgren E, Smekal D, et al. Mechanical chest compressions and simultaneous defibrillation vs conventional cardiopulmonary resuscitation in out-of-hospital cardiac arrest: The LINC randomized trial. JAMA 2014;311(1):53–61.

20. Gates S, Quinn T, Deakin CD, et al. Mechanical chest compression for out of hospital cardiac arrest: Systematic review and meta-analysis. Resuscitation 2015; 94:91–7.
21. Soar J, Callaway CW, Aibiki M, et al. Part 4: advanced life support: 2015 international consensus on cardiopulmonary resuscitation and emergency cardiovascular care science with treatment recommendations. Resuscitation 2015;95: e71–120.
22. Soar J, Donnino MW, Maconochie I, et al. 2018 international consensus on cardiopulmonary resuscitation and emergency cardiovascular care science with treatment recommendations summary. Circulation 2018;138:e714–30.
23. Reades R, Studnek JR, Vandeventer S, et al. Intraosseous versus intravenous vascular access during out-of-hospital cardiac arrest: a randomized controlled trial. Ann Emerg Med 2011;58(6):509–16.
24. Granfeldt A, Avis SR, Lind P, et al. Intravenous vs. intraosseous administration of drugs during cardiac arrest: A systematic review. Resuscitation 2020;149:150–7.
25. Link Mark S, Berkow Lauren C, Kudenchuk Peter J, et al. Part 7: Adult Advanced Cardiovascular Life Support: 2015 American Heart Association guidelines update for cardiopulmonary resuscitation and emergency cardiovascular care. Circulation 2015;132(18_suppl_2):S444–64.
26. Ristagno G, Sun S, Tang W, et al. Effects of epinephrine and vasopressin on cerebral microcirculatory flows during and after cardiopulmonary resuscitation*. Crit Care Med 2007;35(9):2145–9.
27. Loomba RS, Nijhawan K, Aggarwal S, et al. Increased return of spontaneous circulation at the expense of neurologic outcomes: Is prehospital epinephrine for out-of-hospital cardiac arrest really worth it? J Crit Care 2015;30(6):1376–81.
28. Perkins GD, Ji C, Deakin CD, et al. A randomized trial of epinephrine in out-of-hospital cardiac arrest. N Engl J Med 2018;379(8):711–21.
29. Holmberg MJ, Issa MS, Moskowitz A, et al. Vasopressors during adult cardiac arrest: A systematic review and meta-analysis. Resuscitation 2019;139:106–21.
30. Hansen M, Schmicker Robert H, Newgard Craig D, et al. Time to epinephrine administration and survival from nonshockable out-of-hospital cardiac arrest among children and adults. Circulation 2018;137(19):2032–40.
31. Ewy GA, Bobrow BJ, Chikani V, et al. The time dependent association of adrenaline administration and survival from out-of-hospital cardiac arrest. Resuscitation 2015;96:180–5.
32. Homma Y, Shiga T, Funakoshi H, et al. Association of the time to first epinephrine administration and outcomes in out-of-hospital cardiac arrest: SOS-KANTO 2012 study. Am J Emerg Med 2019;37(2):241–8.
33. Wenzel V, Lindner KH, Augenstein S, et al. Intraosseous vasopressin improves coronary perfusion pressure rapidly during cardiopulmonary resuscitation in pigs. Crit Care Med 1999;27(8):1565–9.
34. Lindner KH, Dirks B, Strohmenger H-U, et al. Randomised comparison of epinephrine and vasopressin in patients with out-of-hospital ventricular fibrillation. Lancet 1997;349(9051):535–7.
35. Mukoyama T, Kinoshita K, Nagao K, et al. Reduced effectiveness of vasopressin in repeated doses for patients undergoing prolonged cardiopulmonary resuscitation. Resuscitation 2009;80(7):755–61.
36. Callaway CW, Hostler D, Doshi AA, et al. Usefulness of vasopressin administered with epinephrine during out-of-hospital cardiac arrest. Am J Cardiol 2006;98(10): 1316–21.

37. Gueugniaud P-Y, David J-S, Chanzy E, et al. Vasopressin and epinephrine vs. epinephrine alone in cardiopulmonary resuscitation. N Engl J Med 2008;359: 21–30.
38. Ducros L, Vicaut E, Soleil C, et al. Effect of the addition of vasopressin or vasopressin plus nitroglycerin to epinephrine on arterial blood pressure during cardiopulmonary resuscitation in humans. J Emerg Med 2011;41(5):453–9.
39. Kudenchuk PJ, Cobb LA, Copass MK, et al. Amiodarone for resuscitation after out-of-hospital cardiac arrest due to ventricular fibrillation. N Engl J Med 1999; 341(12):871–8.
40. Dorian P, Cass D, Schwartz B, et al. Amiodarone as compared with lidocaine for shock-resistant ventricular fibrillation. N Engl J Med 2002;346(12):884–90.
41. Kudenchuk PJ, Brown SP, Daya M, et al. Amiodarone, lidocaine, or placebo in out-of-hospital cardiac arrest. N Engl J Med 2016;374(18):1711–22.
42. Ali MU, Fitzpatrick-Lewis D, Kenny M, et al. Effectiveness of antiarrhythmic drugs for shockable cardiac arrest: A systematic review. Resuscitation 2018;132:63–72.
43. Ahrens T, Schallom L, Bettorf K, et al. End-tidal carbon dioxide measurements as a prognostic indicator of outcome in cardiac arrest. Am J Crit Care 2001;10(6): 391–8.
44. Wayne MA, Levine RL, Miller CC. Use of end-tidal carbon dioxide to predict outcome in prehospital cardiac arrest. Ann Emerg Med 1995;25(6):762–7.
45. Levine RL. End-tidal carbon dioxide and outcome of out-of-hospital cardiac arrest. N Engl J Med 1997;337(5):301–6.
46. Paiva EF, Paxton JH, O'Neil BJ. The use of end-tidal carbon dioxide (ETCO 2) measurement to guide management of cardiac arrest: A systematic review. Resuscitation 2018;123:1–7.
47. Sanders AB, Ewy GA, Taft TV. Prognostic and therapeutic importance of the aortic diastolic pressure in resuscitation from cardiac arrest. Crit Care Med 1984;12(10): 871–3.
48. Morgan RW, Kilbaugh TJ, Shoap W, et al. A hemodynamic-directed approach to pediatric cardiopulmonary resuscitation (HD-CPR) improves survival. Resuscitation 2017;111:41–7.
49. Paradis NA, Martin GB, Rivers EP, et al. Coronary perfusion pressure and the return of spontaneous circulation in human cardiopulmonary resuscitation. JAMA 1990;263(8):1106–13.
50. Berg Robert A, Sutton Robert M, Reeder Ron W, et al. Association between diastolic blood pressure during pediatric in-hospital cardiopulmonary resuscitation and survival. Circulation 2018;137(17):1784–95.
51. Callaway Clifton W, Donnino Michael W, Fink Ericka L, et al. Part 8: post–cardiac arrest care. Circulation 2015;132(18_suppl_2):S465–82.
52. Bernard SA, Smith K, Finn J, et al. Induction of therapeutic hypothermia during out-of-hospital cardiac arrest using a rapid infusion of cold saline: the rinse trial (rapid infusion of cold normal saline). Circulation 2016;134(11):797–805.
53. Hypothermia after Cardiac Arrest Study Group. Mild therapeutic hypothermia to improve the neurologic outcome after cardiac arrest. N Engl J Med 2002; 346(8):549–56.
54. Lascarrou J-B, Merdji H, Le Gouge A, et al. Targeted Temperature Management for Cardiac Arrest with Nonshockable Rhythm. N Engl J Med 2019;381(24): 2327–37.
55. Kim T, Paine MG, Meng H, et al. Combined intra- and post-cardiac arrest hypothermic-targeted temperature management in a rat model of asphyxial

cardiac arrest improves survival and neurologic outcome compared to either strategy alone. Resuscitation 2016;107:94–101.

56. Ala N, Peter S, William SS, et al. Critical time window for intra-arrest cooling with cold saline flush in a dog model of cardiopulmonary resuscitation. Circulation 2006;113(23):2690–6.

57. Che D, Li L, Kopil CM, et al. Impact of therapeutic hypothermia onset and duration on survival, neurologic function, and neurodegeneration after cardiac arrest. Crit Care Med 2011;39(6):1423–30.

58. Kim F, Nichol G, Maynard C, et al. Effect of prehospital induction of mild hypothermia on survival and neurological status among adults with cardiac arrest: a randomized clinical trial. JAMA 2014;311(1):45–52.

59. Castrén M, Nordberg P, Svensson L, et al. Intra-arrest transnasal evaporative cooling: a randomized, prehospital, multicenter study (PRINCE: Pre-ROSC Intra-Nasal Cooling Effectiveness). Circulation 2010;122(7):729–36.

60. Nordberg P, Taccone FS, Truhlar A, et al. Effect of trans-nasal evaporative intra-arrest cooling on functional neurologic outcome in out-of-hospital cardiac arrest: the PRINCESS randomized clinical trial. JAMA 2019;321(17):1677–85.

61. Awad A, Silvio TF, Martin J, et al. Time to intra-arrest therapeutic hypothermia in out-of-hospital cardiac arrest patients and its association with neurologic outcome: A propensity matched sub-analysis of the PRINCESS trial. Intensive Care Med 2020;46(7):1361–70.

62. Deakin CD, Morley P, Soar S, et al. Double sequential defibrillation for refractory ventricular fibrillation cardiac arrest: A systematic review. Resuscitation 2020. S0300-9572(20)30244-30246.

63. Cortez E, Krebs W, Davis J, et al. Use of double sequential external defibrillation for refractory ventricular fibrillation during out-of-hospital cardiac arrest. Resuscitation 2016;108:82–6.

64. Cabañas JG, Myers JB, Williams JG, et al. Double sequential external defibrillation in out-of-hospital refractory ventricular fibrillation: a report of ten cases. Prehosp Emerg Care 2015;19(1):126–30.

65. Johnston M, Cheskes S, Ross G, et al. Double sequential external defibrillation and survival from out-of-hospital cardiac arrest: a case report. Prehosp Emerg Care 2016;20(5):662–6.

66. Merlin MA, Tagore A, Bauter R, et al. A case series of double sequence defibrillation. Prehosp Emerg Care 2016;20(4):550–3.

67. Delorenzo A, Nehme Z, Yates J, et al. Double sequential external defibrillation for refractory ventricular fibrillation out-of-hospital cardiac arrest: A systematic review and meta-analysis. Resuscitation 2019;135:124–9.

68. Blaivas M, Fox JC. Outcome in cardiac arrest patients found to have cardiac standstill on the bedside emergency department echocardiogram. Acad Emerg Med 2001;8(6):616–21.

69. Hernandez C, Shuler K, Hannan H, et al. C.A.U.S.E.: Cardiac arrest ultra-sound exam-A better approach to managing patients in primary non-arrhythmogenic cardiac arrest. Resuscitation 2008;76(2):198–206.

70. Flato UAP, Paiva EF, Carballo MT, et al. Echocardiography for prognostication during the resuscitation of intensive care unit patients with non-shockable rhythm cardiac arrest. Resuscitation 2015;92:1–6.

71. Gaspari R, Weekes A, Adhikari S, et al. Emergency department point-of-care ultrasound in out-of-hospital and in-ED cardiac arrest. Resuscitation 2016;109:33–9.

72. Reynolds JC, Nicholson TC, Drennan I, et al. Prognostication with point-of-care echocardiography during cardiac arrest: A systematic review. Resuscitation 2020;152:56–68.
73. Teran F, Dean AJ, Centeno C, et al. Evaluation of out-of-hospital cardiac arrest using transesophageal echocardiography in the emergency department. Resuscitation 2019;137:140–7.

Postarrest Interventions that Save Lives

Alexis Steinberg, MD[a,c], Jonathan Elmer, MD, MSc[a,b,c],*

KEYWORDS

- Percutaneous coronary intervention • Temperature-targeted management • Seizure
- Mechanical circulatory support

KEY POINTS

- A focused diagnostic work-up to identify and reverse the inciting cause of arrest is essential to prevent rearrest and improve outcomes.
- Percutaneous coronary intervention should be considered for all patients after arrest.
- Preventing secondary brain injury by initiating targeted temperature management, maintaining optimal perfusion pressure, optimizing ventilator management, and controlling seizures can further improve outcomes.
- Transfer to specialty care should be considered during initial resuscitation efforts.
- Neurologic prognostication and withdrawal of life-sustaining therapy for perceived poor neurologic prognosis should be delayed in all cases.

INTRODUCTION

Care of patients resuscitated from cardiac arrest is challenging. Mortality and morbidity are common even after return of spontaneous circulation (ROSC). In managing these patients, clinicians must simultaneously address multiple problems. Goals in the early postarrest period include cardiopulmonary stabilization and prevention of secondary brain injury. Given the complexity and importance of the minutes immediately after ROSC, an organized approach is crucial and is associated with demonstrable outcome benefits.[1]

Identifying Causes of Arrest that Require Immediate Intervention

Autopsy series show cardiac causes, particularly coronary artery disease, are the most common cause of out-of-hospital cardiac arrest (OHCA).[2] However, only a minority of patients with OHCA are successfully resuscitated and survive to hospital

a Department of Critical Care Medicine, University of Pittsburgh, 3550 Terrace Street, Pittsburgh, PA 15214, USA; b Department of Emergency Medicine, University of Pittsburgh, Iroquois Building, Suite 400A, 3600 Forbes Avenue, Pittsburgh, PA 15213, USA; c Department of Neurology, University of Pittsburgh, Kauffman Building, 3471 Fifth Avenue, Suite 802, Pittsburgh, PA, 15213, USA
* Corresponding author. Department of Emergency Medicine, University of Pittsburgh, Iroquois Building, Suite 400A, 3600 Forbes Ave, Pittsburgh, PA 15213.
E-mail address: elmerjp@upmc.edu

Emerg Med Clin N Am 38 (2020) 771–782
https://doi.org/10.1016/j.emc.2020.06.001
0733-8627/20/© 2020 Elsevier Inc. All rights reserved.

emed.theclinics.com

care. The demographics of the subgroup seen and evaluated in the emergency department (ED) are distinct from the broader group of patients with OHCA.[3] A recent large cohort study classified the arrest cause after a full inpatient diagnostic work-up, finding only a minority of cases were caused by acute coronary syndrome (ACS) or other cardiac causes.[4] A rapid, directed work-up is needed to evaluate for treatable arrest causes (**Table 1**). A brief history should be obtained from emergency medical services or family regarding the circumstances of the arrest. In some cases, history may suggest the underlying cause (eg, antecedent chest pain followed by ventricular fibrillation may suggest ACS, whereas presence of drug paraphernalia at the scene may suggest overdose). A focused physical examination can evaluate for signs of trauma, gastrointestinal hemorrhage, primary neurologic catastrophes such as intra-cerebral hemorrhage, and so forth.

Table 1
Diagnostic evaluation of patients after cardiac arrest

Underlying Cause	Work-up
Cardiac • ACS • Structural heart disease • Cardiomyopathies • RV failure (eg, pulmonary hypertension, pulmonary embolus) • Arrhythmia	ECG Troponin BNP Point-of-care ultrasonography CXR Cardiac catheterization
Pulmonary • Primary respiratory failure (eg, COPD, asthma) • Large airway obstruction	CXR Blood gas CT angiography of chest Peak and plateau pressures Bronchoscopy
Trauma • Exsanguination • Pneumothorax (rib/sternal fractures) • Cardiac tamponade • Solid organ laceration	Point-of-care ultrasonography Comprehensive cross-sectional imaging (CT chest/abdomen/pelvis) CXR
Neurologic • Stroke • Subarachnoid hemorrhage	CT head CT angiography head/neck CT perfusion
Septic shock	Cultures (blood, urine, ±sputum) CXR Complete blood count Lactate
Metabolic derangements • Diabetic ketoacidosis • Hypoglycemia • Hyperkalemia	Comprehensive metabolic panel
Exposures • Toxicologic • Environmental (eg, electrocution, hypothermia)	Detailed history Urine drug screen (eg, ethanol level, acetaminophen) ECG for intervals

Abbreviations: BNP, brain natriuretic peptide; COPD, chronic obstructive pulmonary disease; CT, computed tomography; CXR, chest radiograph; ECG, electrocardiogram; RV, right ventricle.

Because cardiovascular causes are common, an electrocardiogram (ECG) should be obtained on all patients after arrest. Although the data on emergent cardiac catheterization postarrest are mixed (discussed later), patients with ACSs and survivable neurologic injury likely benefit from early revascularization.[5] Laboratory testing, including a comprehensive metabolic panel, troponin, lactate, arterial blood gas, glucose, complete blood count, and coagulation studies, should be obtained. Severe metabolic disarray, such as hyperkalemia, diabetic emergencies, and hypoglycemia, can result in arrest. Point-of-care ultrasonography may inform initial resuscitation efforts and narrow the differential diagnosis.[6,7]

Chest radiograph can help with endotracheal tube placement and rule out a pneumothorax. In patients with coma or abnormal neurologic findings, early postarrest computed tomography (CT) imaging of the brain obtained in the ED is abnormal in 5% to 10% of patients.[8] Abnormalities include early cerebral edema, an ominous prognostic sign, and acute cerebrovascular disorder responsible for the initial arrest. Chest compressions commonly result in rib or sternal fractures and associated pneumothorax or solid organ injury.[9] For this reason, many centers obtain comprehensive cross-sectional imaging to screen for both causes and consequences of OHCA. Chest imaging is also sensitive and specific for diagnosis of pulmonary embolism (PE).[10] Arrest from PE defines the embolism as high risk, and these patients should be considered for thrombolytic therapy.[11]

Preventing Early Rearrest

One in 5 patients with OHCA that regain pulses rearrest, and rearrest worsens survival.[12-14] The timing is biphasic, occurring both minutes after ROSC and then hours later. Early rearrest can occur when patients shocked out of ventricular fibrillation refibrillate, particularly in the setting of ongoing myocardial ischemia. These patients may benefit from antidysrhythmic agents such as amiodarone or lidocaine. Refractory ventricular arrhythmias can be managed with mechanical circulatory support and coronary revascularization.[15] Recurrence of pulseless electrical activity is also common as bolus dose vasopressors given during cardiopulmonary resuscitation (CPR) are cleared. Administration of vasoactive agents by continuous infusion is commonly needed in the minutes after initial resuscitation. Patients with cardiogenic shock may require inotropic support.[16-18] The median time to delayed rearrest is about 5 hours.[14] Delayed rearrest often results from persistent myocardial dysfunction,[19] systemic inflammation with associated vasoplegia, and multisystem organ failure.[19,20]

Percutaneous Coronary Intervention

Patients with ST-elevations on ECG postarrest require immediate coronary angiography.[5,21-23] High doses of vasopressors, particularly bolus administration during CPR, can cause transient coronary vasospasm and result in a variety of ECG abnormalities, including ST elevation. It is reasonable to obtain a repeat ECG a few minutes after ROSC because many abnormalities rapidly resolve, but cardiac catheterization should typically not be delayed to obtain serial ECGs over time. Centers capable of performing early neurologic risk stratification may consider deferring percutaneous coronary intervention (PCI) in patients with early objective evidence of severe brain injury, because these patients are unlikely to benefit from revascularization.[24] However, given the limited specificity of many early neuroprognostic signs,[25] these decisions should be made with the utmost caution and only by clinicians with special expertise. Public reporting of postprocedural mortality may create a perverse disincentive to offer PCI to critically ill patients, including those resuscitated from OHCA.[26] Medical decision making should optimize care for the individual patient rather than reflecting fear of publicly reported outcomes.

Timing of PCI for patients with OHCA without ST-elevations is controversial. Post-arrest ECG is neither sensitive nor specific for diagnosis of ACS.[27–29] For patients with ACS, revascularization can improve myocardial function and prevent recurrent arrhythmias. Nevertheless, a recent randomized controlled trial failed to find benefit from emergent versus delayed PCI in patients with OHCA without ST-elevations.[30] The overall incidence of culprit lesions was only 15% in this study, reflecting the low incidence of cardiac causes of OHCA in patients who survive to the hospital. Other limitations to the study include delayed initiation of targeted temperature management (TTM) and hemodynamic resuscitation, and lack of baseline risk stratification of neurologic illness.

Overall, if pretest probability for ACS is high based on available data and there are neither contraindications to anticoagulation nor evidence of devastating primary brain injury, early PCI should be considered in discussion with interventional cardiology.

Mechanical Circulatory Support

Use of mechanical circulatory support (MCS) during and after cardiac arrest is steadily increasing.[31,32] MCS can preserve brain and coronary perfusion, buying time for definitive treatment in the event of refractory cardiac arrest. After initial ROSC, MCS can augment or replace inadequate cardiac output and may offer myocardial protection in some settings.[33]

Initiating MCS during CPR (termed extracorporeal CPR [ECPR]) requires venoarterial (VA) extracorporeal membrane oxygenation (ECMO). In the event of refractory ventricular arrhythmias from ACS, VA-ECMO can maintain cerebral perfusion and act as a bridge to coronary revascularization.[34] In the event of massive PE or other causes of acute right ventricular failure, VA-ECMO bypasses the failing right ventricle and pulmonary circulation to maintain systemic perfusion. Use of ECPR is growing worldwide.[35] Institutional protocols, inclusion criteria, and outcomes of ECPR vary widely across centers and regions.[34,36–40] ECPR is an expensive and complex intervention with little high-level evidence supporting its use. Nevertheless, it has reasonable face validity and future randomized trials may show benefit.[41]

ECMO may also be useful in the early postarrest period. VA-ECMO provides biventricular and pulmonary support, so it may have a role in both left and right ventricular failure or refractory hypoxemia. Compared with other MCS devices, VA-ECMO is also the most invasive and has the highest associated procedural risks.[35] Intra-aortic balloon pumps (IABPs) and Impella catheters can also be used in the postarrest period to support patients with significant cardiogenic shock. Despite the physiologic rationale for IABP, among patients with cardiogenic shock from acute myocardial infarction, IABP does not improve outcomes compared with conventional care.[42] In addition, it is unclear whether Impella confers significant outcome benefit compared with IABP or conventional care for patients with cardiogenic shock.[43,44]

Preventing Secondary Brain Injury

Anoxic brain injury is the most common proximate cause of death and disability for patients admitted after OHCA.[45–48] The brain is highly susceptible to ischemia after cardiac arrest. Hypoxic ischemic injury can lead to impaired cerebral autoregulation, cerebral edema, and delayed neurodegeneration.[19] Secondary brain injury can occur in the hours to days following ROSC and worsens outcomes.

Optimal perfusion pressure

Adequate cerebral perfusion is necessary after cardiac arrest to prevent further neuronal damage in the already-injured brain. Hours to days after ROSC, cerebral hypoperfusion can develop.[49] During this time, cerebral autoregulation is often impaired, and a smaller decrease in mean arterial pressure (MAP) can cause drastic changes to cerebral blood flow, with critical opening pressures for the cerebral vasculature exceeding 110 mm Hg.[50] Thus, even in the absence of systemic hypotension, cerebral perfusion may be inadequate.[51,52] The ideal MAP after cardiac arrest is unknown and likely needs to be tailored to patient-specific parameters. Multiple observation studies have shown improved neurologic outcome with maintaining a higher MAP (>80 mm Hg), even if vasopressors are required.[53-55] Two recent randomized control trials comparing an MAP of 65 to 75 mm Hg with 80 to 100 mm Hg showed that higher MAPs were feasible but not associated with secondary outcomes of favorable neurologic status.[56,57] One concern about augmenting postarrest MAP is the potential to decrease cardiac output if there is concomitant myocardial dysfunction. Our local practice is to maintain MAPs greater than 80 mm Hg, if other organ systems are not harmed. In any event, hypotension should be avoided.

The best method used to maintain adequate MAP is also unknown. Fluid resuscitation may be required initially and depends on the clinical scenario and the patient's current volume status. Vasopressor or inotropic medications are also often necessary, but the selection of vasoactive agents depends on the type of underlying shock. There is growing literature suggesting potential for harm when epinephrine infusions are used in patients with cardiogenic shock.[58,59]

Ventilator management: oxygenation and ventilation

Hypoxia is consistently associated with worse outcomes after cardiac arrest.[60] Hyperoxia may also cause secondary brain injury, likely mediated by oxidative stress during reperfusion.[61,62] The optimal range for partial pressure of arterial oxygen (Pao_2) is unknown, but 80 to 200 mm Hg is reasonable and a Pao_2 greater than 300 mm Hg should be avoided. If cooling is ongoing, blood gas results must be temperature corrected.

Cerebral blood flow can be altered through ventilation.[21] Hyperventilation-induced hypocapnia causes cerebral vasoconstriction and can cause cerebral ischemia and secondary brain injury.[63] Mild therapeutic hypercapnia can improve cerebral blood flow and may reduce biomarkers of brain injury,[64] although early-phase trial data are mixed.[56] Cerebral vasodilation also increases cerebral blood volume, which can increase intracranial pressure and worsen ischemia.[65] Current guidelines recommend normocapnia ($Paco_2$ 35–45 mm Hg) in the postarrest period.[5,21]

Targeted temperature management

TTM likely offers neuroprotection after cardiac arrest.[5,21,66] The optimal target temperature is unknown. Earlier trials showed benefit from cooling to 32°C to 34°C compared with either normothermia or no temperature management.[67,68] Subsequently, the large TTM trial showed no difference between 33°C and 36°C.[69] These studies enrolled only or mostly patients with initial shockable rhythms. The TTM study was also limited by a lack of standardization of cooling protocols and used a noninferiority trial design.[69] More recently, a smaller randomized controlled trial showed benefit of cooling to 33°C compared with 37°C for patients with an initial nonshockable rhythm.[70] Fever after cardiac arrest must be avoided; each degree more than 37°C is associated with worse outcome.[71]

TTM should be started immediately, because delays can reduce the benefit of cooling. Timing of TTM initiation must be balanced with need for any lifesaving diagnostic work-up or interventions (eg, PCI) and any contraindications (eg, uncontrolled hemorrhage). The best method for induction is unknown.

Shivering secondary to cooling can result in inability to meet temperature goals, so pharmacologic (sedation with or without neuromuscular blockade) and nonpharmacologic (skin counterwarming) interventions may be necessary. If sedation is required, short-acting medications (fentanyl, propofol, or dexmedetomidine) are preferable, and benzodiazepines should be avoided if possible.[72]

Seizures

Many patients who remain comatose after ROSC have abnormal electroencephalogram (EEG) patterns on the spectrum of seizure activity.[73,74] Seizures may worsen secondary brain injury. However, currently there is little evidence that treating these patterns improves neurologic outcomes.[75] It is reasonable to treat patients after cardiac arrest who have generalized tonic-clonic seizures with antiepileptic drugs, although generalized tonic-clonic seizures are an uncommon manifestation of global anoxic injury.[76] Myoclonus can be observed clinically in the first hours following ROSC, and was historically thought to be ominous. More recent research shows that its presence does not invariably predict poor outcome.[77,78] EEGs can differentiate myoclonus subtypes associated with poor outcome from those that are not ominous.[79,80] Transfer to a center with EEG monitoring should be considered to evaluate for seizures and for prognostication purposes.

Transfer to Specialty Care Center

For resuscitated patients who remain comatose, early transfer to a high-volume specialty care center should be considered.[1] Transport to a cardiac resuscitation center has been associated with increased survival and improved short-term and long-term outcomes.[81–85] These specialty care centers can offer PCI, cardiac and neurologic critical care, and TTM. For unstable patients, active engagement of a critical care transport team is crucial when arranging interfacility transport. Using a critical care transport team has been shown to be safe and feasible.[60] Both secondary prevention (arrhythmia work-up with defibrillator implantation, medication-assisted treatment of opioid addiction) and rehabilitation (neurologic and cardiac) have contributed to better outcomes for cardiac arrest survivors,[86] supporting the importance of transfer to a specialty care center.

Delayed Neuroprognostication

Clinical nihilism and early limitations in care may result in avoidable mortality.[47,48] Overall, quality in post–cardiac arrest neuroprognostication studies is low, and no single sign, symptom, or diagnostic test can accurately predict poor neurologic outcome in the first 24 hours.[25] Validated risk stratification tools exist but are not intended to rule out recoverable disease.[87] Early brain imaging can aid with risk stratification and prognostication but should not be used as a single modality of prognosis in the immediate scenario.[8,88,89] More advanced neuroprognostication tools, such as EEG, MRI, and blood biomarkers, are less useful in the acute postresuscitation period. When the prognosis is unclear, as is common in the acute phase of postarrest care, resuscitation should continue and early withdrawal of life-sustaining therapy should be avoided.

SUMMARY

Postarrest care that improves survival and functional status starts in the prehospital setting and continues to discharge planning. In the ED, parallel postresuscitation efforts should focus on work-up of underlying causes, preventing rearrest, and minimizing secondary brain injury.

DISCLOSURE

Dr. Elmer's research time is supported by the NIH through grant 5K23NS097629.

REFERENCES

1. Panchal AR, Berg KM, Cabañas JG, et al. 2019 American Heart Association Focused Update on Systems of Care: Dispatcher-Assisted Cardiopulmonary Resuscitation and Cardiac Arrest Centers: An Update to the American Heart Association guidelines for cardiopulmonary resuscitation and emergency cardiovascular care. Circulation 2019. https://doi.org/10.1161/CIR.0000000000000733. CIR0000000000000733.
2. Farb A, Tang AL, Burke AP, et al. Sudden coronary death. Frequency of active coronary lesions, inactive coronary lesions, and myocardial infarction. Circulation 1995;92(7):1701–9.
3. Okubo M, Schmicker RH, Wallace DJ, et al. Variation in survival after out-of-hospital cardiac arrest between emergency medical services agencies. JAMA Cardiol 2018;3(10):989–99.
4. Chen N, Callaway CW, Guyette FX, et al. Arrest etiology among patients resuscitated from cardiac arrest. Resuscitation 2018;130:33–40.
5. Callaway CW, Donnino MW, Fink EL, et al. Part 8: post-cardiac arrest care: 2015 American Heart Association guidelines update for cardiopulmonary resuscitation and emergency cardiovascular care. Circulation 2015;132(18 Suppl 2):S465–82.
6. Clattenburg EJ, Wroe P, Brown S, et al. Point-of-care ultrasound use in patients with cardiac arrest is associated prolonged cardiopulmonary resuscitation pauses: A prospective cohort study. Resuscitation 2018;122:65–8.
7. Stickles SP, Carpenter CR, Gekle R, et al. The diagnostic accuracy of a point-of-care ultrasound protocol for shock etiology: a systematic review and meta-analysis. CJEM 2019;21(3):406–17.
8. Metter RB, Rittenberger JC, Guyette FX, et al. Association between a quantitative CT scan measure of brain edema and outcome after cardiac arrest. Resuscitation 2011;82(9):1180–5.
9. Champigneulle B, Haruel PA, Pirracchio R, et al. Major traumatic complications after out-of-hospital cardiac arrest: Insights from the Parisian registry. Resuscitation 2018;128:70–5.
10. Chen Z, Deblois S, Toporowicz K, et al. Yield of CT pulmonary angiography in the diagnosis of acute pulmonary embolism: short report. BMC Res Notes 2019; 12(1):41.
11. Task Force Members, Konstantinides SV, Meyer G, et al. 2019 ESC Guidelines for the diagnosis and management of acute pulmonary embolism developed in collaboration with the European Respiratory Society (ERS): The Task Force for the diagnosis and management of acute pulmonary embolism of the European Society of Cardiology (ESC). Eur Respir J 2019;54(3). https://doi.org/10.1183/13993003.01647-2019.
12. Salcido DD, Sundermann ML, Koller AC, et al. Incidence and outcomes of rearrest following out-of-hospital cardiac arrest. Resuscitation 2015;86:19–24.
13. Salcido DD, Stephenson AM, Condle JP, et al. Incidence of rearrest after return of spontaneous circulation in out-of-hospital cardiac arrest. Prehosp Emerg Care 2010;14(4):413–8.

14. Bhardwaj A, Ikeda DJ, Grossestreuer AV, et al. Factors associated with re-arrest following initial resuscitation from cardiac arrest. Resuscitation 2017;111:90–5.

15. Guerra F, Shkoza M, Scappini L, et al. Role of electrical storm as a mortality and morbidity risk factor and its clinical predictors: a meta-analysis. Europace 2014; 16(3):347–53.

16. Laurent I, Monchi M, Chiche J-D, et al. Reversible myocardial dysfunction in survivors of out-of-hospital cardiac arrest. J Am Coll Cardiol 2002;40(12):2110–6.

17. Huang L, Weil MH, Tang W, et al. Comparison between dobutamine and levosimendan for management of postresuscitation myocardial dysfunction. Crit Care Med 2005;33(3):487–91.

18. Kern KB, Hilwig RW, Berg RA, et al. Postresuscitation left ventricular systolic and diastolic dysfunction. Treatment with dobutamine. Circulation 1997;95(12): 2610–3.

19. Nolan JP, Neumar RW, Adrie C, et al. Post-cardiac arrest syndrome: epidemiology, pathophysiology, treatment, and prognostication. A Scientific Statement from the International Liaison Committee on Resuscitation; the American Heart Association Emergency Cardiovascular Care Committee; the Council on Cardiovascular Surgery and Anesthesia; the Council on Cardiopulmonary, Perioperative, and Critical Care; the Council on Clinical Cardiology; the Council on Stroke. Resuscitation 2008;79(3):350–79.

20. Cerchiari EL, Safar P, Klein E, et al. Visceral, hematologic and bacteriologic changes and neurologic outcome after cardiac arrest in dogs. The visceral post-resuscitation syndrome. Resuscitation 1993;25(2):119–36.

21. Nolan JP, Soar J, Cariou A, et al. European Resuscitation Council and European Society of Intensive Care Medicine 2015 guidelines for post-resuscitation care. Intensive Care Med 2015;41(12):2039–56.

22. O'Gara PT, Kushner FG, Ascheim DD, et al. 2013 ACCF/AHA guideline for the management of ST-elevation myocardial infarction: executive summary: a report of the American College of Cardiology Foundation/American Heart Association Task Force on Practice Guidelines. Circulation 2013;127(4):529–55.

23. Task Force on the management of ST-segment elevation acute myocardial infarction of the European Society of Cardiology (ESC), Steg PG, James SK, et al. ESC Guidelines for the management of acute myocardial infarction in patients presenting with ST-segment elevation. Eur Heart J 2012;33(20):2569–619.

24. Reynolds JC, Callaway CW, El Khoudary SR, et al. Coronary angiography predicts improved outcome following cardiac arrest: propensity-adjusted analysis. J Intensive Care Med 2009;24(3):179–86.

25. Geocadin RG, Callaway CW, Fink EL, et al. Standards for studies of neurological prognostication in comatose survivors of cardiac arrest: A scientific statement from the american heart association. Circulation 2019;140(9):e517–42.

26. Peberdy MA, Donnino MW, Callaway CW, et al. Impact of percutaneous coronary intervention performance reporting on cardiac resuscitation centers: a scientific statement from the American Heart Association. Circulation 2013;128(7):762–73.

27. Stær-Jensen H, Nakstad ER, Fossum E, et al. Post-resuscitation ECG for selection of patients for immediate coronary angiography in out-of-hospital cardiac arrest. Circ Cardiovasc Interv 2015;8(10). https://doi.org/10.1161/CIRCINTERVENTIONS.115.002784.

28. Zanuttini D, Armellini I, Nucifora G, et al. Predictive value of electrocardiogram in diagnosing acute coronary artery lesions among patients with out-of-hospital-cardiac-arrest. Resuscitation 2013;84(9):1250–4.

29. Spaulding CM, Joly LM, Rosenberg A, et al. Immediate coronary angiography in survivors of out-of-hospital cardiac arrest. N Engl J Med 1997;336(23):1629–33.

30. Lemkes JS, Janssens GN, van der Hoeven NW, et al. Coronary Angiography after Cardiac Arrest without ST-segment elevation. N Engl J Med 2019;380(15): 1397–407.

31. Patel NJ, Patel N, Bhardwaj B, et al. Trends in utilization of mechanical circulatory support in patients hospitalized after out-of-hospital cardiac arrest. Resuscitation 2018;127:105–13.

32. Patel NJ, Atti V, Kumar V, et al. Temporal trends of survival and utilization of mechanical circulatory support devices in patients with in-hospital cardiac arrest secondary to ventricular tachycardia/ventricular fibrillation. Catheter Cardiovasc Interv 2019;94(4):578–87.

33. Rihal CS, Naidu SS, Givertz MM, et al. 2015 SCAI/ACC/HFSA/STS Clinical Expert Consensus Statement on the Use of Percutaneous Mechanical Circulatory Support Devices in Cardiovascular Care: Endorsed by the American Heart Assocation, the Cardiological Society of India, and Sociedad Latino Americana de Cardiologia Intervencion; Affirmation of Value by the Canadian Association of Interventional Cardiology-Association Canadienne de Cardiologie d'intervention. J Am Coll Cardiol 2015;65(19):e7–26.

34. Bartos JA, Carlson K, Carlson C, et al. Surviving refractory out-of-hospital ventricular fibrillation cardiac arrest: Critical care and extracorporeal membrane oxygenation management. Resuscitation 2018;132:47–55.

35. ELSO Registry. ECLS registry report: international summary 2017. Available at: https://www.elso.org/Registry/Statistics/InternationalSummary.aspx. Accessed November 21, 2019.

36. Sakamoto T, Morimura N, Nagao K, et al. Extracorporeal cardiopulmonary resuscitation versus conventional cardiopulmonary resuscitation in adults with out-of-hospital cardiac arrest: a prospective observational study. Resuscitation 2014; 85(6):762–8.

37. Bouglé A, Le Gall A, Dumas F, et al. ExtraCorporeal life support for Cardiac ARrest in patients with post cardiac arrest syndrome: The ECCAR study. Arch Cardiovasc Dis 2019;112(4):253–60.

38. Lee H, Sung K, Suh GY, et al. Outcomes of transported and in-house patients on extracorporeal life support: a propensity score-matching study. Eur J Cardiothorac Surg 2019. https://doi.org/10.1093/ejcts/ezz227.

39. Chonde M, Sappington P, Kormos R, et al. The Use of ECMO for the treatment of refractory cardiac arrest or postarrest cardiogenic shock following in-hospital cardiac arrest: a 10-year experience. J Intensive Care Med 2018. https://doi.org/10.1177/0885066617751398. 885066617751398.

40. Stub D, Bernard S, Pellegrino V, et al. Refractory cardiac arrest treated with mechanical CPR, hypothermia, ECMO and early reperfusion (the CHEER trial). Resuscitation 2015;86:88–94.

41. A Comparative Study Between a Pre-hospital and an In-hospital Circulatory Support Strategy (ECMO) in Refractory Cardiac Arrest (APACAR2) - Full Text View - ClinicalTrials.gov. Available at: https://clinicaltrials.gov/ct2/show/NCT02527031. Accessed December 12, 2019.

42. Thiele H, Zeymer U, Neumann F-J, et al. Intraaortic balloon support for myocardial infarction with cardiogenic shock. N Engl J Med 2012;367(14):1287–96.

43. Ouweneel DM, Eriksen E, Sjauw KD, et al. Percutaneous mechanical circulatory support versus intra-aortic balloon pump in cardiogenic shock after acute myocardial infarction. J Am Coll Cardiol 2017;69(3):278–87.

44. Cheng JM, den Uil CA, Hoeks SE, et al. Percutaneous left ventricular assist devices vs. intra-aortic balloon pump counterpulsation for treatment of cardiogenic shock: a meta-analysis of controlled trials. Eur Heart J 2009;30(17):2102–8.
45. Laver S, Farrow C, Turner D, et al. Mode of death after admission to an intensive care unit following cardiac arrest. Intensive Care Med 2004;30(11):2126–8.
46. Mongardon N, Dumas F, Ricome S, et al. Postcardiac arrest syndrome: from immediate resuscitation to long-term outcome. Ann Intensive Care 2011;1(1):45.
47. Elmer J, Torres C, Aufderheide TP, et al. Association of early withdrawal of life-sustaining therapy for perceived neurological prognosis with mortality after cardiac arrest. Resuscitation 2016;102:127–35.
48. May TL, Ruthazer R, Riker RR, et al. Early withdrawal of life support after resuscitation from cardiac arrest is common and may result in additional deaths. Resuscitation 2019;139:308–13.
49. Wolfson SK, Safar P, Reich H, et al. Dynamic heterogeneity of cerebral hypoperfusion after prolonged cardiac arrest in dogs measured by the stable xenon/CT technique: a preliminary study. Resuscitation 1992;23(1):1–20.
50. Pham P, Bindra J, Chuan A, et al. Are changes in cerebrovascular autoregulation following cardiac arrest associated with neurological outcome? Results of a pilot study. Resuscitation 2015;96:192–8.
51. Sundgreen C, Larsen FS, Herzog TM, et al. Autoregulation of cerebral blood flow in patients resuscitated from cardiac arrest. Stroke 2001;32(1):128–32.
52. Iordanova B, Li L, Clark RSB, et al. Alterations in Cerebral Blood Flow after Resuscitation from Cardiac Arrest. Front Pediatr 2017;5:174.
53. Ameloot K, Meex I, Genbrugge C, et al. Hemodynamic targets during therapeutic hypothermia after cardiac arrest: A prospective observational study. Resuscitation 2015;91:56–62.
54. Roberts BW, Kilgannon JH, Hunter BR, et al. Association between elevated mean arterial blood pressure and neurologic outcome after resuscitation from cardiac arrest: results from a multicenter prospective cohort study. Crit Care Med 2019; 47(1):93–100.
55. Russo JJ, Di Santo P, Simard T, et al. Optimal mean arterial pressure in comatose survivors of out-of-hospital cardiac arrest: An analysis of area below blood pressure thresholds. Resuscitation 2018;128:175–80.
56. Jakkula P, Pettilä V, Skrifvars MB, et al. Targeting low-normal or high-normal mean arterial pressure after cardiac arrest and resuscitation: a randomised pilot trial. Intensive Care Med 2018;44(12):2091–101.
57. Ameloot K, De Deyne C, Eertmans W, et al. Early goal-directed haemodynamic optimization of cerebral oxygenation in comatose survivors after cardiac arrest: the Neuroprotect post-cardiac arrest trial. Eur Heart J 2019;40(22):1804–14.
58. Léopold V, Gayat E, Pirracchio R, et al. Epinephrine and short-term survival in cardiogenic shock: an individual data meta-analysis of 2583 patients. Intensive Care Med 2018;44(6):847–56.
59. Levy B, Clere-Jehl R, Legras A, et al. Epinephrine Versus Norepinephrine for Cardiogenic Shock After Acute Myocardial Infarction. J Am Coll Cardiol 2018; 72(2):173–82.
60. Hartke A, Mumma BE, Rittenberger JC, et al. Incidence of re-arrest and critical events during prolonged transport of post-cardiac arrest patients. Resuscitation 2010;81(8):938–42.
61. Roberts BW, Kilgannon JH, Hunter BR, et al. Association Between Early Hyperoxia Exposure After Resuscitation From Cardiac Arrest and Neurological

Disability: Prospective Multicenter Protocol-Directed Cohort Study. Circulation 2018;137(20):2114–24.

62. Wang C-H, Chang W-T, Huang C-H, et al. The effect of hyperoxia on survival following adult cardiac arrest: a systematic review and meta-analysis of observational studies. Resuscitation 2014;85(9):1142–8.

63. McKenzie N, Williams TA, Tohira H, et al. A systematic review and meta-analysis of the association between arterial carbon dioxide tension and outcomes after cardiac arrest. Resuscitation 2017;111:116–26.

64. Eastwood GM, Schneider AG, Suzuki S, et al. Targeted therapeutic mild hypercapnia after cardiac arrest: A phase II multi-centre randomised controlled trial (the CCC trial). Resuscitation 2016;104:83–90.

65. Helmerhorst HJF, Roos-Blom M-J, van Westerloo DJ, et al. Associations of arterial carbon dioxide and arterial oxygen concentrations with hospital mortality after resuscitation from cardiac arrest. Crit Care 2015;19:348.

66. Geocadin RG, Wijdicks E, Armstrong MJ, et al. Practice guideline summary: Reducing brain injury following cardiopulmonary resuscitation: Report of the Guideline Development, Dissemination, and Implementation Subcommittee of the American Academy of Neurology. Neurology 2017;88(22):2141–9.

67. Bernard SA, Gray TW, Buist MD, et al. Treatment of comatose survivors of out-of-hospital cardiac arrest with induced hypothermia. N Engl J Med 2002;346(8):557–63.

68. Hypothermia after Cardiac Arrest Study Group. Mild therapeutic hypothermia to improve the neurologic outcome after cardiac arrest. N Engl J Med 2002;346(8):549–56.

69. Nielsen N, Wetterslev J, Cronberg T, et al. Targeted temperature management at 33°C versus 36°C after cardiac arrest. N Engl J Med 2013;369(23):2197–206.

70. Lascarrou J-B, Merdji H, Le Gouge A, et al. Targeted temperature management for cardiac arrest with nonshockable rhythm. N Engl J Med 2019;381(24):2327–37.

71. Zeiner A, Holzer M, Sterz F, et al. Hyperthermia after cardiac arrest is associated with an unfavorable neurologic outcome. Arch Intern Med 2001;161(16):2007–12.

72. Paul M, Bougouin W, Dumas F, et al. Comparison of two sedation regimens during targeted temperature management after cardiac arrest. Resuscitation 2018;128:204–10.

73. Rittenberger JC, Popescu A, Brenner RP, et al. Frequency and timing of nonconvulsive status epilepticus in comatose post-cardiac arrest subjects treated with hypothermia. Neurocrit Care 2012;16(1):114–22.

74. Faro J, Coppler PJ, Dezfulian C, et al. Differential association of subtypes of epileptiform activity with outcome after cardiac arrest. Resuscitation 2019;136:138–45.

75. Ruijter BJ, van Putten MJAM, Horn J, et al. Treatment of electroencephalographic status epilepticus after cardiopulmonary resuscitation (TELSTAR): study protocol for a randomized controlled trial. Trials 2014;15:433.

76. Brophy GM, Bell R, Claassen J, et al. Guidelines for the evaluation and management of status epilepticus. Neurocrit Care 2012;17(1):3–23.

77. Aicua Rapun I, Novy J, Solari D, et al. Early Lance-Adams syndrome after cardiac arrest: Prevalence, time to return to awareness, and outcome in a large cohort. Resuscitation 2017;115:169–72.

78. Elmer J, Rittenberger JC, Faro J, et al. Clinically distinct electroencephalographic phenotypes of early myoclonus after cardiac arrest. Ann Neurol 2016;80(2):175–84.

79. Rossetti AO, Urbano LA, Delodder F, et al. Prognostic value of continuous EEG monitoring during therapeutic hypothermia after cardiac arrest. Crit Care 2010; 14(5):R173.

80. Westhall E, Rossetti AO, van Rootselaar A-F, et al. Standardized EEG interpretation accurately predicts prognosis after cardiac arrest. Neurology 2016;86(16): 1482–90.

81. Lipe D, Giwa A, Caputo ND, et al. Do Out-of-Hospital Cardiac Arrest Patients Have Increased Chances of Survival When Transported to a Cardiac Resuscitation Center? J Am Heart Assoc 2018;7(23):e011079.

82. Schober A, Sterz F, Laggner AN, et al. Admission of out-of-hospital cardiac arrest victims to a high volume cardiac arrest center is linked to improved outcome. Resuscitation 2016;106:42–8.

83. Elmer J, Callaway CW, Chang C-CH, et al. Long-Term Outcomes of Out-of-Hospital Cardiac Arrest Care at Regionalized Centers. Ann Emerg Med 2019; 73(1):29–39.

84. Elmer J, Rittenberger JC, Coppler PJ, et al. Long-term survival benefit from treatment at a specialty center after cardiac arrest. Resuscitation 2016;108:48–53.

85. Matsuyama T, Kiyohara K, Kitamura T, et al. Hospital characteristics and favourable neurological outcome among patients with out-of-hospital cardiac arrest in Osaka, Japan. Resuscitation 2017;110:146–53.

86. Antiarrhythmics versus Implantable Defibrillators (AVID) Investigators. A comparison of antiarrhythmic-drug therapy with implantable defibrillators in patients resuscitated from near-fatal ventricular arrhythmias. N Engl J Med 1997; 337(22):1576–83.

87. Coppler PJ, Elmer J, Calderon L, et al. Validation of the Pittsburgh Cardiac Arrest Category illness severity score. Resuscitation 2015;89:86–92.

88. Torbey MT, Selim M, Knorr J, et al. Quantitative analysis of the loss of distinction between gray and white matter in comatose patients after cardiac arrest. Stroke 2000;31(9):2163–7.

89. Yanagawa Y, Un-no Y, Sakamoto T, et al. Cerebral density on CT immediately after a successful resuscitation of cardiopulmonary arrest correlates with outcome. Resuscitation 2005;64(1):97–101.

Fluid Resuscitation
History, Physiology, and Modern Fluid Resuscitation Strategies

David Gordon, MD[a], Rory Spiegel, MD[b],*

KEYWORDS

- Crystalloid • Colloid • Balanced solutions • Fluid resuscitation • Fluid administration

KEY POINTS

- Balanced crystalloid offers theoretic benefits over normal saline, but to date large studies demonstrate only minimal benefits. Rather than the choice of crystalloid, clinicians should focus on the volume of fluid administered.
- The use of colloids has never been found to improve patient-centered outcomes. Initial volume repletion in the emergency department should be performed primarily with intravenous crystalloids.
- Fluid administration should be seen in the greater scheme of a patient resuscitation, modeled after trauma resuscitation, damage control resuscitation with the primary goal of controlling the underlying cause of the patients' shock.
- Although fluids can play a pivotal role in resuscitating patients, patients should be evaluated for potential harms of additional fluids prior to their administration.
- Early use of low-dose vasopressors has the potential to increase venous tone, limiting the volume of fluid required during initial resuscitative efforts.

INTRODUCTION

The repletion of patients' intravascular volume through the use of an intravenous (IV) electrolyte solution was first described by a young Irish physician, William Brooke O'Shaughnessy, in 1831. Immersing himself in the middle of a cholera outbreak in Sutherland, England, O'Shaughnessy observed that large amounts of water, sodium, chloride, and bicarbonate were being lost in these patients' stool.

The indications of cure … are two in number –first to restore the blood to its natural specific gravity; second to restore its deficient saline matters[1] … The first of these can only be affected by absorption, by imbibition, or by the injection of aqueous fluid into the veins.[1]

[a] Department of Medicine, University of Maryland Medical Center, 110 South Paca Pratt Street, Baltimore, MD 21201, USA; [b] Attending Emergency Medicine, Georgetown University Hospital, Washington Hospital Center, Faculty Critical Care, 110 Irving Street, East Building Room 3124, Washington, DC 20010, USA
* Corresponding author.
E-mail address: Rory.j.Spiegel@medstar.net

Emerg Med Clin N Am 38 (2020) 783–793
https://doi.org/10.1016/j.emc.2020.06.004
0733-8627/20/© 2020 Elsevier Inc. All rights reserved.

Since these humble beginnings, IV fluid therapy has become a key component of the initial management of shock in the emergency department. This article will discuss types of fluid, their physiologic effects, and current strategies on how best to utilize fluids when resuscitating patients in shock.

THE GREAT FLUID DEBATE
Normal Saline Versus Balanced Solutions

Lactated Ringers (LR), was discovered by Sydney Ringer and his laboratory assistant in 1883, when a saline solution mistakenly made with tap water rather than a distilled solution was used while studying frog hearts.[2] They noted cardiac activity was sustained for longer periods with the fortuitous tap water solution.[2] This prompted Ringer to further investigate the inorganic compounds present in the water, and to create his own solution.[2] His solution has undergone multiple revisions, the most famous of which was made by Alexis Hartmann, who in 1930 added lactate in the hopes of limiting the acidosis observed with previous iterations.[2]

Normal saline (NS) in its current form seems to originate from Joseph Hamburger, a Dutch physiologist, who in 1896 observed that a 0.9% sodium-chloride (NaCl) solution was more similar to human blood's freezing point than fluids of alternate tonicities.[3]

The debate over the appropriate crystalloid has been going on since Hartman first proposed his modified sodium-lactate solution as a means of preventing the acidosis observed with large-volume infusions of normal saline.[4–6] Because of its high chloride (Cl) content, normal saline is an acidotic solution with a pH of 5.6.[7] Solutions such as LR or PlasmaLyte replace a portion of their chloride content with an alternative anion that is metabolized to bicarbonate after its administration (**Table 1**). These chloride poor solutions are considered balanced solutions because of their more neutral effects on the acid-base physiology and chemical composure more similar to plasma.

Although the administration of NS will lead to a hyperchloremic, nonanion gap metabolic acidosis, it is unclear whether this acidosis has detrimental effects clinically.

Table 1
Electrolyte concentrations of various crystalloid solutions

	0.9% NS	0.45% NS	3% NS[a]	Lactate Ringers	PlasmaLyte	D5+ 0.9% NS[a]	D5+ 0.45% NS[a]
Na mEq/L	154	77	513	130	140	154	77
Cl mEq/L	154	77	513	109	93	154	77
K mEq/L	—	—	—	4	5	—	—
Ca mEq/L	—	—	—	217	—	—	—
Mg mEq/L	—	—	—	—	3	—	—
Acetate	—	—	—	—	27	—	—
Gluconate	—	—	—	—	23	—	—
Glucose g	—	—	—	—	—	50	50
Lactate mEq/L	—	—	—	—28	—	—	—
Glucose	—	—	—	—	—	—	—
mOsm/L	308	154	1027	273	294	560	406
SID	0	0	0	21	12	0	0
pH	5.6	5.6	50	6.5	7.4	4.0	4.0

[a] Specifically for Baxter products.

Several small nonrandomized and animal studies have found increased inflammation, impaired kidney function, increased pressor requirement, higher transfusion requirements, and even increased mortality associated with the administration of high chloride solutions.[8] The SPLIT Trial, a large, multicenter, cluster-randomized control trial comparing the use of NS with PlasmaLyte, by Young and colleagues,[9] did not demonstrate these harms.

Recently, 2 large single-center, pragmatic, cluster-randomized, multiple crossover trials were published to evaluate NS versus balanced solutions.[10,11] Both studies demonstrated greater derangement of serum Cl and bicarbonate concentrations in the normal saline groups. The study of noncritically ill emergency department patients also noted an improvement in the rate of major adverse kidney events (MAKE-30), a composite outcome including death, new renal replacement therapy, or persistent renal dysfunction at 30 days in patients randomized to balanced fluids.[10] Similarly, the SMART Trial, enrolling patients admitted to the intensive care unit (ICU), observed a 1.1% absolute decrease in the rate of MAKE-30 in patients who received balanced solutions.[11] Importantly, while both studies found a statistical difference in the rate of MAKE-30, the absolute difference was small (approximately 1% in either study), and no single individual endpoint was significantly different, including mortality.[11] A subgroup analysis reported a statistically significant improvement in both the composite outcome MAKE-30 and mortality in isolation in the cohort of patients admitted with sepsis.[12] Although interesting, this subgroup analysis should be viewed as hypothesis generating, requiring further validation. A recent Cochrane review examining over 20,000 patients in randomized controlled trials (RCTs) comparing normal saline with balanced solutions identified no difference in the rate of renal failure or death at 30 days.[13] Although the acid-base consequences of normal saline may indeed be real, the patient-centered consequences of using normal saline instead of a more balanced solution seems to be mostly a theoretic concern.

Colloid Versus Crystalloid

The second major consideration when determining what fluid to administer is whether to use a crystalloid or colloid solution. Colloids are defined as: "protein or polysaccharide solution that can be used to increase or maintain osmotic (oncotic) pressure in the intravascular compartment such as albumin, dextran, Hetastarch; or certain blood components such as plasma and platelets."[14] This discussion of colloids as resuscitative fluids will focus on albumin, as studies examining Hetastarch found an associated risk of renal failure and death.[15] Additionally, specific indications for albumin beyond resuscitation, such as hepatorenal syndrome and spontaneous bacterial peritonitis,[16] are beyond the scope of this article.

The physiologic defense for the use of colloids rests primarily on the Starling equation, or the ability to increase plasma oncotic pressure, increasing fluid reabsorption, thereby increasing circulating volume. The classic teaching is that fluid exchange occurs at the level of the capillary and is governed predominantly by 4 variables: the capillary oncotic pressure, the interstitial oncotic pressure, the capillary hydrostatic pressure, and interstitial hydrostatic pressure.[17,18] Over the course of the capillary, the forces begin to balance out such that the arterial side favors filtration, and the venous side favors reabsorption (**Fig. 1**A).[18]

Recent experimental evidence has challenged this view in favor of the revised Starling equation. In the revised Starling equation, plasma hydrostatic pressure is the dominant force. This results in net filtration occurring throughout the capillary without any reabsorption (**Fig. 1**B).[18] The lymphatic system then serves as the major pathway for filtered fluid to return to the vascular circulation.[18] In this model, the major

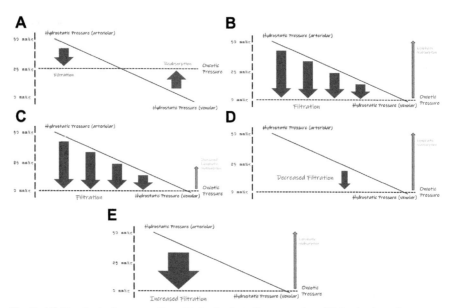

Fig. 1. (*A*) Classic starling equation. (*B*) Revised starling equation. (*C*) Revised starling equation in congestive heart failure patient. (*D*) Revised starling equation in patient in septic shock before resuscitation. (*E*) Revised starling equation in patient in septic shock after resuscitation.

determinants of the of filtration are the plasma hydrostatic pressure and vascular integrity.[18] The dominant forces of reabsorption are the lymphatic tone and right atrial pressure. Because most reabsorption occurs through the lymphatic system, the major determinants of reabsorption are lymphatic tone and right atrial pressure, the eventual basin for the lymphatic system.[18]

Although the lymphatic system can accommodate the volume of fluid filtered out of the vascular beds under normal conditions,[17] a decrease in lymphatic drainage or an increase in vascular filtration can result in interstitial edema. In a patient with congestive heart failure, filtration at the capillaries occurs at a normal rate, but lymphatic drainage is impaired because of elevated right atrial pressure, leading to interstitial edema (**Fig. 1**C). Conversely, in sepsis, because of systemic inflammation, there is a decrease in glycocalyx integrity, leading to the potential for an increase in net filtration.[19] Patients in septic shock are typically hypotensive, leading to a decrease in hydrostatic pressure and vascular filtration (**Fig. 1**D). It is only after the restoration of hydrostatic pressure through aggressive IV fluid administration that the loss of integrity of the glycocalyx becomes evident, and extravascular fluid accumulation is observed (**Fig. 1**E).

RCT data examining the use of colloids as resuscitative fluids have not consistently demonstrated fluid-sparing outcomes that would support the classic Starling theory. These trials observed small differences in overall fluid administration and early improvements in hemodynamic parameters; however, the differences were clinically inconsequential and failed to translate into an improvement in mortality.[20,21]

Outside the confines of specific disease states, where clinically relevant improvements in patient outcomes have been demonstrated, clinicians should limit the use of colloids in their resuscitative efforts. In fact, despite many physiologic theories expounding on the benefits of various fluid choices (both colloids and crystalloids) over others, evidence has failed to identify the existence of an ideal IV fluid. The choice of solution matters far less than the quantity of fluid that is given. Thus, clinicians should feel free to use whichever solution is most convenient to them and refocus their attention on strategies to limit over-resuscitation and the downstream harms of fluid administration.

THE FORGOTTEN PHYSIOLOGY OF VENOUS RETURN

The current management of shock has been focused on the restoration of arterial blood pressure, end-organ perfusion, and oxygen delivery. Most resuscitative models focus on methods for optimizing cardiac output, but this is a limited view of the circulatory system. Venous return physiology plays a large role in determining the cardiac output, and the variables that determine the venous return are often overlooked. Understanding of the determinants of venous return is vital to understanding the safe and effective use of IV fluids.

The 3 variables that determine venous return are the right atrial pressure, the mean systemic filling pressure (Pms), and the vascular resistance. Under most clinical circumstances, vascular resistance minimally influences venous return; thus right atrial pressure and Pms are the major determinants of venous return.[22]

Pms is an elusive concept, primarily because of the difficulties encountered when attempting to measure its existence. Technically it is defined as the pressure in the vascular system if blood flow were to cease.[23] Functionally the Pms is the pressure driving blood back to the heart. It is in direct competition with the right atrial pressure and is determined by the volume of blood in the venous circulation and the intrinsic compliance of the vascular bed. Essentially a certain volume of fluid is required to fill the vascular bed to exert force on the vessel walls. This volume is called the unstressed volume. The volume of blood above this level is the stressed volume, or the volume that will increase Pms and venous return (**Fig. 2**).[23]

For example, in a patient with distributive shock from sepsis, the total volume of blood has not changed. Instead, vasodilation has led to an increase in vascular compliance, shifting a portion of the stressed volume to an unstressed state. This in turn leads to a decrease in the Pms and venous return.[24] Conversely, in a patient with hemorrhagic shock, there is also a decrease in the stressed volume. In this instance, however, it is not because of a change in vascular compliance, but rather a decrease in absolute blood volume. The physiologic response is to increase catecholamine levels, inducing venoconstriction, shifting blood from the unstressed to the stressed volume, increasing the Pms and temporarily maintaining the venous return. If bleeding is not controlled, however, blood loss will outpace venoconstrictive compensation, and further attempts to augment preload through the shifting of unstressed to stressed volume will be futile.

In septic shock, resuscitative efforts typically occur in a 2-stage process. First, adding volume to the system (in the form of a fluid bolus), will increase both the stressed volume and the total volume. Once an appropriate amount of fluid is given, attempts are made to reduce the vessel wall compliance, with the addition of vasopressor agents, causing a change in the ratio of volume in the stressed and unstressed states. In this case the total volume would stay constant, while the unstressed volume decreases, and the stressed volume increases. In contrast, for patients in hemorrhagic shock, intrinsic catecholamines have already constricted the venous system, maximally recruiting unstressed to stressed volume. The administration of IV fluids, in this case blood products, to replace the lost blood, is an attempt to restore the total volume and stressed volume to a more physiologic state.

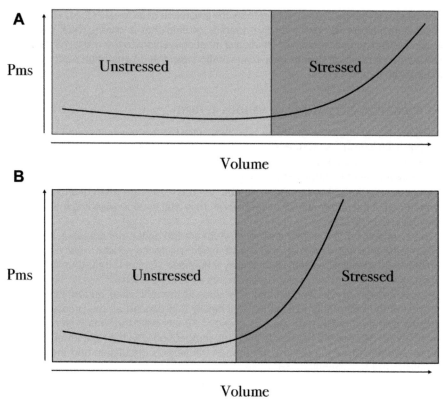

Fig. 2. (A) Unstressed and stressed volume. (B) Unstressed and stressed volume following and increase in vascular compliance.

With these principles in mind, it is important to remember the intended goals of a fluid bolus, to increase cardiac output and oxygen delivery to the end-organs. But it equally important to remember this is only achieved if the fluid bolus results in an augmentation of Pms and increases venous return.

THE CLINICAL REALITY OF A FLUID BOLUS

Traditionally it has been taught that a fluid bolus of 500 to 1000 mL should be rapidly infused into the circulation to assess for an adequate hemodynamic response prior to deciding whether to administer further volume challenges. Studies describing the effects of the administration of IV fluids in a rapid bolus have observed the desired increase in cardiac output lasts for approximately 120 minutes, at which point cardiac function seems to return to prior levels.[25] Studies indicate a more rapid administration of the fluid bolus leads to a shorter period of observed effects on cardiac output.[25] This phenomenon is likely caused by the rapid increase in hydrostatic pressure induced by the bolus, leading to an increase in filtration of fluid from the intravascular space. The central venous pressure (CVP), however, remains elevated for much longer.[25]

A MODERN-DAY RESUSCITATIVE STRATEGY

Typically, a fluid responsiveness strategy is recommended as the gold standard to guide fluid administration, defined as a response of 10% to 15% increase in a patient's cardiac output.[26] Recent data suggest that the use of a passive leg raise and some form of noninvasive cardiac output monitoring (ie ultrasound or pulse pressure variation) is the most accurate measure to predict whether an individual patient will respond to a fluid bolus.[26] Although PLR seems to adequately predict a patient's response to fluid, no data suggest that a fluid responsiveness strategy improves patient-important outcomes. Approximately 90% of healthy volunteers will respond to a fluid bolus by increasing their cardiac output.[27] One may conclude that people exist naturally in a fluid responsive state, and to iatrogenically drive someone to the flat portion of their Frank-Starling curve is by definition over-resuscitation. Because of the effects of a fluid bolus on cardiac output are short-lived, and the effects on CVP and venous congestion are more enduring, a resuscitative strategy that encourages multiple fluid boluses based on the response of cardiac output may cause harm. A growing body of evidence suggests aggressive fluid resuscitative strategies are harmful, leading to increased rates of acute kidney injury (AKI), pulmonary edema, acute respiratory distress syndrome, and even death.[28]

In a trial of African children in septic shock, those randomized to IV fluid bolus therapy resolved shock quicker but died more frequently than those randomized to maintenance fluid alone.[29,30] Despite concerns with this trial's external validity (eg, pediatric patients treated in nonindustrialized countries), similar results have been demonstrated in multiple trials in varied patient populations. Adult septic shock patients in Zambia randomized to a resuscitation strategy of correcting early hemodynamic abnormalities with IV fluid therapy had a more rapid resolution of shock, but this strategy was also associated with increased mortality.[31] Hjortrup and colleagues[32] found that an aggressive response to hemodynamic perturbations led to an increase in the frequency of AKI. Although these vigorous resuscitative strategies were all associated with timelier improvements in early hemodynamic markers, this came at the cost of downstream morbidity and mortality.

It is not hard to imagine the physiologic underpinning of such observations. As discussed, sepsis leads to increases in venodilation, a decrease in stressed volume, and in turn a decrease in venous return and cardiac output. In addition, the inflammatory milieu increases capillary permeability, increasing the filtration at the capillary level. Prior to resuscitative efforts, extravascular fluid accumulation is limited by the decreased hydrostatic pressure of the hypotensive state. Only after active resuscitation with IV fluid boluses is the loss of vascular integrity fully realized, creating a circular feedback loop. IV fluids are administered to increase blood pressure, and this increase in blood pressure leads to an increase in hydrostatic forces, increasing the rate of fluid leaving the capillaries. This capillary leak leads to an increase in tissue edema, a decrease in intravascular volume, and hypotension. In response, more fluids are administered, leading to more third spacing of fluids and tissue edema.

Clearly there are harms associated with the use of IV fluids. Optimal resuscitative strategies take these risks into account when administering IV fluids to patients in shock. The first step is the understanding that resuscitation alone does not correct shock. Studies examining interventions intended to optimize patients' hemodynamic abnormalities, in any type of shock, have failed to demonstrate an improvement in patient outcomes.[33,34] The only beneficial therapies have been ones that focus on the correction of the underlying cause or strategies that seek to limit resuscitative interventions until source control is achieved. Given this understanding, fluids should be viewed as a bridge, intended to support patients until control of the underlying shock state can be achieved.

The concept of damage control resuscitation has been successfully implemented in patients with traumatic injuries leading to hemorrhagic shock.[35] In fact, for patients in hemorrhagic shock, aggressive resuscitation prior to achieving hemorrhage control is detrimental. Rather, a damage control strategy (DCS) focusing on maintaining the minimal blood pressure to maintain end-organ perfusion until hemorrhage control is achieved improves overall survival.[36–38] The authors believe that all resuscitative efforts, no matter the source of shock, should be viewed from a similar perspective. Any resuscitative strategy should attempt to define the cause of the patients' hemodynamic collapse. Once identified, measures to control the etiology of shock should be undertaken in parallel to the hemodynamic resuscitation. Classically in septic shock, a prescribed volume of fluids is administered regardless of the patient's volume status. However, in the authors' view of DCS, fluids would be administered as thoughtfully as vasopressors.

The authors advocate for a fluid tolerance strategy that assesses an individual patient's fluid tolerance by examining the potential benefit or harm associated with additional fluid administration. Unlike fluid responsiveness, fluid tolerance is not based on a single measure, but rather is a holistic approach, examining the patient's history, current presentation, and bedside ultrasound to determine whether a patient is more likely to be helped or harmed from IV fluids. For example, a history of pulmonary hypertension or congestive heart failure would indicate that the patient may be fluid intolerant. Likewise, a patient presenting with septic shock is more likely to have increased capillary leak compared to a patient with hypovolemia caused by diabetic ketoacidosis.

The authors caution against the use of serum lactate as an indicator of a patient's fluid requirements.[39] There is a growing body of evidence that lactate is a poor surrogate for tissue hypoperfusion and hypovolemia. A recently published RCT[40] examining a lactate-guided resuscitation strategy suggested harms associated with this approach. Rather, a nonclearing lactate level should alert clinicians of the ongoing stress experienced by the patient, prompting an inquiry into whether the source of the patient's shock is truly controlled. It is the authors' opinion that the interpretation of lactate should be separate from decisions regarding ongoing fluid resuscitation.

Both physical examination and point of care ultrasound should focus on signs indicating that further fluid administration is likely to be detrimental to the patient. Signs concerning for heart failure, such as jugular vein distension, orthopnea, and decreased pulse pressure are all indicative of potential fluid intolerance, but they are fairly late findings and often not present despite significant volume overload.[26,41] An elevated CVP (a level > 8 mm Hg or a rising level with ongoing fluid administration), although much maligned for its inability to predict fluid responsiveness, is a fairly reliable marker of fluid intolerance.[28,42] Echocardiographic markers of fluid intolerance, including a reduction in left-sided systolic function or ejection fraction,[26] a decrease in right-sided function as indicated by a low tricuspid annular plane excursion,[43] and a large inferior vena cava without respiratory variation are also fairly sensitive markers that further fluid is likely to be harmful.[26,44]

An assessment of fluid tolerance should not be based on cardiac function in isolation, but should also include a determination of capillary integrity and accumulation of extravascular fluid. This includes extremity edema and pulmonary edema seen in a standard chest radiograph or on ultrasound. Ultrasonographic signs of venous congestion present on the hepatic, portal, or intrarenal veins have been demonstrated to be strong markers of fluid intolerance in critically ill patients.[45–48]

Finally, it is important to continue to reassess patients' ultrasonographic and physical examination signs of volume intolerance, as they may be absent during an initial assessment, only to become obvious as the physiology evolves. Similar to fluid responsiveness strategies, assessments of fluid intolerance should be made prior to the administration of each IV fluid bolus and not only during the initial assessment.

SUMMARY

It is important to note that the discovery of IV fluids failed to have a significant impact in limiting the mortality during subsequent cholera outbreaks. It was not until Dr. John Snow discovered that contaminated drinking water from the Broad Street pump was the source of 1 specific deadly outbreak that control of future epidemics was achieved. This observation should serve as a clear reminder that IV fluid therapy is not a cure but rather a bridge until definitive control of the patient's source of shock can be controlled. Moreover, there are clear harms associated with the aggressive use IV fluid administration. Clinicians should strive to identify signs of these harms and limit fluid administration in patients when fluid intolerance is present.

DISCLOSURE

The authors have nothing to disclose.

REFERENCES

1. Cosnett JE. The origins of intravenous fluid therapy. Lancet 1989;1(8641):768–71.
2. Baskett TF. The resuscitation greats: Sydney Ringer and lactated Ringer's solution. Resuscitation 2003;58(1):5–7.
3. Awad S, Allison SP, Lobo DN. The history of 0.9% saline. Clin Nutr 2008;27(2): 179–88.
4. Hartmann AF, Senn MJ. Studies in the metabolism of sodium r-lactate. I. Response of normal human subjects to the intravenous injection of sodium r-lactate. J Clin Invest 1932;11(2):327–35.
5. Hartmann AF, Senn MJ. Studies in the metabolism of sodium r-lactate. II. Response of human subjects with acidosis to the intravenous injection of sodium r-lactate. J Clin Invest 1932;11(2):337–44.
6. Hartmann AF, Senn MJ. Studies in the metabolism of sodium r-lactate. III. Response of human subjects with liver damage, disturbed water and mineral balance, and renal insufficiency to the intravenous injection of sodium r-lactate. J Clin Invest 1932;11(2):345–55.
7. 0.9% Sodium Chloride Injection, USP VisIV Container. Hospira, Inc. 2014. Available at: https://www.accessdata.fda.gov/drugsatfda_docs/label/2017/016366s214lbl. pdf. Accessed November 16, 2019.
8. Semler MW, Kellum JA. Balanced Crystalloid Solutions. Am J Respir Crit Care Med 2019;199(8):952–60.
9. Young P, Bailey M, Beasley R, et al. Effect of a buffered crystalloid solution vs saline on acute kidney injury among patients in the intensive care unit: The SPLIT randomized clinical trial. JAMA 2015;314(16):1701–10.
10. Self WH, Semler MW, Wanderer JP, et al. Balanced crystalloids versus saline in noncritically ill adults. N Engl J Med 2018;378(9):819–28.
11. Semler MW, Self WH, Rice TW. Balanced crystalloids versus saline in critically ill adults. N Engl J Med 2018;378(20):1951.
12. Brown RM, Wang L, Coston TD, et al. Balanced crystalloids versus saline in sepsis: a secondary analysis of the SMART trial. Am J Respir Crit Care Med 2019;200(12):1487–95.

13. Antequera Martín AM, Barea Mendoza JA, Muriel A, et al. Buffered solutions versus 0.9% saline for resuscitation in critically ill adults and children. Cochrane Database Syst Rev 2019;(7):CD012247.

14. Title 21- food and drugs chapter I –Food and Drug Administration Department of Health and Human Services. Subchapter L- regulations under certain other acts Administered by the Food and Drug Administration. Part 1270 human tissue intended for transplantation. Subpart A- general provisions ec 1270.3 Definitions. 2019. Available at: https://www.accessdata.fda.gov/scripts/cdrh/cfdocs/cfcfr/CFRSearch.cfm?fr=1270.3. Accessed November 16, 2019.

15. Perner A, Haase N, Guttormsen AB, et al. Hydroxyethyl Starch 130/0.42 versus Ringer's Acetate in Severe Sepsis. N Engl J Med 2012;367(2):124–34.

16. Vincent JL, Russell JA, Jacob M, et al. Albumin administration in the acutely ill: what is new and where next? Crit Care 2014;18(4):231.

17. Taylor AE. Capillary fluid filtration. Starling forces and lymph flow. Circ Res 1981; 49(3):557–75.

18. Woodcock TE, Woodcock TM. Revised Starling equation and the glycocalyx model of transvascular fluid exchange: an improved paradigm for prescribing intravenous fluid therapy. Br J Anaesth 2012;108(3):384–94.

19. Chelazzi C, Villa G, Mancinelli P, et al. Glycocalyx and sepsis-induced alterations in vascular permeability. Crit Care 2015;19:26.

20. Caironi P, Tognoni G, Masson S, et al. Albumin replacement in patients with severe sepsis or septic shock. N Engl J Med 2014;370(15):1412–21.

21. Finfer S, Bellomo R, Boyce N, et al. A comparison of albumin and saline for fluid resuscitation in the intensive care unit. N Engl J Med 2004;350(22):2247–56.

22. Guyton AC. Determination of cardiac output by equating venous return curves with cardiac response curves. Physiol Rev 1955;35(1):123–9.

23. Funk DJ, Jacobsohn E, Kumar A. The role of venous return in critical illness and shock-part I: physiology. Crit Care Med 2013;41(1):255–62.

24. Funk DJ, Jacobsohn E, Kumar A. Role of the venous return in critical illness and shock: part II-shock and mechanical ventilation. Crit Care Med 2013;41(2):573–9.

25. Glassford NJ, Eastwood GM, Bellomo R. Physiological changes after fluid bolus therapy in sepsis: a systematic review of contemporary data. Crit Care 2014; 18(6):696.

26. Bentzer P, Griesdale DE, Boyd J, et al. Will this hemodynamically unstable patient respond to a bolus of intravenous fluids? JAMA 2016;316(12):1298–309.

27. Miller J, Ho CX, Tang J, et al. Assessing fluid responsiveness in spontaneously breathing patients. Acad Emerg Med 2016;23(2):186–90.

28. Wiedemann HP, Wheeler AP, Bernard GR, et al. Comparison of two fluid-management strategies in acute lung injury. N Engl J Med 2006;354(24):2564–75.

29. Maitland K, Kiguli S, Opoka RO, et al. Mortality after fluid bolus in African children with severe infection. N Engl J Med 2011;364(26):2483–95.

30. Maitland K, George EC, Evans JA, et al. Exploring mechanisms of excess mortality with early fluid resuscitation: insights from the FEAST trial. BMC Med 2013; 11:68.

31. Andrews B, Semler MW, Muchemwa L, et al. Effect of an early resuscitation protocol on in-hospital mortality among adults with sepsis and hypotension: a randomized clinical trial. JAMA 2017;318(13):1233–40.

32. Hjortrup PB, Haase N, Bundgaard H, et al. Restricting volumes of resuscitation fluid in adults with septic shock after initial management: the CLASSIC randomised, parallel-group, multicentre feasibility trial. Intensive Care Med 2016; 42(11):1695–705.

33. Gattinoni L, Brazzi L, Pelosi P, et al. A trial of goal-oriented hemodynamic therapy in critically ill patients. N Engl J Med 1995;333(16):1025–32.
34. Shoemaker WC. Goal-oriented hemodynamic therapy. N Engl J Med 1996; 334(12):799–800 [author reply: 800].
35. Ball CG. Damage control resuscitation: history, theory and technique. Can J Surg 2014;57(1):55–60.
36. Morrison CA, Carrick MM, Norman MA, et al. Hypotensive resuscitation strategy reduces transfusion requirements and severe postoperative coagulopathy in trauma patients with hemorrhagic shock: preliminary results of a randomized controlled trial. J Trauma 2011;70(3):652–63.
37. Dutton RP, Mackenzie CF, Scalea TM. Hypotensive resuscitation during active hemorrhage: impact on in-hospital mortality. J Trauma 2002;52(6):1141–6.
38. Bickell WH, Wall MJ Jr, Pepe PE, et al. Immediate versus delayed fluid resuscitation for hypotensive patients with penetrating torso injuries. N Engl J Med 1994; 331(17):1105–9.
39. Spiegel R, Gordon D, Marik PE. The origins of the Lacto-Bolo reflex: the mythology of lactate in sepsis. J Thorac Dis 2020;12(Suppl 1):S48–53.
40. Hernandez G, Ospina-Tascon GA, Damiani LP, et al. Effect of a resuscitation strategy targeting peripheral perfusion status vs serum lactate levels on 28-day mortality among patients with septic shock: the ANDROMEDA-SHOCK randomized clinical trial. JAMA 2019;321(7):654–64.
41. Wang CS, FitzGerald JM, Schulzer M, et al. Does this dyspneic patient in the emergency department have congestive heart failure? JAMA 2005;294(15): 1944–56.
42. Mullens W, Abrahams Z, Francis GS, et al. Importance of venous congestion for worsening of renal function in advanced decompensated heart failure. J Am Coll Cardiol 2009;53(7):589–96.
43. Vallabhajosyula S, Kumar M, Pandompatam G, et al. Prognostic impact of isolated right ventricular dysfunction in sepsis and septic shock: an 8-year historical cohort study. Ann Intensive Care 2017;7(1):94.
44. Corl KA, George NR, Romanoff J, et al. Inferior vena cava collapsibility detects fluid responsiveness among spontaneously breathing critically-ill patients. J Crit Care 2017;41:130–7.
45. Beaubien-Souligny W, Benkreira A, Robillard P, et al. Alterations in portal vein flow and intrarenal venous flow are associated with acute kidney injury after cardiac surgery: a prospective observational cohort study. J Am Heart Assoc 2018; 7(19):e009961.
46. Beaubien-Souligny W, Eljaiek R, Fortier A, et al. The Association between pulsatile portal flow and acute kidney injury after cardiac surgery: a retrospective cohort study. J Cardiothorac Vasc Anesth 2018;32(4):1780–7.
47. Eljaiek R, Cavayas YA, Rodrigue E, et al. High postoperative portal venous flow pulsatility indicates right ventricular dysfunction and predicts complications in cardiac surgery patients. Br J Anaesth 2019;122(2):206–14.
48. Iida N, Seo Y, Sai S, et al. Clinical implications of intrarenal hemodynamic evaluation by Doppler ultrasonography in heart failure. JACC Heart Fail 2016;4(8): 674–82.

Emergency Transfusions

Michael S. Farrell, MD, MS[a,b], Woon Cho Kim, MD, MPH[a,b],
Deborah M. Stein, MD, MPH[a,b,*]

KEYWORDS

- Transfusion • Blood • Resuscitation • Coagulopathy

KEY POINTS

- In the setting of bleeding, crystalloid should be limited and blood transfusions should be initiated early.
- Blood products should be utilized in a balanced ratio and should be guided by viscoelastic assays and endpoints of resuscitation.
- It is essential to urgently address the cause of the hemodynamic instability or coagulopathy to maximize the benefit of any transfusion.

INTRODUCTION

Trauma is the leading cause of life-years lost throughout the world, with hemorrhage accounting for 30% to 40% of trauma mortalities.[1–3] The ability to recognize and treat acute blood loss and trauma-induced coagulopathy (TIC) is a skill for all emergency providers. There are numerous approaches to emergency transfusion resuscitation but they each center on the early utilization of blood products while allowing for permissive hypotension and minimizing crystalloid administration. Together, these factors have been shown to improve outcomes and decrease complications.[4,5] This article approaches the major principles of emergency transfusions, starting with obtaining access and advancing through resuscitation approaches and concluding with special considerations and endpoints of resuscitation.

CONSIDERATIONS IN EMERGENT TRANSFUSION

Once a patient is identified as needing an emergent transfusion, the focus should be on establishing hemostasis and correcting coagulopathy in a timely manner. The time to hemostasis consistently has been associated with outcome and, therefore, must be a primary focus alongside initial stabilization maneuvers and airway securement.[6]

a Department of Surgery, University of California San Francisco, 1001 Potrero Avenue, Ward 3A, San Francisco, CA 94110, USA; b Zuckerberg San Francisco General Hospital, San Francisco, CA, USA
* Corresponding author. 1001 Potrero Avenue, Ward 3A, San Francisco, CA 94110.
E-mail address: Deborah.Stein@ucsf.edu
Twitter: @mfarrellmd (M.S.F.)

Emerg Med Clin N Am 38 (2020) 795–805
https://doi.org/10.1016/j.emc.2020.06.005
0733-8627/20/© 2020 Elsevier Inc. All rights reserved.
emed.theclinics.com

The decision to transfuse a patient should coincide with multiple other considerations (**Box 1**).

OBTAINING ACCESS

Intravenous (IV) access is a critical first step in addressing emergency transfusions. Although obtaining large-bore IVs is taught in courses, such as advanced trauma life support (ATLS), it is easily overlooked until it is difficult to obtain.[7] This article addresses 4 different approaches: prehospital IV placement, central venous catheter (CVC), intraosseous (IO) access, and rapid infusion catheter.

Prehospital Intravenous Access

Obtaining IV access prior to decompensation can be life-saving. Large-bore peripheral IVs are the preferred access for rapid delivery of resuscitative fluids in an unstable patient. One unique situation that warrants special attention is in the prehospital setting. Paramedics are very capable of placing IVs under difficult situations; however, prehospital IV placement does not appear to improve patient outcomes significantly.[8] When assessed in a study of 200 participants, prehospital time was prolonged in patients when IV access was obtained in the prehospital setting.[9] Additionally, there was no improvement in the time to transfusion upon hospital arrival.[9] Therefore, it is recommend that, particularly in situations with short prehospital times, the goal should be to expedite transportation, with a scoop-and-run approach.

Central Venous Catheter

CVC placement is a viable option in the emergent setting, particularly when placed under ultrasound guidance.[10] On average, placing a CVC requires more than 3 minutes to place; however, this may take longer based on operator experience, collapsed vessels from hypovolemic shock, and variant anatomy.[11] When selecting the type of CVC, a CVC with an 8-French or 9-French sheath is preferred because larger diameter and shorter catheter length limit resistance and facilitate rapid infusion.[12]

Box 1
Considerations in resuscitation

Does the patient have sufficient IV access?
  Does the patient require additional access? If so, what resources are available?

Will the patient benefit from blood transfusion?
  How much blood loss occurred in the prehospital setting?
  Is the patient currently bleeding? If so, what is the safest method to achieve hemostasis?

How urgent is this transfusion?
  Is it appropriate to use uncrossmatched or type-specific blood?
  Are multiple units of blood expected? If so, is massive transfusion anticipated?

What other factors are contributing to ongoing bleeding or hemodynamic instability?
  Is the patient on anticoagulation or antiplatelet therapy?
  Are there signs and symptoms of coagulopathy from other causes, such as acute hemorrhagic or septic shock?
  Are these factors correctable?

What are the endpoints of resuscitation?
  Is the patient hemodynamically stable after the resuscitation?
  What laboratory values are available to determine resuscitation status?

Not all CVCs are compatible for contrast power injectors for computed tomography scans, if that is deemed necessary. It is important that providers are familiar with their available equipment to help expedite patient care. With respect to patient complications, there is a risk of unintended arterial injury, line infection, and deep venous thrombosis, especially when placed in an urgent situation. It generally is recommended that these lines should be replaced under sterile conditions within 48 hours.[13,14]

Intraosseous Device

IO device placement offers a rapid alternative to IV access that most physicians, nurses, and paramedics are trained to place.[15,16] The timing for the placement of an IO device is equivalent to the timing for a peripheral IV and is faster than placement of a CVC.[11] Although an IO device does have a slower transfusion rate compared with an IV, in animal models, the time to return blood pressure to baseline is comparable. Furthermore, IO devices have been shown to be safe for administration of blood products.[17]

Rapid Infuser Catheter

A rapid infuser catheter can be a valuable tool to secure adequate access for massive transfusion when a CVC or IO is not readily available. This initially requires a 20-gauge IV access in a superficial peripheral vein, typically in the upper or lower extremities, which then can be exchanged into a large bore sheath over wire.[18]

PERMISSIVE HYPOTENSION

Most patients who require emergency transfusions have some degree of hemodynamic instability. It is important that this is not corrected too abruptly, because it can result in platelet disruption and ongoing bleeding. There are numerous studies that have demonstrated the importance of permissive hypotension. Bickell and colleagues[19] showed that delaying fluid resuscitation in patients with a systolic blood pressure (SBP) less than or equal to 90 mm Hg until they reached the operating room for penetrating torso injuries resulted in an 8% improved survival. Morrison and colleagues[20] demonstrated that targeting a mean arterial pressure of 50 mm Hg, rather than 65 mm Hg, resulted in lower rates of death and coagulopathy in the early postoperative setting. Schreiber and colleagues performed a feasibility study in patients with prehospital SBPs of less than or equal to 90 mm Hg. This study compared administering 2 L of crystalloid initially and additional fluid to maintain an SBP greater than or equal to 110 mm Hg to those patients who received 250-mL boluses of crystalloid to maintain a radial pulse of an SBP greater than or equal to 70 mm Hg. This study demonstrated a 10% improvement in mortality in the permissive hypotension group.[21]

MASSIVE TRANSFUSION AND CRITICAL ADMINISTRATION THRESHOLD

The American College of Surgeons Committee on Trauma (ACS-COT) mandates that trauma centers develop a massive transfusion protocol (MTP). The goal of the MTP should be to meet the transfusion requirements of the patient rapidly. The MTP is centered on identifying triggers for activation of MTP, product availability and delivery, continuation of the MTP during procedures and in the intensive care unit (ICU), transfusion targets, and termination of the MTP.[22]

There are numerous criteria that may be used to trigger an MTP, ranging from blood transfusion requirement in the trauma bay to the Assessment of Blood Consumption (ABC) score (**Box 2**). The ABC score assigns a score of either 0 or 1 to 4

Box 2
Assessment of blood consumption

Penetrating mechanism (no = 0 points; yes = 1 point)

Heart rate ($\leq$120 = 0 points; >120 = 1 point)

SBP ($\geq$90 = 0 points; <90 = 1 point)

FAST examination (negative = 0 points; positive = 1 point)

Abbreviation: FAST, focused assessment with sonography for trauma.

Data from Nunez TC, Voskresensky IV, Dossett LA, Shinall R, Dutton WD, Cotton BA. Early prediction of massive transfusion in trauma: simple as ABC (assessment of blood consumption)?. J Trauma. 2009;66(2):346-352. https://doi.org/10.1097/TA.0b013e3181961c35.

---

components that are easily assessed in the trauma bay. The ABC score has been validated in a multicenter study, with a score of 2 or more resulting in a sensitivity of 75% to 90% and a specificity of 67% to 88% for predicting the need for massive transfusion.[23]

The initiation of the MTP must be accompanied by a plan for administering blood products and recognizing when the MTP may be discontinued (described later); uncrossed blood products should be utilized until group-matched products are available. The ACS-COT recommends the MTP should be administered in a ratio-driven fashion until all surgical bleeding is controlled in the operating room or there is radiographic and physiologic evidence of bleeding control after angioembolization.[22]

Massive transfusion historically has been defined as administration of 10 U of packed red blood cells (pRBCs) over a 24-hour period. This definition can be problematic, because it does not account for patients who die early within this fixed time period and fails to recognize the difference between patients who are acutely unstable and those who require transfusions from slow persistent bleeding.[24,25] Alternatively, the critical administration threshold, defined as requiring 3 U of pRBC transfusion per hour, is believed to better reflect the severity of hemorrhagic shock and a better predictor of mortality.[26]

FIXED RATIO RESUSCITATION

Over the past decade, there has been increased focus on how to deliver blood products in the order and ratio that are best suited to meet the physiologic demands associated with hemorrhagic shock. In general, the goal is to "replace what the patient is losing." In other words, the bleeding patient is losing red blood cells as well as clotting factors and platelets, and the resuscitation plan must account for each component.

The Prospective, Observational, Multicenter, Major Trauma Transfusion (PROMMTT) study was a landmark trial looking at transfusion ratios. This was a prospective cohort study that included 10 level 1 trauma centers. All patients were adult trauma patients who survived at least the first 30 minutes after admission and who received at least 1 U of pRBCs within the first 6 hours and at least total 3 U of blood products within 24 hours. The primary outcome was in-hospital mortality with a focus on the number and type of transfusions as well as the timing they were administered. The PROMMTT study highlighted that at 30 minutes after admission, 67% of patients had not received plasma and 99% had not received platelets. Although the resuscitation was more likely to become balanced with more time after admission, across multiple level 1 trauma centers, there was no constant ratio of blood products administered during the period of active resuscitation. It also recognized that higher plasma and platelet ratios were associated with decreased 6-hour mortality.[27]

The follow-up Pragmatic, Randomized Optimal Platelet and Plasma Ratios (PROPPR) trial was designed to address the effectiveness of using plasma:platelets:pRBC ratios, 1:1:1 versus 1:1:2. This phase 3 multicenter trial compared 24-hour and 30-day mortality between patients who received platelets first and then alternative plasma and pRBCs in either a 1:1 or a 1:2 ratio. The PROPPR trial showed the 1:1:1 group achieved hemostasis and experienced fewer deaths related to exsanguination by 24 hours. There was no difference found between the groups with respect to 24-hour and 30-day mortality. This study recognized that 1:1:1 resulted in hemostasis and fewer deaths within the first 24 hours.[5]

VISCOELASTIC ASSAY GOAL-DIRECTED THERAPY

The use of viscoelastic assays (VHAs), such as thromboelastography (TEG) and rotational thromboelastometry, has offered an alternative to the use of traditional coagulation laboratory panels. Unlike conventional coagulation assays, such as the international normalized ratio and partial thromboplastic time, VHAs give more insight into which steps of coagulation are either deficient or hyperactive. In this way, VHAs allow for early recognition of TIC and provide a goal-directed path to the correction of TIC.[28,29] VHA-guided resuscitation has resulted in improved survival with decreased transfusion requirements compared with MTP resuscitation guided by the more conventional coagulation assays.[30,31] There is an ongoing debate about the use of VHA versus fixed ratio transfusions.[32]

TRANSFUSION CONSIDERATIONS AND ADJUNCTS
Limiting Crystalloid Infusions

Crystalloids are relatively inexpensive and convenient fluid of choice for resuscitation. For this reason, ATLS recommends judicious administration of no more than 1 L of crystalloid while allowing permissive hypotension during the initial phase of emergent resuscitation.[7] Aggressive crystalloid resuscitation fell out of favor, however, because it is associated with several complications. One major concern is that crystalloid can worsen the trauma triad that consists of acidosis, hypothermia, and coagulopathy. Specifically, most crystalloid solutions have a low pH resulting in metabolic acidosis and are not sufficiently warmed, which contributes to hypothermia. Additionally, because crystalloid solutions do not contain clotting factors, dilution coagulopathy may develop. Although crystalloid infusions may be more easily available, liberal use of crystalloid can be detrimental to patients.[4,33]

Aggressive early fluid resuscitation also has been associated with numerous complications beyond the initial mortality. In a prospective multicenter study that contained approximately 2000 patients, the volume of crystalloid resuscitation was associated with ventilator days as well as both days in ICU and hospital length of stay.[34] Additionally, crystalloid volume was associated, in a dose-dependent fashion, with the development of acute lung injury, acute respiratory distress syndrome, multiple organ failure, bloodstream infections, surgical site infections, and abdominal and extremity compartment syndromes.[34]

Plasma First

Damage control resuscitation in trauma is based on the premise of preventing and correcting coagulopathy. Given that plasma has been shown to decrease coagulopathy and limit endothelial inflammatory response, it is reasonable to consider starting resuscitation efforts with plasma, as opposed to pRBCs.[35] The Prehospital Plasma during Air Medical Transport in Trauma Patients at Risk for Hemorrhagic Shock (PAMPer) study evaluated approximately 500 patients in a multicenter phase 3 superiority trial. This study compared prehospital use of thawed plasma with standard care. In this case, the standard-care group may have received crystalloid solution, which was available at all sites, and/or pRBCs, which were available at 13 of 27 sites. The PAMPer study showed a 9.8% decrease in 30-day mortality for patients who received plasma.[36]

Unfortunately, not all studies have shown a clear improvement in patient outcomes. One study in an urban setting with short prehospital times was stopped early due to the lack of improvement in the setting of a high financial burden of providing prehospital plasma.[37] A separate study that included a large number of air transport showed an improvement in TEG studies but failed to show a significant outcome improvement.[38]

Uncrossmatched Blood

In the emergency setting where crossmatched blood is not immediately available uncrossmatched type O blood should be used for resuscitation.[39] The goal in these instances is to provide blood that is compatible, even if not type-specific. Ideally, uncrossmatched O blood should be available in the emergency department to allow for an effective way to transfuse pRBCs.[40] In settings where there is a high rate of injury recidivism in the trauma population, frequent use of uncrossmatched blood transfusion may increase the likelihood of receiving multiple transfusions over the course of their lifetime, increasing the risk of hemolytic transfusion reactions (HTRs). Approximately 30% to 40% of patients who receive uncrossmatched blood meet some criteria for HTRs, although it is rare for a patient to develop clinically significant adverse effects.[41,42] A high index of suspicion should be maintained for HTRs when transfusing an unstable patient with acute hemorrhage nonetheless.

One area of concern with using uncrossmatched blood is the development of anti-Rh antibodies. This is a concern especially in women of childbearing age. Women with Rh-negative or unknown Rh status should receive Rh-negative blood. Alloimmunization occurs in approximately 20% of Rh-negative patients who receive Rh-positive blood. Most of these patients develop anti-D antibodies with transfusions of 2 U to 4 U of blood.[43] Although RhD alloimmunization may not pose immediate risks during the acute transfusion period, this may affect a woman's subsequent pregnancy or future transfusion. It is recommended that Rh-negative women who receive Rh-positive transfusions should receive treatment. One option is to administer Rh immunoglobulin (RhIg) within 72 hours of the initial transfusion. One vial of RhIg contains 300 μg of the immunoglobulin and is effective at neutralizing 15 mL of erythrocytes. Approximately 14 vials of RhIg are required to neutralize a single pRBC transfusion, but a single vial is sufficient to neutralize a single Rh-positive platelet transfusion.[44–46]

Whole Blood

The goal with all resuscitation is to restore physiologic balance, resulting in a hemodynamically stable patient. One way to do this is to transfuse whole blood. Recently, there has been an increase in civilian research assessing the safety and feasibility of whole blood. In multiple studies, whole-blood has shown similar or improved survival compared with traditional ratio-based MTP resuscitation. Additionally, patients who received whole blood have required fewer transfusions to obtain higher hemoglobin goals. Importantly, low-titer whole blood has shown either similar or decreased transfusion reaction profiles.[47–51] Taken together, this suggests a benefit to using whole blood but most studies at this point are relatively small and additional work is required before its clinical utility and safety can be fully endorsed.

Tranexamic Acid

Tranexamic acid (TXA) is an adjunct to massive transfusion in the setting of hyperfibrinolysis. The Clinical Randomisation of an Antifibrinolytic in Significant Haemorrhage 2 (CRASH-2) trial concluded that TXA safely reduces the risk of death in bleeding trauma patients without significantly increasing the risk of vascular occlusive events.[52] As understanding of the variations of fibrinolysis continues to develop, there has been ongoing work to assess outcomes related to TXA administration. CRASH-2 presumed a hyperfibrinolytic state occurred in severely injured trauma patients, but with VHAs it is now recognized that patients may be in a hyperfibrinolytic, physiologic fibrinolytic, or shutdown fibrinolytic state. There is no known benefit for TXA use in patients in a physiologic fibrinolytic state.[53]

COMPLICATIONS OF MASSIVE TRANSFUSIONS

Massive transfusion carries risks similar to routine transfusions while also having complications associated with large-volume resuscitations.[54] Management of these conditions is beyond the scope of this article but should be considered (**Box 3**).

SPECIAL CONSIDERATIONS

Emergent transfusion must be tailored to individual patients' comorbid conditions. In addition to traumatic causes of hemorrhage, gravid patients with obstetric hemorrhage may impose further challenges in management. Patients with advanced heart failure or end-stage renal disease undergoing large-volume resuscitation are highly susceptible to hypervolemia-induced respiratory and cardiac failure. Patients with advanced liver failure present with variety of hemostatic abnormalities, which increases risks for both bleeding and thrombotic events.[55]

ENDPOINTS OF RESUSCITATION

It is important to be able to recognize when the goals of a resuscitation have been met. A key component of this requires that any ongoing bleeding has been addressed.

Box 3
Complications of massive transfusion

Acute complications
- Acute transfusion reactions
- Transfusion-related acute lung injury
- Transfusion-associated circulatory overload
- Dilutional coagulopathy
- Electrolyte abnormalities, including hypocalcemia
- Metabolic alkalosis
- Bacterial sepsis
- Hypothermia

Delayed complications
- Delayed transfusion reactions
- Transfusion-related immunomodulation
- Microchimerism

Once satisfied, there are numerous endpoints that include hemodynamic findings (eg, mean arterial pressure, central venous pressure, and cardiac output) as well as chemical markers (eg, base deficit and/or lactate), or end-organ function (eg, urine output).[22] VHA is a newer tool that also may serve a role to demonstrate correction of any coagulopathy.[56]

SUMMARY

Successful emergency transfusions require early recognition and activation of resources to minimize delays in treatment. Obtaining access fast is key to allow efficient delivery of resuscitative fluids. The initial goals should focus on replacement of blood in a balanced fashion. There is an ongoing debate regarding the best approach to transfusions, with some advocating for resuscitation with a fixed ratio of blood products and others preferring to use VHAs to guide transfusions. Whole-blood transfusion also is a debated strategy. It generally is accepted that transfusions should be started early and crystalloid infusions should be limited. As hemodynamic stability is restored, endpoints of resuscitation should be used to guide the resuscitation.

DISCLOSURE

The authors have nothing to disclose.

REFERENCES

1. Krug EG, Sharma GK, Lozano R. The global burden of injuries. Am J Public Health 2000;90(4):523–6.
2. Curry N, Hopewell S, Dorée C, et al. The acute management of trauma hemorrhage: a systematic review of randomized controlled trials. Crit Care 2011; 15(2):R92.
3. Kauvar DS, Lefering R, Wade CE. Impact of hemorrhage on trauma outcome: an overview of epidemiology, clinical presentations, and therapeutic considerations. J Trauma 2006;60(6 Suppl):S3–11.
4. Cantle PM, Cotton BA. Balanced resuscitation in trauma management. Surg Clin North Am 2017;97(5):999–1014.
5. Holcomb JB, Tilley BC, Baraniuk S, et al. Transfusion of plasma, platelets, and red blood cells in a 1:1:1 vs a 1:1:2 ratio and mortality in patients with severe trauma: the PROPPR randomized clinical trial. JAMA 2015;313(5):471–82.
6. Chang R, Kerby JD, Kalkwarf KJ, et al. Earlier time to hemostasis is associated with decreased mortality and rate of complications: Results from the Pragmatic Randomized Optimal Platelet and Plasma Ratio trial. J Trauma Acute Care Surg 2019;87(2):342–9.
7. Trauma ACoSCo. ATLS, advanced trauma life support student course manual. 10th edition. Chicago: American College of Surgeons; 2018.
8. Prottengeier J, Maier JN, Gall C, et al. Does it matter who places the intravenous? An inter-professional comparison of prehospital intravenous access difficulties between physicians and paramedics. Eur J Emerg Med 2017;24(6):443–9.
9. Engels PT, Passos E, Beckett AN, et al. IV access in bleeding trauma patients: a performance review. Injury 2014;45(1):77–82.
10. Taylor RW, Palagiri AV. Central venous catheterization. Crit Care Med 2007;35(5): 1390–6.

11. Chreiman KM, Dumas RP, Seamon MJ, et al. The intraosseous have it: A prospective observational study of vascular access success rates in patients in extremis using video review. J Trauma Acute Care Surg 2018;84(4):558–63.
12. Reddick AD, Ronald J, Morrison WG. Intravenous fluid resuscitation: was Poiseuille right? Emerg Med J 2011;28(3):201–2.
13. Marik PE, Flemmer M, Harrison W. The risk of catheter-related bloodstream infection with femoral venous catheters as compared to subclavian and internal jugular venous catheters: a systematic review of the literature and meta-analysis. Crit Care Med 2012;40(8):2479–85.
14. Hamada SR, Fromentin M, Ronot M, et al. Femoral arterial and central venous catheters in the trauma resuscitation room. Injury 2018;49(5):927–32.
15. Anson JA. Vascular access in resuscitation: is there a role for the intraosseous route? Anesthesiology 2014;120(4):1015–31.
16. Engels PT, Erdogan M, Widder SL, et al. Use of intraosseous devices in trauma: a survey of trauma practitioners in Canada, Australia and New Zealand. Can J Surg 2016;59(6):374–82.
17. Plewa MC, King RW, Fenn-Buderer N, et al. Hematologic safety of intraosseous blood transfusion in a swine model of pediatric hemorrhagic hypovolemia. Acad Emerg Med 1995;2(9):799–809.
18. Hulse EJ, Thomas GO. Vascular access on the 21st century military battlefield. J R Army Med Corps 2010;156(4 Suppl 1):385–90.
19. Bickell WH, Wall MJ, Pepe PE, et al. Immediate versus delayed fluid resuscitation for hypotensive patients with penetrating torso injuries. N Engl J Med 1994; 331(17):1105–9.
20. Morrison CA, Carrick MM, Norman MA, et al. Hypotensive resuscitation strategy reduces transfusion requirements and severe postoperative coagulopathy in trauma patients with hemorrhagic shock: preliminary results of a randomized controlled trial. J Trauma 2011;70(3):652–63.
21. Schreiber MA, Meier EN, Tisherman SA, et al. A controlled resuscitation strategy is feasible and safe in hypotensive trauma patients: results of a prospective randomized pilot trial. J Trauma Acute Care Surg 2015;78(4):687–95 [discussion: 695–7].
22. Surgeons CoTotACo. ACS TQIP massive transfusion in trauma guidelines. Chicago: American College of Surgeons; 2015.
23. Cotton BA, Dossett LA, Haut ER, et al. Multicenter validation of a simplified score to predict massive transfusion in trauma. J Trauma 2010;69(Suppl 1):S33–9.
24. Mitra B, Cameron PA, Gruen RL, et al. The definition of massive transfusion in trauma: a critical variable in examining evidence for resuscitation. Eur J Emerg Med 2011;18(3):137–42.
25. Savage SA, Sumislawski JJ, Zarzaur BL, et al. The new metric to define large-volume hemorrhage: results of a prospective study of the critical administration threshold. J Trauma Acute Care Surg 2015;78(2):224–9 [discussion: 229–30].
26. Savage SA, Zarzaur BL, Croce MA, et al. Redefining massive transfusion when every second counts. J Trauma Acute Care Surg 2013;74(2):396–400 [discussion: 400–2].
27. Holcomb JB, del Junco DJ, Fox EE, et al. The prospective, observational, multi-center, major trauma transfusion (PROMMTT) study: comparative effectiveness of a time-varying treatment with competing risks. JAMA Surg 2013;148(2):127–36.
28. Kornblith LZ, Moore HB, Cohen MJ. Trauma-induced coagulopathy: The past, present, and future. J Thromb Haemost 2019;17(6):852–62.

29. Stettler GR, Moore EE, Nunns GR, et al. Rotational thromboelastometry thresholds for patients at risk for massive transfusion. J Surg Res 2018;228:154–9.
30. Coleman JR, Moore EE, Chapman MP, et al. Rapid TEG efficiently guides hemostatic resuscitation in trauma patients. Surgery 2018;164(3):489–93.
31. Gonzalez E, Moore EE, Moore HB, et al. Goal-directed hemostatic resuscitation of trauma-induced coagulopathy: a pragmatic randomized clinical trial comparing a viscoelastic assay to conventional coagulation assays. Ann Surg 2016;263(6): 1051–9.
32. Howley IW, Haut ER, Jacobs L, et al. Is thromboelastography (TEG)-based resuscitation better than empirical 1:1 transfusion? Trauma Surg Acute Care Open 2018;3(1):e000140.
33. Wise R, Faurie M, Malbrain MLNG, et al. Strategies for intravenous fluid resuscitation in trauma patients. World J Surg 2017;41(5):1170–83.
34. Kasotakis G, Sideris A, Yang Y, et al. Aggressive early crystalloid resuscitation adversely affects outcomes in adult blunt trauma patients: an analysis of the Glue Grant database. J Trauma Acute Care Surg 2013;74(5):1215–21 [discussion: 1221–2].
35. Pati S, Potter DR, Baimukanova G, et al. Modulating the endotheliopathy of trauma: Factor concentrate versus fresh frozen plasma. J Trauma Acute Care Surg 2016;80(4):576–84 [discussion: 584–5].
36. Sperry JL, Guyette FX, Brown JB, et al. Prehospital plasma during air medical transport in trauma patients at risk for hemorrhagic shock. N Engl J Med 2018; 379(4):315–26.
37. Moore HB, Moore EE, Chapman MP, et al. Plasma-first resuscitation to treat haemorrhagic shock during emergency ground transportation in an urban area: a randomised trial. Lancet 2018;392(10144):283–91.
38. Henriksen HH, Rahbar E, Baer LA, et al. Pre-hospital transfusion of plasma in hemorrhaging trauma patients independently improves hemostatic competence and acidosis. Scand J Trauma Resusc Emerg Med 2016;24(1):145.
39. Dutton RP, Shih D, Edelman BB, et al. Safety of uncrossmatched type-O red cells for resuscitation from hemorrhagic shock. J Trauma 2005;59(6):1445–9.
40. Harris CT, Totten M, Davenport D, et al. Experience with uncrossmatched blood refrigerator in emergency department. Trauma Surg Acute Care Open 2018;3(1): e000184.
41. Miraflor E, Yeung L, Strumwasser A, et al. Emergency uncrossmatched transfusion effect on blood type alloantibodies. J Trauma Acute Care Surg 2012;72(1): 48–52 [discussion: 52–3].
42. Flommersfeld S, Mand C, Kühne CA, et al. Unmatched type O RhD+ red blood cells in multiple injured patients. Transfus Med Hemother 2018;45(3):158–61.
43. Gonzalez-Porras JR, Graciani IF, Perez-Simon JA, et al. Prospective evaluation of a transfusion policy of D+ red blood cells into D- patients. Transfusion 2008; 48(7):1318–24.
44. Zipursky A, Israels LG. The pathogenesis and prevention of Rh immunization. Can Med Assoc J 1967;97(21):1245–57.
45. Cid J, Harm SK, Yazer MH. Platelet transfusion - the art and science of compromise. Transfus Med Hemother 2013;40(3):160–71.
46. Yazer MH, Waters JH, Spinella PC, et al. Use of uncrossmatched erythrocytes in emergency bleeding situations. Anesthesiology 2018;128(3):650–6.
47. Yazer MH, Jackson B, Sperry JL, et al. Initial safety and feasibility of cold-stored uncrossmatched whole blood transfusion in civilian trauma patients. J Trauma Acute Care Surg 2016;81(1):21–6.

48. Cotton BA, Podbielski J, Camp E, et al. A randomized controlled pilot trial of modified whole blood versus component therapy in severely injured patients requiring large volume transfusions. Ann Surg 2013;258(4):527–32 [discussion: 532–3].

49. Seheult JN, Anto V, Alarcon LH, et al. Clinical outcomes among low-titer group O whole blood recipients compared to recipients of conventional components in civilian trauma resuscitation. Transfusion 2018;58(8):1838–45.

50. Williams J, Merutka N, Meyer D, et al. Safety profile and impact of low-titer group o whole blood for emergency use in trauma. J Trauma Acute Care Surg 2020; 88(1):87–93.

51. Hazelton JP, Cannon JW, Zatorski C, et al. Cold-stored whole blood: A better method of trauma resuscitation? J Trauma Acute Care Surg 2019;87(5):1035–41.

52. Shakur H, Roberts I, Bautista R, et al. Effects of tranexamic acid on death, vascular occlusive events, and blood transfusion in trauma patients with significant haemorrhage (CRASH-2): a randomised, placebo-controlled trial. Lancet 2010;376(9734):23–32.

53. Moore HB, Moore EE, Huebner BR, et al. Tranexamic acid is associated with increased mortality in patients with physiological fibrinolysis. J Surg Res 2017; 220:438–43.

54. Sihler KC, Napolitano LM. Complications of massive transfusion. Chest 2010; 137(1):209–20.

55. Intagliata NM, Argo CK, Stine JG, et al. Concepts and controversies in haemostasis and thrombosis associated with liver disease: proceedings of the 7th international coagulation in liver disease conference. Thromb Haemost 2018;118(8): 1491–506.

56. Connelly CR, Schreiber MA. Endpoints in resuscitation. Curr Opin Crit Care 2015; 21(6):512–9.

Updates in Sepsis Resuscitation

Timothy Ellender, MD*, Nicole Benzoni, MD, MPHS

KEYWORDS

- Sepsis • Septic shock • Bacteremia

KEY POINTS

- Sepsis care has trended toward earlier, less invasive interventions over the past 20 years.
- Fluid resuscitation, antibiotics, source control, and vasopressor support form the cornerstones of sepsis care.
- Skilled ventilator management, nutritional support, and glucose control are less emphasized but still important in the first 24 to 48 hours of septic shock care.
- Balanced fluids are preferred over normal saline, with a few notable exceptions.
- New areas of research include vitamin supplementation, β-blockade, and immunomodulation.

INTRODUCTION

Sepsis is a life-threatening, dysregulated response to infection characterized by intravascular hypovolemia, impaired hemodynamics, and end-organ damage. Although understanding of sepsis has changed profoundly over the past 20 years, it remains a critical illness with high mortality. This article provides a brief background on early goal-directed therapy (EGDT) and the Surviving Sepsis Campaign (SSC) and then focuses on recent literature, trends, and controversies in sepsis resuscitation specific to the emergency department (ED).

EARLY GOAL-DIRECTED THERAPY AND THE SURVIVING SEPSIS CAMPAIGN

EGDT traces its origins to a study by Rivers and colleagues,[1] a highly influential and controversial randomized controlled trial (RCT). The EGDT trial revolutionized sepsis care by initiating intensive care interventions for patients with septic shock in the ED within 6 hours of sepsis identification. Some elements of the study are still recognizable in current sepsis care.

Department of Emergency Medicine, Indiana University, 1701 North Senate Avenue, Indianapolis, IN 46202, USA
* Corresponding author.
E-mail address: tellende@iu.edu

Emerg Med Clin N Am 38 (2020) 807–818
https://doi.org/10.1016/j.emc.2020.06.006
0733-8627/20/© 2020 Elsevier Inc. All rights reserved.
emed.theclinics.com

In the EGDT trial, both the EGDT and standard therapy groups were monitored with central venous pressure (CVP), mean arterial pressure (MAP), and urine output (UOP) to guide resuscitation. Management in the standard therapy group was largely left to provider discretion with respect to hemodynamic support, blood cultures, and antibiotics. Importantly, there were no hemodynamic or metabolic targets for patients in the standard therapy group. In contrast, the EGDT group had protocoled resuscitation to optimize hemodynamic variables and also targeted central venous oxygen saturation ($Scvo_2$). Intravenous fluid (IVF) boluses were used to achieve a goal CVP of 8 mm Hg to 12 mm Hg. Once the CVP goal was attained, vasopressors were added if the MAP was less than 65 mm Hg. Vasodilators were initiated if the MAP remained greater than 90 mm Hg. Any patients with $Scvo_2$ less than 70% after these initial steps underwent packed red blood cell (pRBC) transfusion to achieve a 30% hematocrit. If $Scvo_2$ remained less than 70% after these interventions, a dobutamine infusion was started to augment cardiac output.

Using this protocoled sepsis resuscitation approach, EGDT patients had decreased vasopressor requirements, decreased need for mechanical ventilation, and absolute 16% decrease in mortality, both in hospital and at 28 days.[1] The remarkable results of this trial led to a paradigm shift in sepsis resuscitation that focused on early, hemodynamic-targeted interventions.

Following the EGDT trial, the SSC was formed as a collaborative effort between the Society of Critical Care Medicine (SCCM), European Society of Intensive Care Medicine (ESICM), and the International Sepsis Forum to provide comprehensive recommendations for the management of sepsis. SSC guidelines have consistently focused on an early, protocoled, and intensive approach to sepsis care, though select recommendations have changed. For example, EGDT therapy no longer requires routine administration of dobutamine, liberal pRBC transfusion, or a reliance on pulmonary arterial or central venous monitoring.[2] The SSC's most recent guidelines were published in 2016, with an update published in 2018.[3,4]

CURRENT CONTROVERSIES
Challenges to Early Goal-Directed Therapy

Around the time the SSC released its 2016 guidelines, 3 large RCTs (ProCESS, ARISE, and PROMISE) were published and brought into question the efficacy of EGDT.[5–7] These large randomized trials, and a subsequent meta-analysis, failed to show a mortality reduction with EGDT.[8] Importantly, these studies were conducted approximately 10 years after the initial EGDT trial. As such, many investigators propose that the paradigm shift created by Rivers and colleagues[1] made usual sepsis care in these 3 larger sepsis trials more closely resemble EGDT. Thus, outcome differences may have been harder to prove.

Defining and Identifying Sepsis

Despite the importance of early sepsis detection, no single test or strategy perfectly identifies when an infection transitions to sepsis. Shortly before the 2016 SSC guidelines were released, a task force from SCCM and ESICM published revised sepsis definitions entitled The Third International Consensus Definitions for Sepsis and Septic Shock (Sepsis-3) (**Table 1**).[9]

In Sepsis-3, the Sequential Organ Failure Assessment (SOFA) score was applied to help identify organ dysfunction and replace the systemic inflammatory response syndrome (SIRS)-based criteria. SIRS scoring proved neither sufficiently sensitive nor

Table 1
Sepsis-3 definitions

Systemic Inflammatory Response Syndrome Category	Sepsis-3 Definition
Sepsis	Life-threatening organ dysfunction originating from a patient's dysregulated infection response
Severe sepsis	N/A*
Septic shock	MAP ≥65 mm Hg and serum lactate >2 mmol/L (28 mg/dL) despite adequate volume resuscitation

* not applicable, "severe sepsis" was removed after being deemed redundant terminology.
Data from Singer M, Deutschman CS, Seymour CW, et al. The third international consensus definitions for sepsis and septic shock (Sepsis-3). Jama 2016;315:801-10.

specific for clinical use.[9–11] The SOFA score identifies dysfunction across 6 organ systems and is designed to stratify mortality risk in critically ill patients. A simplified Quick SOFA (qSOFA) score has been validated for ED use and more accurately identifies patients at increased risk for in-hospital mortality than SIRS (**Table 2**).[12]

Because the 2016 SSC guidelines were published shortly after Sepsis-3 was released, SIRS was maintained. A subsequent SSC update, however, supports the adoption of the SOFA score.[4] Despite these new recommendations, there is continued controversy over the optimal method for early identification of sepsis.

Table 2
Quick Sequential Organ Failure Assessment Scoring System

	Value	Points
Glasgow Coma Scale score	<15	1
Respiratory rate	≥22 per minute	1
Systolic blood pressure	≤100 mm Hg	1

Score 2 to 3: high risk for in-hospital mortality.
Data from Freund Y, Lemachatti N, Krastinova E, et al. Prognostic Accuracy of Sepsis-3 Criteria for In-Hospital Mortality Among Patients With Suspected Infection Presenting to the Emergency Department. JAMA 2017;317:301-8.

The One-Hour Bundle

The 2018 SSC update also combined the previous 3-hour and 6-hour care bundles into a single 1-hour bundle, with the goal of immediately initiating sepsis resuscitation. This bundle included blood culture collection, antibiotic administration, IVF administration, lactate level, and the administration of vasopressor medications as needed, within 1 hour of a patient's arrival to the ED.[4] Given the practical limitations of this recommendation, SCCM and the American College of Emergency Physicians (ACEP) released a joint policy statement recommending against implementation of the bundle. The American Academy of Emergency Medicine (AAEM) released a statement outlining similar concerns.

At present, the SSC continues to endorse the 1-hour bundle but notes that not all components are expected to be completed within that time period. Both ACEP and AAEM are developing guidelines to address concerns and, while recognizing the severity of sepsis and the need to quickly initiate care, recommend against hospital implementation of the 1-hour bundle at the time of this article's publication.

KEY COMPONENTS OF EMERGENCY DEPARTMENT SEPSIS MANAGEMENT
Antibiotics, Source Control, and Blood Cultures

Antibiotics are crucial in sepsis care, with a goal of initiation within 1 hour of identification. Empiric combination antibiotics (2 or more antibiotic classes) are recommended initially for septic shock of unclear origin.[3] Antibiotics targeted toward the likely source are recommended for sepsis without shock, including neutropenia or bacteremia.[3] Antibiotics should be narrowed to a simplified regimen as soon as sensitivities result or the patient improves. An antibiotic course of 7 days to 10 days typically is adequate.[3]

Blood culture sensitivity in septic shock is imperfect and drops significantly (10.6% absolute decrease in 1 study) shortly after antibiotic administration.[13] Blood cultures should be obtained if possible prior to antibiotic administration, but antibiotics should not be delayed if cultures cannot be drawn. Source control (eg, removal of contaminated lines and abscess drainage) should be attained as soon as clinically feasible.[3]

Mechanical Ventilation

Sepsis is a major cause of acute respiratory distress syndrome (ARDS), and a lung-protective strategy is recommended in all intubated septic patients.[3,14] A lower tidal volume (6–8 mL/kg of ideal body weight) is preferred, with a plateau pressure target of less than 30 cm H_2O. In patients who develop moderate to severe ARDS ($Pao_2/Fio_2 \leq 200$ mm Hg), clinicians should target a higher positive end-expiratory pressure (PEEP). Higher PEEP, titrated to a driving pressure less than 12 cm H_2O to 15 cm H_2O (plateau pressure minus PEEP), may stent open small airways to improve gas exchange without increasing oxygen exposure or barotrauma risk.[15] This can be achieved in moderate to severe ARDS patients in the ED by setting a low tidal volume and increasing PEEP to a plateau pressure of 28 cm H_2O. Prone positioning is another effective intervention for severe ARDS if staff are properly trained.[16]

Intravenous Fluids

Although the need for IVF administration in sepsis is not controversial, the optimal amount and type of fluid are still debated. Current SSC guidelines recommend resuscitation with at least 30 mL/kg of IV crystalloid fluid within 3 hours (unless there is clear evidence of pulmonary edema or volume overload), with additional fluid boluses based on continued hemodynamic monitoring.[3]

In recent years, the use of balanced crystalloid fluids instead of 0.9% normal saline (NS) have been advocated for sepsis resuscitation. Balanced fluids contain sodium, potassium, and chloride in concentrations that more closely mimic plasma levels than NS. Observational and small RCTs suggest balanced fluid resuscitation is associated with decreased in-hospital mortality in intensive care unit (ICU) patients with septic shock and decreased acute kidney injury (AKI) in the general ICU population.[17,18]

The Isotonic Solutions and Major Adverse Renal Events Trial (SMART) compared balanced crystalloids with NS in approximately 15,800 patients enrolled after medical or surgical ICU admission. The primary composite outcome was major adverse kidney events, defined as death from any cause, any renal replacement therapy, or persistent renal dysfunction (creatinine level $\geq 200\%$ from baseline) within 30 days or until hospital discharge. The balanced fluid group had significantly fewer major adverse kidney events, although it was a small (0.9%) absolute difference.[19] The difference in the composite outcome was driven primarily by 30-day in-hospital mortality differences in septic patients although mortality differences alone missed statistical significance.

Given the results of SMART and previous smaller trials, many investigators recommend balanced solutions over NS, unless specifically indicated by situations where NS may benefit patients (eg, ICP control or metabolic alkalosis).

MONITORING THE SEPTIC EMERGENCY DEPARTMENT PATIENT
Fluid Responsiveness

Early resuscitation requires an appropriate amount of fluid administration to optimize cardiac output and prevent volume overload. Fluid responsiveness is demonstrated by the change in stroke volume to a bolus of fluid. This can be assessed by dynamic or static indicators. When EGDT was developed, static indicators, such as CVP monitoring, commonly were used to guide fluid resuscitation. CVP is affected, however, by thoracic, pericardial, and abdominal pressures as well as liver and renal impairment.[20] Studies of correlation between CVP and fluid responsiveness have shown it has an overall poor predictive value.[21]

A recent meta-analysis affirmed a simpler and less invasive test, the passive leg raise (PLR), as an accurate and useful measurement to predict fluid responsiveness. A PLR requires rapidly transitioning a patient from a semirecumbent position to supine and placing a patient's legs at 45°. This results in a transient (300–500 mL) bolus of peripheral venous blood to the patient's central circulation. Response is measured after 30 seconds to 90 seconds and requires either a cardiac output monitor or arterial line to measure pulse pressure for accurate assessment.[22] Current SSC guidelines recommend dynamic markers (eg, systolic pressure variation and PLR) rather than static measurements (eg, CVP).[3]

Peripheral Perfusion

Rivers and colleagues' EGDT protocol relied heavily on invasive monitoring to guide sepsis care, including peripheral perfusion assessment by $Scvo_2$.[1] An ED-based study of 300 patients investigated whether serum lactate was a reasonable alternative to invasive measures of tissue hypoxia. Researchers used IVF and vasopressors to target a goal $Scvo_2$ greater than or equal to 70% or a lactate clearance greater than or equal to 10%. Although it did not reach statistical significance, mortality was lower in the lactate clearance group.[23] After this study, serial lactates were heralded as a noninvasive method to monitor septic patients' peripheral perfusion. Although lactate can accumulate due to tissue hypoxia and anaerobic metabolism, it is important to recognize that lactate levels can be elevated for many other reasons. Lactate levels increase in the setting of liver or renal disease (due to decreased clearance), medication effects, or adrenergic stimulation.[24]

More recently, capillary refill time (CRT) has been studied as a marker of perfusion and resuscitation status. A small cohort in Chile suggested that CRT less than 4 seconds were predictive of mortality and adverse outcomes.[25] The recent ANDROMEDA-SHOCK trial compared lactate and CRT-driven resuscitation strategies in patients with septic shock. In this trial, patients managed with a CRT-guided resuscitation strategy had improved SOFA scores and decreased mortality, although the latter just missed statistical significance.[26] Although this study is insufficient to recommend a current practice change, CRT does offer a viable alternative to monitor peripheral perfusion of septic patients in resource-limited settings.

HEMODYNAMIC SUPPORT FOR THE SEPTIC EMERGENCY DEPARTMENT PATIENT

Current SSC guidelines recommend a target MAP of 65 mm Hg for patients with sepsis.[3] Vasopressor medications should be initiated in patients who do not meet this MAP goal after adequate fluid resuscitation. Norepinephrine is recommended as the first-line vasopressor medication. If patients fail to achieve the MAP target with norepinephrine, vasopressin or epinephrine is recommended as a second-line agent to increase the MAP to target. Epinephrine may be preferable in patients that would benefit from its inotropic effects, although clinicians should be aware of the associated risk for tachyarrhythmias and that it may complicate serial lactate monitoring. Elevated lactate in response to epinephrine is actually a good prognostic sign.[27]

Determining MAP Target

A recent trial randomized patients to a standard (65–70 mm Hg) or a higher (80–85 mm Hg) MAP target. Results of this trial demonstrated that patients with chronic hypertension had decreased renal replacement therapy requirements with higher MAP targets, although there was no difference in survival seen between the 2 groups. There were similar adverse events between the groups, with the exception that atrial fibrillation occurred more commonly in the higher MAP target group.[28] In patients with septic shock and a history of chronic hypertension, it, therefore, may be reasonable to target a higher MAP if there are persistent signs of insufficient organ perfusion (eg, low urine output despite adequate fluid resuscitation).

Catecholamine Alternatives

Vasopressin, or antidiuretic hormone, functions primarily to resorb water at renal nephrons. In shock states, vasopressin supports blood pressure by increasing vascular resistance. There is a corresponding decrease in heart rate and cardiac output. Digital, limb, and myocardial ischemia are known risks of high vasopressin infusion rates. As such, only low-dose vasopressin ($\leq$0.03 U/min) is recommended as a possible second-line agent in refractory septic shock.[29] The Vasopressin and Septic Shock Trial (VASST) randomized patients with septic shock with persistent hypotension (despite low-dose norepinephrine) to low-dose vasopressin or continued norepinephrine titration. Patients with unstable coronary disease or advanced heart failure were excluded. No significant difference was seen in mortality or in in adverse event rates.[30] The Ventricular Tachycardia Ablation versus Escalated Antiarrhythmic Drug Therapy in Ischemic Heart Disease (VANISH) trial randomized vasopressin versus norepinephrine as an early vasopressor and found no difference in their primary outcome of kidney failure-free days or a secondary outcome of mortality.[31]

Angiotensin II targets a different mechanism—the renin-angiotensin-aldosterone system—to affect blood pressure.[32] The Angiotensin II for the Treatment of Vasodilatory Shock (ATHOS-3) trial evaluated patients in vasodilatory shock in a high-output state ($Scvo_2$ >70% and CVP >8 or cardiac index >2.3 L/min) receiving norepinephrine for MAP support. Compared with placebo, angiotensin II was significantly more likely to achieve the primary endpoint of increased MAP within 3 hours.[33] Despite significant limitations of ATHOS-3, the Food and Drug Administration (FDA) approved angiotensin II for clinical use. The FDA also reported an increased incidence of combined arterial and venous thromboembolic events among those receiving angiotensin II (12.9% vs 5.1%, respectively).[34]

Both vasopressin and angiotensin II seem to have norepinephrine-sparing effects, although no improvement in patient-centered outcomes has been demonstrated with either agent. Vasopressin is established in current SSC guidelines for catecholamine-resistant septic shock management, whereas angiotensin II is a newer agent with a safety profile that needs further investigation.

IMMUNOMODULATION IN SEPSIS: CORTICOSTEROID USE

Immune system dysregulation in septic shock results from a complex interaction between autonomic, metabolic, and molecular variables. Anti-inflammatory agents may help normalize this response. In laboratory studies, corticosteroids act more as anti-inflammatory agents rather than immunosuppressants, which may contribute to the beneficial signal seen with their use in sepsis.[35]

A 2015 Cochrane review found decreased mortality rates in patients receiving a low-dose (less than 400 mg IV hydrocortisone daily), prolonged course (3 or more days before tapering) of steroids. Survival benefits were dependent on illness severity and a lower dose and longer duration of corticosteroids. Short courses of high-dose steroids were not beneficial and may be associated with harm.[36] A 2018 meta-analysis did not find a mortality benefit with corticosteroid use but still demonstrated an association with decreased shock duration, need for mechanical ventilation, and ICU length of stay. Select adverse events (hyperglycemia and viral infections) were increased in the corticosteroid group.[37]

The Adjunctive Corticosteroid Treatment in Critically Ill Patients with Septic Shock (ADRENAL) trial is the largest RCT of corticosteroids in sepsis to date. Investigators randomized patients with septic shock to receive either hydrocortisone (200 mg IV daily for 7 days) or placebo. There was no change in mortality, but median time on the ventilator, time to shock resolution, and ICU length of stay were all significantly shorter in patients on corticosteroids. There was no difference in complications, bacteremia recurrence, 28-day mortality, or renal replacement therapy rate.[38]

Current research suggests corticosteroid use improves several patient-related outcomes, although not mortality. SSC guidelines recommend hydrocortisone (200 mg IV daily) if adequate IVF and vasopressors fail to restore hemodynamic stability.[3]

SEPTIC CARDIOMYOPATHY

Septic cardiomyopathy is a global, reversible myocardial dysfunction. It is thought to result in part from ventricular-arterial decoupling, which is worsened by tachycardia.[39] At present, no targeted intervention has been developed specifically for myocardial depression in sepsis. Focus largely has been on supportive care with IVF, vasopressors, and inotropic agents.[39]

Dobutamine

Dobutamine is a synthetic catecholamine that primarily affects β_1 receptors, and secondarily β_2 and α_1 receptors, resulting in increased cardiac output with minimal effects on blood pressure. It is an inotropic agent recommended for use in patients with cardiac dysfunction as a means of improving cardiac index. Dobutamine, when used in combination with norepinephrine, performs similarly to epinephrine alone in patients with septic shock.[40]

Esmolol

Although catecholamines are used as vasopressor support, adrenergic overstimulation is associated with multiple adverse effects, including metabolic derangement, hypercoagulability, and cardiopulmonary dysfunction.[41,42] Esmolol, a short-acting β_1-selective blocker, may counteract overstimulation and myocardial dysfunction.[43] In an Italian RCT of septic shock patients on norepinephrine infusions, using esmolol to achieve heart rate control improved stroke volume index and decreased fluid and vasopressor requirements. Surprisingly, there was also decreased 28-day mortality rate in the esmolol group (49.4% mortality) versus patients receiving vasopressors alone (80.4%), although the implications are unclear because the control group had uncharacteristically high mortality.[44]

Importantly, this study excluded patients with significant cardiac dysfunction or underlying valvular disease. Furthermore, its conclusions cannot be extrapolated to early sepsis resuscitation, when intravascular volume depletion rather than catecholamine overstimulation is the likely etiology of tachycardia. Blocking that response may lead to worsened hemodynamic compromise. Although intriguing, β-blockade in septic shock cannot yet be recommended for routine use.

NUTRITIONAL AND METABOLIC SUPPORT
Glucose Control

Metabolic derangements play a significant role in sepsis, and glucose levels can vary widely. The SSC recommends a target of serum glucose less than 180 mg/dL, with avoidance of hypoglycemia.[3]

Nutrition

Early enteral nutrition (within 24–48 hours) has been linked to reduced infectious complications in critically ill patients. Although nutrition support is usually started in the ICU, if patients remain in ED for a prolonged period, enteral nutrition should be initiated once hemodynamically stable and vasopressors are being withdrawn.[45]

Ascorbic Acid (Vitamin C)

Vitamin C may prevent reactive oxygen species overproduction, which contributes to microvascular and alveolar dysfunction and is utilized in catecholamine synthesis.[46,47] A retrospective observational study of 94 patients by Marik and colleagues[48] garnered significant attention to vitamin supplementation in septic patients. Infusion of hydrocortisone, thiamine, and vitamin C was associated with markedly decreased in-hospital mortality (8.5%) in patients who had received the infusion as compared to patients who had not (40.4% in-hospital mortality) as well as more rapid vasopressor weaning.[48]

A follow-up RCT, the Vitamin C Infusion for Treatment in Sepsis Induced Acute Lung Injury (CITRIS-ALI) trial, randomized septic patients with ARDS to either IV vitamin C or placebo (5% dextrose in water) within 48 hours of ARDS onset. There was no difference in either coprimary endpoint (modified SOFA score or C-reactive protein and thrombomodulin levels). Patients receiving vitamin C had lower mortality.[49] The recently published Vitamin C, Hydrocortisone and Thiamine In Patients With Septic Shock Trial (VITAMINS) randomized patients with septic shock to vitamin C, thiamine, and hydrocortisone versus hydrocortisone alone. There were no differences in the primary outcome of time alive and free of vasopressor administration over 7 days. Nor was there improvement in 9 of 10 secondary outcomes, including mortality.[50] Given the conflicting research, the authors recommend that fundamental components of ED sepsis care take priority over routine ascorbic acid administration.

SUMMARY

Sepsis care has evolved significantly since Rivers and colleagues[1] highlighted EGDT's benefits with early antibiotics, fluid resuscitation, and close monitoring. Overall understanding is more nuanced, particularly regarding fluid selection, vasopressor, inotropic, and ventilator support. Other components, such as nutrition therapy and glucose control, tend to receive less attention but also are important

Table 3
Emergency department sepsis response—critical actions

Screening cues	Utilize screening tools to drive warning cues: SIRS, qSOFA, National Early Warning Score Does clinical data make sepsis a possibility? Is an infectious cause likely? Should escalation of care be triggered?
Bedside actions	Administer oxygen to maintain Spo_2 >94% (88%–92% if at risk of CO_2 retention [eg, chronic obstructive pulmonary disease]). Draw blood cultures and consider infective source. Think source control (eg, cerebrospinal fluid, urine, sputum, and chest radiograph)! Administer intravenous antibiotics (consider broad-spectrum coverage). Consider local resistance patterns and allergies prior to administration. Consider IVF resuscitation (30 mL/kg) using balanced crystalloid (delivered rapidly in divided aliquots) in patients with sepsis who are (1) hypotensive, (2) have a serum lactate >2 mmol/L, or (3) show signs of AKI. Check serial lactates. Consider hourly urine output measurement. May require urinary catheter.

to sepsis care. Further research has led to the exploration of new therapies including immunomodulation, β-blockade, and vitamin supplementation. At its core, however, EGDT emphasizes the importance of the first few hours for these critically ill patients, reaffirming the importance of ED providers skilled in sepsis management (**Table 3**).

DISCLOSURE

The authors have nothing to disclose.

REFERENCES

1. Rivers E, Nguyen B, Havstad S, et al. Early goal-directed therapy in the treatment of severe sepsis and septic shock. N Engl J Med 2001;345:1368–77.
2. Holst LB, Haase N, Wetterslev J, et al. Lower versus higher hemoglobin threshold for transfusion in septic shock. N Engl J Med 2014;371:1381–91.
3. Rhodes A, Evans LE, Alhazzani W, et al. Surviving sepsis campaign: international guidelines for management of sepsis and septic shock: 2016. Crit Care Med 2017;45:486–552.
4. Levy MM, Evans LE, Rhodes A. The surviving sepsis campaign bundle: 2018 update. Intensive Care Med 2018;44:925–8.
5. Peake SL, Delaney A, Bailey M, et al. Goal-directed resuscitation for patients with early septic shock. N Engl J Med 2014;371:1496–506.
6. Yealy DM, Kellum JA, Huang DT, et al. A randomized trial of protocol-based care for early septic shock. N Engl J Med 2014;370:1683–93.
7. Mouncey PR, Osborn TM, Power GS, et al. Trial of early, goal-directed resuscitation for septic shock. N Engl J Med 2015;372:1301–11.
8. Rowan KM, Angus DC, Bailey M, et al. Early, goal-directed therapy for septic shock - a patient-level meta-analysis. N Engl J Med 2017;376:2223–34.
9. Singer M, Deutschman CS, Seymour CW, et al. The third international consensus definitions for sepsis and septic shock (Sepsis-3). JAMA 2016;315:801–10.

10. Churpek MM, Zadravecz FJ, Winslow C, et al. Incidence and prognostic value of the systemic inflammatory response syndrome and organ dysfunctions in ward patients. Am J Respir Crit Care Med 2015;192:958–64.
11. Kaukonen KM, Bailey M, Pilcher D, et al. Systemic inflammatory response syndrome criteria in defining severe sepsis. N Engl J Med 2015;372:1629–38.
12. Freund Y, Lemachatti N, Krastinova E, et al. Prognostic accuracy of sepsis-3 criteria for in-hospital mortality among patients with suspected infection presenting to the emergency department. JAMA 2017;317:301–8.
13. Cheng MP, Stenstrom R, Paquette K, et al. Blood culture results before and after antimicrobial administration in patients with severe manifestations of sepsis: a diagnostic study. Ann Intern Med 2019;171:547–54.
14. Frutos-Vivar F, Nin N, Esteban A. Epidemiology of acute lung injury and acute respiratory distress syndrome. Curr Opin Crit Care 2004;10:1–6.
15. Amato MB, Meade MO, Slutsky AS, et al. Driving pressure and survival in the acute respiratory distress syndrome. N Engl J Med 2015;372:747–55.
16. Guérin C, Reignier J, Richard J-C, et al. Prone positioning in severe acute respiratory distress syndrome. N Engl J Med 2013;368:2159–68.
17. Yunos NM, Bellomo R, Hegarty C, et al. Association between a chloride-liberal vs chloride-restrictive intravenous fluid administration strategy and kidney injury in critically ill adults. JAMA 2012;308:1566–72.
18. Raghunathan K, Shaw A, Nathanson B, et al. Association between the choice of IV crystalloid and in-hospital mortality among critically ill adults with sepsis*. Crit Care Med 2014;42:1585–91.
19. Semler MW, Self WH, Wanderer JP, et al. Balanced crystalloids versus saline in critically ill adults. N Engl J Med 2018;378:829–39.
20. Legrand M, Dupuis C, Simon C, et al. Association between systemic hemodynamics and septic acute kidney injury in critically ill patients: a retrospective observational study. Crit Care 2013;17:R278.
21. Marik PE, Baram M, Vahid B. Does central venous pressure predict fluid responsiveness? A systematic review of the literature and the tale of seven mares. Chest 2008;134:172–8.
22. Monnet X, Marik P, Teboul JL. Passive leg raising for predicting fluid responsiveness: a systematic review and meta-analysis. Intensive Care Med 2016;42: 1935–47.
23. Jones AE, Shapiro NI, Trzeciak S, et al. Lactate clearance vs central venous oxygen saturation as goals of early sepsis therapy: a randomized clinical trial. JAMA 2010;303:739–46.
24. Wardi G, Brice J, Correia M, et al. Demystifying lactate in the emergency department. Ann Emerg Med 2020;75:287–98.
25. Lara B, Enberg L, Ortega M, et al. Capillary refill time during fluid resuscitation in patients with sepsis-related hyperlactatemia at the emergency department is related to mortality. PLoS One 2017;12:e0188548.
26. Hernandez G, Ospina-Tascon GA, Damiani LP, et al. Effect of a resuscitation strategy targeting peripheral perfusion status vs serum lactate levels on 28-day mortality among patients with septic shock: the ANDROMEDA-SHOCK randomized clinical trial. JAMA 2019;321:654–64.
27. Wutrich Y, Barraud D, Conrad M, et al. Early increase in arterial lactate concentration under epinephrine infusion is associated with a better prognosis during shock. Shock 2010;34:4–9.
28. Asfar P, Meziani F, Hamel JF, et al. High versus low blood-pressure target in patients with septic shock. N Engl J Med 2014;370:1583–93.

29. Dunser MW, Mayr AJ, Tur A, et al. Ischemic skin lesions as a complication of continuous vasopressin infusion in catecholamine-resistant vasodilatory shock: incidence and risk factors. Crit Care Med 2003;31:1394–8.

30. Russell JA, Walley KR, Singer J, et al. Vasopressin versus norepinephrine infusion in patients with septic shock. N Engl J Med 2008;358:877–87.

31. Gordon AC, Mason AJ, Thirunavukkarasu N, et al. Effect of early vasopressin vs norepinephrine on kidney failure in patients with septic shock: the VANISH randomized clinical trial. JAMA 2016;316:509–18.

32. Dandona P, Dhindsa S, Ghanim H, et al. Angiotensin II and inflammation: the effect of angiotensin-converting enzyme inhibition and angiotensin II receptor blockade. J Hum Hypertens 2007;21:20–7.

33. Khanna A, English SW, Wang XS, et al. Angiotensin II for the treatment of vasodilatory shock. N Engl J Med 2017;377:419–30.

34. Senatore F, Jagadeesh G, Rose M, et al. FDA Approval of Angiotensin II for the Treatment of Hypotension in Adults with Distributive Shock. Am J Cardiovasc Drugs 2019;19:11–20.

35. Keh D, Boehnke T, Weber-Cartens S, et al. Immunologic and hemodynamic effects of "low-dose" hydrocortisone in septic shock: a double-blind, randomized, placebo-controlled, crossover study. Am J Respir Crit Care Med 2003;167:512–20.

36. Annane D, Bellissant E, Bollaert PE, et al. Corticosteroids for treating sepsis. Cochrane Database Syst Rev 2015;(12):CD002243.

37. Rygard SL, Butler E, Granholm A, et al. Low-dose corticosteroids for adult patients with septic shock: a systematic review with meta-analysis and trial sequential analysis. Intensive Care Med 2018;44:1003–16.

38. Venkatesh B, Finfer S, Cohen J, et al. Adjunctive glucocorticoid therapy in patients with septic shock. N Engl J Med 2018;378:797–808.

39. Guarracino F, Ferro B, Morelli A, et al. Ventriculoarterial decoupling in human septic shock. Crit Care 2014;18:R80.

40. Annane D, Vignon P, Renault A, et al. Norepinephrine plus dobutamine versus epinephrine alone for management of septic shock: a randomised trial. Lancet 2007;370:676–84.

41. Dunser MW, Hasibeder WR. Sympathetic overstimulation during critical illness: adverse effects of adrenergic stress. J Intensive Care Med 2009;24:293–316.

42. Schmittinger CA, Torgersen C, Luckner G, et al. Adverse cardiac events during catecholamine vasopressor therapy: a prospective observational study. Intensive Care Med 2012;38:950–8.

43. Suzuki T, Morisaki H, Serita R, et al. Infusion of the beta-adrenergic blocker esmolol attenuates myocardial dysfunction in septic rats. Crit Care Med 2005;33:2294–301.

44. Morelli A, Ertmer C, Westphal M, et al. Effect of heart rate control with esmolol on hemodynamic and clinical outcomes in patients with septic shock: a randomized clinical trial. JAMA 2013;310:1683–91.

45. McClave SA, Taylor BE, Martindale RG, et al. Guidelines for the Provision and Assessment of Nutrition Support Therapy in the Adult Critically Ill Patient: Society of Critical Care Medicine (SCCM) and American Society for Parenteral and Enteral Nutrition (A.S.P.E.N.). JPEN J Parenter Enteral Nutr 2016;40:159–211.

46. Biesalski HK, McGregor GP. Antioxidant therapy in critical care–is the microcirculation the primary target? Crit Care Med 2007;35:S577–83.

47. Fisher BJ, Seropian IM, Kraskauskas D, et al. Ascorbic acid attenuates lipopolysaccharide-induced acute lung injury. Crit Care Med 2011;39:1454–60.

48. Marik PE, Khangoora V, Rivera R, et al. Hydrocortisone, Vitamin C, and thiamine for the treatment of severe sepsis and septic shock: a retrospective before-after study. Chest 2017;151:1229–38.

49. Fowler AA III, Truwit JD, Hite RD, et al. Effect of Vitamin C infusion on organ failure and biomarkers of inflammation and vascular injury in patients with sepsis and severe acute respiratory failure: the CITRIS-ALI randomized clinical trial. JAMA 2019;322:1261–70.

50. Fujii T, Luethi N, Young PJ, et al. Effect of vitamin c, hydrocortisone, and thiamine vs hydrocortisone alone on time alive and free of vasopressor support among patients with septic shock: the VITAMINS randomized clinical trial. JAMA 2020; 323(5):423–31.

Pediatric Cardiac Arrest Resuscitation

Nathan W. Mick, MD[a,b,*], Rachel J. Williams, MD[b,c]

KEYWORDS

• Pediatric • Cardiac arrest • Epidemiology • Treatment • Prognosis

KEY POINTS

• Cardiac arrest in children is a rare but devastating presentation that is almost always due to a primary respiratory event that progresses to cardiac failure.

• Early recognition and resuscitation of patients in the "prearrest" states of shock or respiratory failure are critical to successful outcomes.

• As respiratory illness is frequently a precursor to cardiac arrest, meticulous support of oxygenation and ventilation is essential in the critically ill infant or child.

• Both targeted temperature management and extracorporeal membrane oxygenation are not associated with marked improvement in outcome in out-of-hospital cardiac arrest in the pediatric population.

INTRODUCTION

Pediatric cardiac arrest is a rare clinical scenario and has profound impacts on both families and clinical care teams. Current evidence-based resuscitation recommendations and research are focused on intervening in the pre–cardiac arrest phase of critical illness, because of the unique causes that occur in the pediatric population. Knowledge of the anatomic and physiologic differences across the pediatric age spectrum is critical to successful management of these challenging situations. This article focuses on the initial assessment of pediatric patients in the prearrest states of respiratory distress or shock, cardiac arrest management, treatment of special circumstances that lead to cardiac arrest, post–cardiac arrest care, and treatment of select underlying causes of cardiac arrest in the pediatric patient.

[a] Department of Emergency Medicine, Pediatric Emergency Medicine, Maine Medical Center, 22 Bramhall Street, Portland, ME 04102, USA; [b] Tufts University School of Medicine, Boston, MA, USA; [c] Pediatric Emergency Medicine, Maine Medical Center, 22 Bramhall Street, Portland, ME 04102, USA
* Corresponding author. Department of Emergency Medicine, Pediatric Emergency Medicine, Maine Medical Center, 22 Bramhall Street, Portland, ME 04102.
E-mail address: mickn@mmc.org
Twitter: @NateMickMD (N.W.M.)

Emerg Med Clin N Am 38 (2020) 819–839
https://doi.org/10.1016/j.emc.2020.06.007
0733-8627/20/© 2020 Elsevier Inc. All rights reserved.

EPIDEMIOLOGY

The incidence of pediatric cardiac arrest follows a bimodal distribution, with the first peak in infancy (2.1 cases per 100,000 person-years) and the second peak in adolescence (1.44 cases per 100,000 person-years).[1] Mortality for out-of-hospital cardiac arrest (OHCA) in the pediatric population is 90% or greater and likely reflects the differences in pathologic condition compared with adults that lead to the arrest.[2]

CAUSE

In contrast to adults, whereby cardiac arrest is typically due to a primary arrhythmia, pediatric patients more commonly experience a respiratory event that leads to hypoxia, acidosis, bradycardia, and arrest. Pulmonary causes of respiratory decompensation that may lead to cardiac arrest are numerous and include acquired conditions (eg, bronchiolitis, pertussis, sepsis, pneumonia, hypoventilation from seizures/status epilepticus) and respiratory failure owing to ingested toxins or nonaccidental trauma. Because of the frequency of respiratory causes of pediatric cardiac arrest, guidelines from the American Heart Association (AHA) and the Pediatric Life Support Task Force of the International Liaison Committee on Resuscitation (ILCOR) continue to emphasize support of oxygenation and ventilation.[3]

Primary arrhythmias do occur in infants and children, particularly those with underlying congenital or structural heart disease, or those with acquired heart conditions (eg, myocarditis). Channelopathies, congenital prolonged QT syndrome, Wolff-Parkinson-White syndrome, Brugada syndrome, and complex congenital heart disease (eg, Tetralogy of Fallot, transposition of the great arteries, hypoplastic left heart syndrome) have all been implicated in cases of pediatric sudden cardiac death. In up to 50% of cases of arrhythmogenic cardiac arrest, patients report warning or prodromal symptoms that include syncope, presyncope, chest pain, or exercise fatigue.[4–6] Patients also may report a family history of early, unexpected, or unexplained death.

INITIAL ASSESSMENT

The goal of the initial assessment of a critically ill child is to quickly identify life-threatening respiratory failure and shock to prevent the onset of cardiac arrest. Current AHA Guidelines for Cardiopulmonary Resuscitation and Emergency Cardiovascular Care recommend a systematic approach to assessing the ill or injured child using the Pediatric Advanced Life Support (PALS) algorithm.[7] This systematic approach consists of the initial impression, primary assessment, and secondary assessment. If cardiac arrest is identified at any point during this initial assessment, immediately start cardiopulmonary resuscitation (CPR) with high-quality chest compressions and proceed with the Pediatric Cardiac Arrest Algorithm.[8] Chest compressions in children should occur at a rate of 100 to 120 per minute, compress at least one-third of the anterior-posterior chest diameter, and interruptions should be avoided.

If CPR is not immediately required, a primary assessment consisting of a hands-on evaluation of the patient's cardiopulmonary and neurologic function using the "ABCDE" model should be performed (**Table 1**).[9] Importantly, vital signs, such as heart rate, blood pressure, and respiratory rate, vary by age (**Table 2**).[10] Any life threat identified during the primary assessment (ie, impending respiratory failure) should be addressed immediately.

After a primary assessment, a secondary assessment consisting of a focused history and thorough physical examination should be performed. Diagnostic laboratory

Table 1
"ABCDE" primary assessment model

	Primary Assessment	Signs of a Life-Threatening Condition
A: Airway	Is the airway patent? Is there movement of the chest and abdomen? Are there breath sounds?	Increased inspiratory effort with retractions Snoring or stridor Lack of airway sounds or phonation
B: Breathing	What is the respiratory rate and pulse oximetry? Is there increased work of breathing? Is there chest expansion and air movement? Are there breath sounds? Are they abnormal?	Apnea or bradypnea Significant increased work of breathing (tachypnea, retractions, nasal flaring, head bobbing or seesaw respirations, grunting) Abnormal or absent breath sounds Hypoxia
C: Circulation	What is the heart rate and rhythm? Are peripheral and central pulses present? What is the capillary refill time? What is the skin color and temperature? What is the blood pressure?	Cardiac arrest Poor perfusion (delayed capillary refill, cyanosis, cool skin, mottling) Hypotension Arrhythmia
D: Disability	What is the patient's Glasgow Coma Scale (GCS)? What is the patient's level of consciousness? What is the pupillary response to light?	Unresponsive or depressed GCS Seizures Abnormal pupils (unequal size or poor response to light)
E: Exposure	Is there fever or hypothermia? Are there skin findings to suggest trauma? Is there significant bleeding? Is there a suggestive rash?	Hypothermia Hemorrhage/significant bruising Petechia/purpura

Data from Thim T, Krarup NH, Grove EL, Rohde CV, Løfgren B. Initial assessment and treatment with the Airway, Breathing, Circulation, Disability, Exposure (ABCDE) approach. Int J Gen Med. 2012;5:117-121. https://doi.org/10.2147/IJGM.S28478.

studies (ie, chemistries, complete blood count, cultures), an electrocardiogram, point-of-care ultrasound, and diagnostic imaging studies (eg, radiograph, computed tomography) may be warranted to further evaluate and identify life-threatening conditions. Some laboratory and imaging studies may need to be repeated to assess the clinical response to interventions (eg, preintubation and postintubation arterial blood gases).

PRECARDIAC ARREST STATES
Respiratory Distress

Basic airway maneuvers for the patient with a patent airway include supplemental oxygen (nasal cannula, oxygen masks), suctioning, and noninvasive positive pressure ventilation. These techniques may be used in spontaneously breathing patients with hypoxemia or respiratory distress.[11] If these prove inadequate, then assisted

Table 2
Normal vital signs by age

Age	Respiratory Rate (10th–90th Percentile)	Heart Rate (10th–90th Percentile)
0–3 mo	34–57	123–164
3–6 mo	33–55	120–159
6–9 mo	31–52	114–152
9–12 mo	30–50	109–145
12–18 mo	28–46	103–140
18–24 mo	25–40	98–135
2–3 y	22–34	92–128
3–4 y	21–29	86–123
4–6 y	20–27	81–117
6–8 y	18–24	74–111
8–12 y	16–22	67–103
12–15 y	15–21	62–96
15–18 y	13–19	58–92

Data from Fleming S, Thompson M, Stevens R, et al. Normal ranges of heart rate and respiratory rate in children from birth to 18 years of age: a systematic review of observational studies. Lancet 2011; 377:1011.

respirations with bag-valve-mask (BVM), insertion of supraglottic airway devices, or intubation may be required. Indications for assisted respirations include severe respiratory distress, depressed mental status, upper-airway obstruction (eg, oropharyngeal burns, anaphylaxis, epiglottitis), or refractory hypoxemia.[12]

Shock

Shock in pediatric patients can have many causes (**Table 3**). Shock can be characterized as compensated or uncompensated with uncompensated typically defined as the presence of poor perfusion with hypotension.

Compensated shock

Patients with inadequate organ perfusion who maintain adequate blood pressure are said to have "compensated" shock. Early physical examination and laboratory signs of compensated shock include the following:

- Tachycardia
- Tachypnea
- Delayed capillary refill
- Cool extremities
- Orthostatic vital signs
- Decreased urine output
- Depressed mental status (eg, sleepiness or irritability)
- Elevated blood lactate level, acidosis, or increased base deficit

Uncompensated shock

Hypotensive or "uncompensated" shock occurs when compensatory mechanisms fail. In addition to hypotension, patients with uncompensated shock may exhibit worsening tachycardia, mottled extremities, markedly delayed capillary refill, worsening tachypnea (compensatory respiratory alkalosis), and altered mental status. Laboratory

Table 3
Mechanism, cause, features, and treatments of shock

Type of Shock	Mechanism	Common Causes	Features	Treatment
Cardiogenic	Decreased cardiac contractility leading to decreased cardiac output	Arrhythmia Congenital heart disease (ALCAPA) Myocarditis Drug ingestions (eg, cocaine) Metabolic derangements (eg, hypoglycemia)	Elevated HR Decreased BP Delayed capillary refill with cool extremities	Inotropes Cautious use of fluid (functional rather than absolute circulating volume deficit) ECMO
Dissociative	Impaired cellular oxygen delivery or utilization due to presence of a toxic metabolite or drug	Carbon monoxide poisoning Cyanide poisoning Methemoglobinemia	Elevated HR Normal or elevated BP Normal capillary refill	Specific antidotes (call local poison control center) Hyperbaric oxygen therapy
Distributive	Inappropriate vasodilation and peripheral pooling of blood	Sepsis Anaphylaxis Drug ingestion (eg, atypical antipsychotics)	Elevated HR Decreased BP Capillary refill may be flash or delayed Extremities may be warm or cool	Fluid resuscitation Antibiotics if infection suspected Vasopressors Epinephrine for anaphylaxis
Hypovolemic (most common cause of shock in children)	Decreased circulating blood volume	Dehydration (diarrhea, vomiting) Osmotic diuresis (hyperglycemia/DKA) Plasma losses (burns) Hemorrhage	Elevated HR Decreased BP Delayed capillary refill with cool extremities	Fluid resuscitation or transfusion Cessation of bleeding (may require operating room)
Neurogenic	Severely reduced systemic vascular resistance from disrupted sympathetic nerve stimulation	Spinal cord injury Traumatic brain injury	Depressed HR and BP Warm extremities	Fluid resuscitation Vasopressors
Obstructive	Mechanical obstruction to ventricular outflow	Cardiac tamponade Tension pneumothorax Massive pulmonary embolism Left-sided congenital heart disease (HLHS, aortic coarctation, critical aortic valve stenosis)	Elevated HR Decreased BP Delayed capillary refill with cool extremities	Pericardiocentesis for tamponade Needle decompression and chest tube for pneumothorax Prostaglandins (for ductal-dependent congenital cardiac lesions)

Abbreviations: ALCAPA, anomalous left coronary artery arising from the pulmonary artery; BP, blood pressure; DKA, diabetic ketoacidosis; HLHS, hypoplastic left heart syndrome; HR, heart rate.

studies may show signs of progressive end-organ failure, including worsening metabolic acidosis, renal failure, coagulopathy, thrombocytopenia, hyperbilirubinemia, or transaminitis. If uncompensated shock is not addressed, it may rapidly progress into cardiopulmonary failure and arrest. Treatment is specific to the cause of the shock and reversal of the underlying cause (see **Table 3**).

Rapid sequence intubation

Intubation and mechanical ventilation may be necessary in shock states for airway protection and to reduce work of breathing. Caution must be taken in the patient who requires mechanical ventilation in the setting of shock, because positive pressure ventilation may lead to depressed venous return and cardiovascular collapse. The patient may require intravenous (IV) fluid resuscitation or vasopressor administration to maintain cardiac output. These therapies should ideally be administered before rapid sequence intubation (RSI) if time allows. Aggressive fluid resuscitation with balanced crystalloid in 20 mL/kg aliquots before intubation may help mitigate the physiologic perturbations that occur with the transition from negative to positive pressure ventilation. In the absence of contraindications, ketamine is the preferred sedative for RSI in pediatric patients with shock.[13]

CARDIAC ARREST

If a critically ill pediatric patient is noted to be unresponsive with apnea or gasping respirations, feel a pulse for no more than 10 seconds. If no pulse is detected, immediately begin chest compression and proceed with the PALS Cardiac Arrest Algorithm.[14] Refer to the AHA Guidelines for Cardiopulmonary Resuscitation and Emergency Cardiovascular Care for the complete Pediatric Advanced Life Support Algorithm. A link to the current guideline is provided here: https://www.ahajournals.org/doi/pdf/10.1161/CIRCULATIONAHA.110.971101.

Airway Management

In the pediatric patient with OHCA, BVM followed by intubation conferred no survival benefit when compared with BVM alone.[15] Decreased survival to hospital discharge has also been shown in cases of in-hospital cardiac arrest that are intubated compared with those that receive only BVM.[16] It is therefore reasonable to continue BVM through the duration of the resuscitation if effective oxygenation and ventilation are achieved. If BVM ventilation is ineffective, advanced airway interventions, such as supraglottic airway devices or intubation, should be considered. While managing the airway during cardiac arrest, it is important to avoid excessive ventilation because this may lead to decreased cardiac output and decreased coronary perfusion pressure. Excessive ventilation via BVM may also cause gastric distension, which can impede diaphragmatic excursion and impair ventilation. Gastric decompression with an orogastric or nasogastric tube may be necessary if BVM ventilation is prolonged. When ventilating with a mask, it is important to maintain the recommended ratio of 2 breaths for every 15 compressions, and to give each breath more than 1 second with just enough volume to make the chest rise.[14]

Rhythm Analysis

After the initiation of chest compressions, attach defibrillator pads or a cardiac monitor to analyze the rhythm. Ventricular tachycardia (VT) and ventricular fibrillation (VF) are considered "shockable" rhythms.[14,17]

Nonshockable rhythms, such as asystole and pulseless electrical activity (PEA), are the most common presenting rhythms in both in-hospital and out-of-hospital pediatric cardiac arrest.[12,14] Rhythms in PEA may have a fast, slow, or normal rate and may be associated with other abnormalities, including conduction delays, prolonged PR or QT intervals, and a widened QRS complex. Potentially reversible causes of cardiac arrest to consider in patients with PEA are known as the "H's and T's" (**Box 1**).

Primary VF is rare in pediatric patients and may quickly degenerate into asystole. VF may be secondary to a cardiac abnormality, channelopathy, sudden impact to the chest, or the "H's and T's."

Patients with VT may present with or without a pulse. Pulseless VT often degenerates into VF and then ultimately asystole. Patients presenting with cardiac arrest whose initial rhythm is shockable (VF or VT) have improved survival and outcome compared with their "nonshockable" counterparts.[13]

Defibrillation

When the presenting rhythm is VF or pulseless VT, early defibrillation is critical to survival. Outcomes are improved when defibrillation is coupled with early, high-quality CPR. An initial defibrillation dose of 2 to 4 J/kg should be administered as soon as the rhythm is deemed shockable. Resume chest compressions immediately after the shock is delivered. If VF or pulseless VT persists at the next rhythm check, the second shock should be given at a dose of 4 J/kg, with increasing doses as needed for refractory shockable rhythms up to a maximum of 10 J/kg and not to exceed the maximum adult dose (200 J biphasic, 360 J monophasic).[18,19]

Pharmacology

CPR should not be interrupted for the administration of medications during cardiac arrest resuscitation. Current AHA guidelines recommend delivery of resuscitation drugs during chest compressions immediately before, or after, shock delivery to allow these agents to circulate before the next rhythm check. Resuscitation medications are calculated based on the child's weight (if known), or with the use of a length-based tape with precalculated dosages. Length-based systems have been shown to reduce the cognitive burden of pediatric resuscitation.[20] Epinephrine increases aortic diastolic pressure and coronary perfusion pressure and is the main pharmacologic agent used to treat cardiac arrest. Epinephrine can be given via the IV or intraosseous route

Box 1
Reversible cause of cardiac arrest (H's and T's)
Hypovolemia
Hypoxia
Hydrogen ion excess (metabolic acidosis)
Hypoglycemia
Hypokalemia or hyperkalemia
Hypothermia or hyperthermia
Tension pneumothorax
Tamponade (cardiac)
Toxin
Thrombosis (pulmonary or coronary)
Trauma

at a dose of 0.01 mg/kg or via the endotracheal tube at a dose of 0.1 mg/kg. In patients with a nonshockable rhythm, epinephrine should be given as soon as PEA or asystole is identified (see PALS algorithm for Pediatric Cardiac Arrest step 10). In patients with a shockable rhythm, the same dose of epinephrine is used and should be administered after the delivery of 2 shocks and CPR (see PALS algorithm for Pediatric Cardiac Arrest step 6). Regardless of the rhythm, epinephrine can be repeated every 3 to 5 minutes. **Table 4** provides a summary of additional resuscitation medications that can be used in the treatment of pediatric cardiac arrest and dysrhythmias.[21]

SPECIAL CIRCUMSTANCES
Hypothermic Arrest

Patients with severe hypothermia may be unresponsive to resuscitative efforts until the core body temperature is rewarmed to at least 30°C. CPR should continue until the body is rewarmed to at least this temperature before terminating resuscitation. Active external rewarming techniques include electric blankets, hot water bottles, warm IV fluids, and overhead warmers. Although simple to deploy, these methods may not have a large or rapid effect on rewarming.[22] Body cavity irrigation with warm fluids is a more invasive, yet more effective, technique for rewarming. Extracorporeal circulation is the most rapid and effective technique for rewarming severely hypothermic patients with cardiac arrest. Transfer to a facility with pediatric extracorporeal membrane oxygenation (ECMO) or cardiopulmonary bypass capabilities should be considered.[22] Survival has been described in patients with prolonged cold-water submersion and resuscitation times up to 40 and 120 minutes, respectively.[14]

Extracorporeal Membrane Oxygenation and Extracorporeal Cardiopulmonary Resuscitation

Beyond its use in hypothermic cardiac arrest, there has been growing interest in ECMO as a method of circulatory rescue in cases of cardiac arrest from other causes and is commonly used in the pediatric population after surgery for congenital heart disease.[23,24] Extracorporeal cardiopulmonary resuscitation (eCPR) is the rapid deployment of venoarterial ECMO during active CPR or for patients with intermittent return of spontaneous circulation (ROSC). In patients who experience an in-hospital arrest, there is an association with favorable neurologic outcomes in the group who received eCPR versus those who were treated with conventional PALS protocols.[25] The ILCOR states that eCPR can be considered for "pediatric patients with cardiac diagnosis who have in-hospital cardiac arrest in settings with existing ECMO protocols, expertise and equipment (Class 2b; Level of evidence C-LD)."[3] Patients who present with OHCA, or those in whom a noncardiac cause for arrest is suspected, should not be considered candidates for eCPR based on the current body of literature.

POSTRESUSCITATION MANAGEMENT

In the early postresuscitation period, the patient should be monitored closely for hypotension and/or arrhythmias that may be a harbinger of recurrent cardiopulmonary collapse. Other goals of postresuscitation care are to preserve neurologic function, prevent secondary end-organ damage, and stabilize the patient for transport to a pediatric tertiary-care facility. Postresuscitation care includes airway management, treatment of shock, glucose management, electroencephalogram (EEG) monitoring, and targeted temperature management (TTM). During this time, the clinician should

Table 4
Drugs of pediatric resuscitation

Medication	Cardiovascular Effects	Indication	Dose	Additional Information
Adenosine	AV nodal conduction block	SupraVT	First dose: 0.1 mg/kg IV or IO (maximum dose 6 mg) Second dose: 0.2 m/kg IV or IO (maximum dose 12 mg)	Follow dose with rapid saline flush Administer in IV as close to the heart as possible (avoid hand or lower extremity)
Amiodarone	Class III antiarrhythmic Slows AV and ventricular conduction Prolongs AV refractory period and QT interval	Cardiac arrest with refractory VF/pulseless VT Stable supraventricular or VT	5 mg/kg IV or IO (maximum dose 300 mg) May repeat dose twice	IV push during cardiac arrest Given over 20–60 min with perfusing rhythm (expert consultation recommended) Do not give with other QT prolonging agents
Atropine	Accelerates sinus or atrial pacemakers Increases speed of AV conduction	Symptomatic bradycardia	0.02 mg/kg IV or IO OR 0.04–0.06 mg/kg ET Minimum dose: 0.1 mg Maximum single dose: 0.5 mg	May repeat dose once if needed
Calcium chloride 10%	Enhanced cardiac automaticity and contractility	Documented hypocalcemia Calcium channel blocker overdose Hypermagnesemia Hyperkalemia	20 mg/kg IV or IO Maximum single dose: 2 g	Administer slowly Not recommended for routine use in cardiac arrest without clear indication
Epinephrine	A1 receptors: increases peripheral vascular resistance B1 receptors: positive chronotropy and inotropy	Cardiac arrest	0.01 mg/kg (0.1 mL/kg 1:10,000) IV or IO 0.1 mg/kg (0.1 mL/kg 1:1000) ET Maximum dose: 1 mg IV/IO or 2.5 mg ET	Repeat every 3–5 min as needed per PALS algorithm
Lidocaine	Class I antiarrhythmic Decreases automaticity Suppresses ventricular arrhythmia	Cardiac arrest with refractory VF/pulseless VT	1 mg/kg IV/IO bolus 20–50 μg/kg/min infusion	Not shown to improve survival to hospital discharge

(continued on next page)

Table 4
(continued)

Medication	Cardiovascular Effects	Indication	Dose	Additional Information
Magnesium sulfate	Inhibits calcium channels leading to smooth muscle relaxation	Torsades de pointes Hypomagnesemia	25–50 mg/kg IV or IO over 10–20 min Maximum dose: 2 g	Give faster in torsades de pointes Insufficient evidence to recommend for or against routine administration during cardiac arrest
Procainamide	Prolongs refractory periods Depresses conduction velocity	VT with a pulse Supraventricular tachycardia Atrial fibrillation/flutter	15 mg/kg IV or IO	Expert consultation recommended Do not give with other QT prolonging agents

Abbreviations: ET, endotracheal tube; IO, intraosseous.

also continue to investigate and treat the underlying cause of the patient's cardiac arrest.[26]

Airway Management

Postresuscitation airway management includes continuous monitoring of oxygenation and ventilation, and placement of a gastric tube to reduce distention of the stomach (**Table 5**). Sudden decompensation of the intubated child may be due to a DOPE (Dislodged endotracheal tube, endotracheal tube Obstruction, Pneumothorax, or Equipment failure).[26]

Extrapolating from adult studies, recent pediatric resuscitation guidelines advocate that oxygen saturation should be maintained between 94% and 99% after ROSC, with the goal of maintaining normoxia (defined as Pao_2 between 60 mm Hg and 300 mm Hg).[19,27] Although smaller studies of the pediatric population have failed to demonstrate a connection between arterial oxygenation and mortality, a large retrospective study suggests that both hypoxia, and to a lesser extent, hyperoxia are associated with increased mortality in cardiac arrest patients who survive to pediatric intensive care unit admission.[28–31] Given that an oxygen saturation of 100% may correlate with Pao_2 elevations up to 500 mm Hg, it is reasonable to titrate inspired oxygen concentration to maintain the saturations within the target range.

Overventilation after pediatric intubation is common in the prehospital and hospital setting.[32,33] Limited observational data suggest that both severe postresuscitation hypocapnia and hypercapnia may be associated with higher mortality.[29] Unless contraindicated by the patient's condition, current guidelines recommend that $Paco_2$ be closely monitored and kept within the target range of 30 mm Hg to 50 mm Hg once ROSC has been achieved.

Treatment of Shock

After ROSC, recurrent shock owing to myocardial dysfunction and vascular instability is common.[34,35] Early derangements in heart rate, blood pressure, urine output, and cardiac rhythm are associated with increased morbidity and mortality.[36–39] Prompt treatment with IV fluids and vasopressors is critical to improve survival and neurologic outcome (**Table 6**). Close monitoring of vital signs, perfusion, and mental status are used to guide fluid and vasoactive medication administration, with the goal to maintain systolic blood pressure above the fifth percentile for age. Currently, there are no studies comparing specific vasoactive agents after ROSC in the pediatric population.

Table 5	
Postresuscitation airway monitoring techniques	
Postresuscitation Airway Monitoring	**Confirmation**
Endotracheal tube position	Bilateral chest wall movement
	Chest radiograph
	Auscultation of bilateral breath sounds
	Absent sounds over the stomach
	Condensation in endotracheal tube
	Exhaled Co_2
Oxygenation	Continuous pulse oximetry
Ventilation	Continuous $Etco_2$ monitoring
	Intermittent blood gas measurements

Table 6
Vasoactive agents for postresuscitaiton management of shock

Vasoactive Agent	Dose Range	Indication
Dopamine	2–20 µg/kg/min IV or IO	First line for fluid refractory shock
Epinephrine	0.05–1 µg/kg/min IV or IO	First line for fluid refractory shock
Norepinephrine	0.05–2 µg/kg/min IV or IO	First line for fluid refractory shock
Vasopressin	0.0002–0.004 units/kg/min IV (maximum rate 0.04 units/min IV)	Catecholamine-resistant shock
Dobutamine	2–20 µg/kg/min IV or IO	Shock with normal BP Second-line agent for hypotensive shock
Milrinone	Load: 50 µg/kg IV or IO over 10–60 min (may cause hypotension) Infusion: 0.25–1 µg/kg/min IV or IO	Shock with normal BP

Glucose Management

Hyperglycemia should be avoided after resuscitation, and studies suggest that both peak blood glucose level and duration of hyperglycemia are predictors of mortality in the critically ill child.[40,41] In addition, hyperglycemia may lead to an osmotic diuresis that can exacerbate hemodynamic instability. Conversely, there is increased mortality after cardiac arrest in nondiabetic patients with hypoglycemia (blood glucose <70 mg/dL). Therefore, low blood glucose should also be corrected.[42]

Electroencephalogram Monitoring

Hypoxic ischemic brain injury secondary to cardiac arrest may lead to seizures, status epilepticus, and even brain death. Seizures and the absence of reactivity on EEG are associated with increased odds of death and unfavorable neurologic outcomes at hospital discharge.[43] To decrease the risk of secondary neurologic injury, EEG should be used in the comatose child to evaluate for seizure activity. Postischemic seizures should be treated aggressively in the same way that seizures are treated in the non-arrest patient.[44–46]

Targeted Temperature Management

TTM refers to the induction of hypothermia in patients after cardiac arrest and has become standard therapy in adults after ROSC and in newborns with hypoxic-ischemic encephalopathy. It is thought that TTM treats reperfusion syndrome that occurs after cardiac arrest by decreasing metabolic demand and free radical production. Current studies have generally focused on 2 temperature ranges: 32°C to 34°C and 36°C to 37.5°C (so-called controlled normothermia). Hypoxic-ischemic injury in the setting of arrest is frequently associated with fever, and elevated body temperature is associated with worse outcomes in most studies. Early research in TTM in children was limited by varied treatment protocols, which made definitive recommendations about efficacy difficult. Two recent pediatric studies (Therapeutic Hypothermia After Pediatric Cardiac Arrest Out-of-Hospital and Therapeutic Hypothermia After Pediatric Cardiac Arrest In-Hospital) examined the efficacy of TTM at 32°C to 34°C and 36°C to 37.5°C for 120 hours (5 days) in both out-of-hospital and in-hospital cardiac arrest.[47,48] Both studies failed to show a significant difference in the primary endpoint of favorable neurobehavioral outcome at 1 year or a difference in the secondary outcomes of survival at 1 year and change in neurobehavioral outcome. Despite these negative outcomes, the 2019 International Consensus on Cardiopulmonary Resuscitation and Emergency Cardiovascular Care Science with Treatment Recommendations from ILCOR considers TTM at either 32°C to 34°C and 36°C to 37.5°C to be reasonable for infants and children between 24 hours and 18 years of age who remain comatose after out-of-hospital or in-hospital cardiac arrest.[3] Despite clinical equipoise in the pediatric cardiac arrest literature, TTM can be considered, although it is imperative to avoid temperatures greater than 37.5°C in the immediate postarrest period.

TREATMENT OF UNDERLYING CAUSE
Sepsis

Sepsis should be considered in all patients presenting with cardiovascular collapse. Early volume resuscitation is a key component to the treatment of septic shock. Although 0.9% saline (normal saline) has been used for volume resuscitation for years, there is a growing body of literature, both in adults and in pediatric patients, that use of balanced crystalloid fluids may be preferable.[49–51] Patients suspected of septic shock should receive an initial 20 mL/kg fluid bolus, followed by a clinical reassessment to determine if further fluid resuscitation is warranted. The total amount of fluid given to patients in septic shock should be determined on a case-by-case basis, taking into consideration patient status and available critical care resources. The PALS guideline also recommends monitoring of the central venous oxygen saturation ($Scvo_2$), if able, with a target $Scvo_2$ ≥70%, and consideration of early assisted ventilation in patients with septic shock and severe sepsis. Etomidate may cause transient adrenal suppression for up to 24 hours after single-dose use when used during RSI in pediatric patients with sepsis.[52] Despite this physiologic fact, there are no well-done studies demonstrating an outcome difference attributable to etomidate usage. Ketamine is a reasonable alternative in pediatric patients with severe sepsis, understanding that reduced dosing may be required to mitigate the hemodynamic effects of induction in shock states regardless of agent chosen.[53]

Structural Heart Disease

Cyanotic congenital heart disease may lead to cardiogenic or obstructive shock and cardiac arrest. As more patients undergo palliative surgical procedures, they may require resuscitation during their preoperative or postoperative course or at times of critical illness. In general, these patients should undergo standard PALS resuscitation practices. Additional prearrest, intraarrest, and postarrest considerations in this special pediatric population include the following:

- Prearrest:
  - Infants with single-ventricle physiology and elevated pulmonary-to-systemic flow ratio before stage I repair may benefit from elevated $Paco_2$ levels of 50 to 60 mm Hg.
  - Infants with single-ventricle physiology who have undergone stage I repair may benefit from systemic vasodilators, such as phenoxybenzamine, milrinone, or nitroprusside.
  - Central venous oxygen saturation ($Scvo_2$) monitoring should be considered to detect hemodynamic changes in the periarrest patient.

- Hypoventilation and negative pressure ventilation may improve oxygen delivery and cardiac output, respectively, in patients with Fontan or hemi-Fontan/bidirectional Glenn physiology.
- Intraarrest:
  - ECMO should be considered for patients with single-ventricle anatomy who have undergone stage I palliation and for patients with Fontan physiology.
  - Occlusion is a known complication of systemic-pulmonary artery or right ventricular-pulmonary artery shunts, and therefore, heparin may be considered adjunctive therapy to the PALS algorithm in these patients.
  - Differences in pulmonary physiology make end-tidal Co_2 is an unreliable indicator of CPR quality in the single-ventricle patient.
- Postarrest:
  - Unlike the previously healthy patient, children with cyanotic congenital heart disease should have a target postresuscitation oxygen saturation of 80%.

A recent AHA scientific statement regarding resuscitation of infants and children with cardiac disease is also available for further review of this complex topic.[54]

Respiratory Causes

Respiratory failure is a leading cause of pediatric cardiac arrest.[55] Upper-airway obstruction, lower-airway obstruction, intrinsic lung disease, and disordered control of breathing can all precipitate respiratory failure (**Table 7**).

Trauma and Abuse

In the patient with undifferentiated shock or cardiac arrest, it is important to consider intentional or accidental traumatic injuries, such as intraabdominal trauma, tension pneumothorax, pericardial tamponade, spinal cord injury, and intracranial hemorrhage, even in the absence of external findings. Proper management of the "ABC's" may prevent or reverse cardiopulmonary collapse in this patient population. Cervical spine precautions may need to be maintained while managing the airway. Consider maneuvers, such as recessing the occiput or elevating the child's torso, to avoid unwanted neck flexion in the younger patient.[56] Trauma to the chest (pneumothorax, hemothorax, pulmonary contusion) can cause respiratory failure. In children with severe head injuries and impending brain herniation, a trial of hyperventilation may be used as a temporizing measure.[57] Resuscitative thoracotomy can be considered in pediatric patients with penetrating trauma and arrest, although outcomes are poor.[58]

Toxic/Metabolic

Accidental or intentional overdose may lead to swift cardiopulmonary collapse and cardiac arrest in pediatric patients. It is important to consider toxic ingestion in the otherwise healthy pediatric patient with cardiac arrest of unknown cause. Treatment of common and/or harmful toxic exposures is provided in **Table 8**.[59–61]

PARENTAL PRESENCE DURING RESUSCITATION

Offering caregivers the option to be present at the bedside is becoming a common practice during pediatric resuscitations and should be encouraged.[62] Research indicates that parents who were present during resuscitation would choose to be present again and would recommend being present to others in a similar situation.[63] Caregivers who were present were also noted to have more constructive grief behaviors and less distress than those who were not present. If family is present, a staff member

Table 7
Cause and management of respiratory failure

Type of Respiratory Distress	Examples	Treatment
Upper-airway obstruction	Infection (croup, epiglottitis) Edema (anaphylaxis) Foreign body	Allowing child to assume position of comfort Jaw thrust or head tilt–chin lift Foreign body removal Suctioning Medications to reduce airway edema (steroids, epinephrine) Minimizing patient agitation Possible disposition to the operating room for advanced airway management
Lower-airway obstruction	Bronchiolitis Asthma	Supplemental oxygen Suctioning Medications (albuterol, ipratropium bromide, steroids, magnesium, ketamine, epinephrine, terbutaline, Heliox)[a] High-flow nasal cannula or BIPAP Endotracheal intubation[b]
Lung tissue disease	Pneumonia (infectious, chemical, aspiration) Cardiogenic pulmonary edema ARDS Traumatic pulmonary contusion	Supplemental oxygen Positive expiratory pressure (noninvasive ventilation such as CPAP or BIPAP, mechanical ventilation with PEEP) Medications as indicated (antibiotics, vasoactive agents, diuretics)
Disordered control of breathing	Increased intracranial pressure Neuromuscular disease Depressed mental status (CNS infection, seizures, metabolic derangement, overdose)	Avoid hypoxemia, hypercarbia, hyperthermia for patients with increased ICP Antidote for overdose Noninvasive or invasive ventilatory support as mental status dictates

Abbreviations: ARDS, acute respiratory distress syndrome; BIPAP, bilevel positive airway pressure; CNS, central nervous system; CPAP, continuous positive airway pressure; ICP, intracranial pressure; PEEP, positive end expiratory pressure.

[a] Medications listed are possible treatments for asthma. Albuterol trial may be indicated in patients with bronchiolitis; however, per American Academy of Pediatrics guidelines no additional medications are shown to be beneficial in patients with bronchiolitis.[42]

[b] If assisted ventilation is required in this population use a low respiratory rate to allow adequate time for exhalation.

should be assigned to convey clinical information and provide comfort, and all team members must be mindful of their presence while remaining focused on the patient.

TERMINATION OF RESUSCITATION

Survival rates for pediatric cardiac arrest remain low.[64,65] The decision to cease resuscitation efforts is multifactorial because no single variable is predictive of

Table 8
Common pediatric toxic exposures, symptoms, and treatments

Overdose	Signs and Symptoms	Treatment
Local anesthetics (topical, IV, epidural)	Altered mental status Seizures Arrhythmia and cardiac arrest	Lipid emulsion therapy: 1.5 mL/kg up to 70 kg 100 mL ≥70 kg[36]
Cocaine	Sympathomimetic toxidrome Acute coronary syndrome Cardiac dysrhythmia	Normalize core temperature Nitroglycerin, benzodiazepines, or phentolamine for coronary vasospasm Sodium bicarbonate 1–2 mEq/kg for ventricular arrhythmia Lidocaine bolus followed by infusion to prevent arrhythmia secondary to myocardial infarction AVOID unopposed α-adrenergic stimulation; do not give β-adrenergic blockers
Tricyclic antidepressants	Hypotension Seizure Altered mental status Cardiovascular effects (IVCD, bradycardia, heart block, prolonged QT interval, ventricular dysrhythmia)	1–2 mEq/kg IV sodium bicarbonate boluses until arterial pH >7.45 followed by sodium bicarbonate infusion to maintain alkalosis 10 mL/kg boluses of normal saline for first-line treatment of hypotension; consider epinephrine or norepinephrine as second-line treatment Consider ECMO if persistent hypotension despite vasopressors AVOID class IA, class IC, and class III antiarrhythmics
Calcium channel blockers[37]	Seizures Altered mental status Hypotension Cardiovascular effects (prolonged QT interval, wide QRS, bradycardia, RBBB, SVT, tornados de pointes, ventricular dysrhythmia)	5–10 mL/kg IV boluses of normal saline for hypotension IV CaCl 10% 20 mg/kg over 10–15 min, may repeat every 10–15 min or follow with infusion of 20–50 mg/kg/h High-dose IV insulin bolus of 0.5–1 unit/kg, followed with 0.5–1 unit/kg/h (titrate every 15–20 min as needed for hemodynamic stability) IV dextrose infusion to maintain euglycemia Potassium repletion as needed Norepinephrine and/or epinephrine as first-line vasopressors. Atropine 0.02 mg/kg IV/IO (maximum dose 0.5 mg) for bradycardia If refractory to above measures consider: • Lipid emulsion therapy • Pacemaker • ECMO

(continued on next page)

Table 8 (continued)		
Overdose	Signs and Symptoms	Treatment
β-adrenergic blockers	Cardiovascular effects (bradycardia, heart block, decreased cardiac contractility)	Epinephrine infusion Consider glucagon in adolescents Consider infusion of glucose and insulin Consider IV calcium administration if cardiovascular effects are refractory to glucagon and catecholamines
Opioids	Hypoventilation/apnea Bradycardia Hypotension Depressed mental status	Support oxygenation/ventilation with BVM and/or intubation Naloxone • 0.1 mg/kg/dose IV/IM/SC/IO (IV preferred), maximum dose 2 mg; repeat every 2–3 min as needed[38] • Alternate dosing for intranasal or endotracheal routes available

Abbreviations: IM, intramuscular; IVCD, interventricular conduction delay; RBBB, right bundle branch block; SC, subcutaneous; SVT, supraventricular tachycardia.

outcome after pediatric cardiac arrest. Duration of CPR, number of doses of epinephrine, age of the patient, presenting cardiac rhythm, cause of arrest, and the likelihood of reversible causes are all factors. Meaningful survival after prolonged resuscitation has been described in the setting of poisoning, hypothermia, recurring or refractory shockable rhythm, and patients with isolated heart disease resuscitated with ECMO.

SUMMARY

Pediatric cardiac arrest is most commonly caused by an initial respiratory insult that progresses to cardiovascular collapse as hypoventilation and hypoxia lead to acidosis. Although relatively rare, it is accompanied by a high degree of stress for caregivers because of the myriad of conditions that must be considered as well as the unique anatomy and physiology of pediatric patients. The range of drug doses and equipment sizes can be daunting, and this cognitive burden can be lessened by length-based resuscitation aids. Aggressive treatment of respiratory distress and shock before arrest is essential given the poor outcome associated with cardiac arrest.

DISCLOSURE

The authors have nothing to disclose.

REFERENCES

1. Meyer L, Stubbs B, Fahrenbruch C, et al. Incidence, causes, and survival trends from cardiovascular-related sudden cardiac arrest in children and young adults 0 to 35 years of age: a 30-year review. Circulation 2012;126:1363.

2. Young KD, Gausche-Hill M, McClung CD, et al. A prospective, population based study of the epidemiology and outcome of out-of-hospital pediatric cardiopulmonary arrest. Pediatrics 2004;114(1):157.

3. Duff JP, Topjian AA, Berg MD, et al. 2019 American Heart Association focused update on pediatric advanced life support: an update to the American Heart Association guidelines for cardiopulmonary resuscitation and emergency cardiovascular care. Pediatrics 2020;145:1.

4. Ilina MV, Kepron CA, Taylor GP, et al. Undiagnosed heart disease leading to sudden unexpected death in childhood: a retrospective study. Pediatrics 2011;128: e513.

5. Liberthson RR. Sudden death from cardiac causes in children and young adults. N Engl J Med 1996;334:1039.

6. Drezner JA, Fudge J, Harmon KG, et al. Warning symptoms and family history in children and young adults with sudden cardiac arrest. J Am Board Fam Med 2012;25:408.

7. Olasveengen TM, de Caen AR, Mancinia ME, et al. 2017 International consensus on cardiopulmonary resuscitation and emergency cardiovascular care science with treatment recommendations summary. Resuscitation 2017;121:201.

8. Part 2: systematic approach to the seriously ill or injured child. In: Chameides L, Samson RA, Schexnayder SM, et al, editors. Pediatric advanced life support provider manual. Dallas (TX): American Heart Association; 2011. p. 7–28.

9. Dieckmann RA, Brownstein D, Gausche-Hill M. The pediatric assessment triangle: a novel approach for the rapid evaluation of children. Pediatr Emerg Care 2010;26(4):312.

10. Fleming S, Thompson M, Stevens R, et al. Normal ranges of heart rate and respiratory rate in children from birth to 18 years of age: a systematic review of observational studies. Lancet 2011;377:1011.

11. Donoghue A, Nagler J, Yamamoto LG. Airway. In: Shaw KN, Bachur RG, editors. Fleisher & Ludwig's textbook of pediatric emergency medicine. 7th edition. Philadelphia: Wolters Kluwer; 2016. p. 20–6.

12. Myers SR, Schinasi DA, Nadel FM. Cardiopulmonary resuscitation. In: Shaw KN, Bachur RG, editors. Fleisher & Ludwig's textbook of pediatric emergency medicine. 7th edition. Philadelphia: Wolters Kluwer; 2016. p. 27–44, 51-52.

13. Balamuth F, Fitzgerald J, Weiss SL. Shock. In: Shaw KN, Bachur RG, editors. Fleisher & Ludwig's textbook of pediatric emergency medicine. 7th edition. Philadelphia: Wolters Kluwer; 2016. p. 55–66.

14. Part 10: recognition and management of cardiac arrest. In: Chameides L, Samson RA, Schexnayder SM, et al, editors. Pediatric advanced life support provider manual. Dallas (TX): American Heart Association; 2011. p. 141–67.

15. Gausche M, Lewis RJ, Stratton SJ, et al. Effect of out-of-hospital pediatric endotracheal intubation on survival and neurological outcome: a controlled clinical trial. JAMA 2000;283:783.

16. Andersen LW, Raymond TT, Berg RA, et al. American Heart Association's Get With The Guidelines-Resuscitation Investigators. Association between tracheal intubation during pediatric in-hospital cardiac arrest and survival. JAMA 2016; 316:1786.

17. Kleinman ME, Chameides L, Schexnayder SM, et al. Part 14: pediatric advanced life support: 2010 American Heart Association Guidelines for Cardiopulmonary Resuscitation and Emergency Cardiovascular Care. Circulation 2010;122(18 suppl 3):S876–908.

18. Link MS, Atkins DL, Passman RS, et al. Part 6: electrical therapies: automated external defibrillators, defibrillation, cardioversion,and pacing: 2010 American Heart Association Guidelines for Cardiopulmonary Resuscitation and Emergency Cardiovascular Care. Circulation 2010;122(18 Suppl 3):S706–19.

19. de Caen AR, Berg MD, Chameides L, et al. Part 12: pediatric advanced life support: 2015 American Heart Association guidelines update for cardiopulmonary resuscitation and emergency cardiovascular care. Circulation 2015;132(18 Suppl 2):S526–42.

20. Luten R, Wears R, Broselow J, et al. Managing the unique size related issues of pediatric resuscitation: reducing cognitive load with resuscitation aids. Acad Emerg Med 2002;9:840.

21. Duff JP, Topjian A, Berg MD, et al. 2018 American Heart Association Focused Update on Pediatric Advanced Life Support: an update to the American Heart Association Guidelines for Cardiopulmonary Resuscitation and Emergency Cardiovascular Care. Circulation 2018;138(23):e731–9.

22. Seeyave DM, Brown KM. Environmental emergencies, radiological emergencies, bites and stings. In: Shaw KN, Bachur RG, editors. Fleisher & Ludwig's textbook of pediatric emergency medicine. 7th edition. Philadelphia: Wolters Kluwer; 2016. p. 718–20, 728–32.

23. Bartlett RH, Gazzaniga AB, Fong SW, et al. Extracorporeal membrane oxygenator support for cardiopulmonary failure. Experience in 28 cases. J Thorac Cardiovasc Surg 1977;73:375.

24. Barbaro RP, Paden ML, Guner YS, et al. ELSO member centers. Pediatric extracorporeal life support organization registry international report 2016. ASAIO J 2017;63:456.

25. Torres-Andres F, Fink EL, Bell MJ, et al. Survival and long-term functional outcomes for children with cardiac arrest treated with extracorporeal cardiopulmonary resuscitation. Pediatr Crit Care Med 2018;19(5):451.

26. Part 11: Postresuscitation Management. In: Chameides L, Samson RA, Schexnayder SM, et al, editors. Pediatric advanced life support provider manual. Dallas (TX): American Heart Association; 2011. p. 171–94.

27. Topjian AA, de Caen A, Wainwright MS, et al. Pediatric post-cardiac arrest care: a scientific statement from the American Heart Association. Circulation 2019; 140(6):e194.

28. Ferguson LP, Durward A, Tibby SM. Relationship between arterial partial oxygen pressure after resuscitation from cardiac arrest and mortality in children. Circulation 2012;126(3):335.

29. Del Castillo J, Lopez-Herce J, Matamoros M, et al. Hyperoxia, hypocapnia and hypercapnia as outcome factors after cardiac arrest in children. Resuscitation 2012;83(12):1456.

30. Guerra-Wallace MM, Casey FL 3rd, Bell MJ, et al. Hyperoxia and hypoxia in children resuscitated from cardiac arrest. Pediatr Crit Care Med 2013;14(3):e143.

31. Bennett KS, Clark AE, Meert KL, et al. Early oxygenation and ventilation measurements after pediatric cardiac arrest: lack of association with outcome. Crit Care Med 2013;41(6):1534.

32. McInnes AD, Sutton RM, Orioles A, et al. The first quantitative report of ventilation rate during in-hospital resuscitation of older children and adolescents. Resuscitation 2011;82(8):1025.

33. Aufderheide TP, Lurie KG. Death by hyperventilation: a common and life-threatening problem during cardiopulmonary resuscitation. Crit Care Med 2004;32(9 Suppl):S345.

34. Conlon TW, Falkensammer CB, Hammond RS, et al. Association of left ventricular systolic function and vasopressor support with survival following pediatric out-of-hospital cardiac arrest. Pediatr Crit Care Med 2015;16(2):146–54.
35. Checchia PA, Sehra R, Moynihan J, et al. Myocardial injury in children following resuscitation after cardiac arrest. Resuscitation 2003;57(2):131–7.
36. Topjian AA, French B, Sutton RM, et al. Early postresuscitation hypotension is associated with increased mortality following pediatric cardiac arrest. Crit Care Med 2014;42(6):1518–23.
37. Lin YR, Li CJ, Wu TK, et al. Post-resuscitative clinical features in the first hour after achieving sustained ROSC predict the duration of survival in children with non-traumatic out-of-hospital cardiac arrest. Resuscitation 2010;81(4):410–7.
38. Lin YR, Wu HP, Chen WL, et al. Predictors of survival and neurologic outcomes in children with traumatic out-of-hospital cardiac arrest during the early postresuscitative period. J Trauma Acute Care Surg 2013;75(3):439–47.
39. Topjian AA, Telford R, Holubkov R, et al. Association of early postresuscitation hypotension with survival to discharge after targeted temperature management for pediatric out-of-hospital cardiac arrest: secondary analysis of a randomized clinical trial. JAMA Pediatr 2018;172(2):143.
40. Srinivasan V, Spinella PC, Drott HR, et al. Association of timing, duration, and intensity of hyperglycemia with intensive care unit mortality in critically ill children. Pediatr Crit Care Med 2004;5(4):329–36.
41. Kong MY, Alten J, Tofil N. Is hyperglycemia really harmful? A critical appraisal of "Persistent hyperglycemia in critically ill children" by Faustino and Apkon (J Pediatr 2005; 146:30-34). Pediatr Crit Care Med 2007;8(5):482–5.
42. Beiser DG1, Carr GE, Edelson DP, et al. Derangements in blood glucose following initial resuscitation from in-hospital cardiac arrest: a report from the national registry of cardiopulmonary resuscitation. Resuscitation 2009;80(6):624–30.
43. Topjian AA1, Sánchez SM, Shults J, et al. Early electroencephalographic background features predict outcomes in children resuscitated from cardiac arrest. Pediatr Crit Care Med 2016;17(6):547–57.
44. Abend NS, Topjian A, Ichord R, et al. Electroencephalographic monitoring during hypothermia after pediatric cardiac arrest. Neurology 2009;72(22):1931–40.
45. Kirkham F. Cardiac arrest and post resuscitation of the brain. Eur J Paediatr Neurol 2011;15(5):379–89.
46. Murdoch-Eaton D, Darowski M, livingston J. Cerebral function monitoring pediatric intensive care: useful features for predicting outcome. Dev Med Child Neurol 2001;43(2):91–6.
47. Moler FW, Silverstein FS, Holubkov R, et al, THAPCA Trial Investigators. Therapeutic hypothermia after out-of-hospital cardiac arrest in children. N Engl J Med 2015;372:1898.
48. Moler FW, Silverstein FS, Holubkov R, et al, THAPCA Trial Investigators. Therapeutic hypothermia after in-hospital cardiac arrest in children. N Engl J Med 2017;376:318.
49. Upadhyay M, Singhi S, Murlidharan J, et al. Randomized evaluation of fluid resuscitation with crystalloid and colloid in pediatric septic shock. Indian Pediatr 2005;42(3):223–31.
50. Ngo NT1, Cao XT, Kneen R, et al. Acute management of dengue shock syndrome: a randomized double-blind comparison of 4 intravenous fluid regimens in the first hour. Clin Infect Dis 2001;32(2):204–13.

51. Emrath ET, Fortenberry JD, Travers C, et al. Resuscitation with balanced fluids is associated with improved survival in pediatric severe sepsis. Crit Care Med 2017; 45:1177.

52. den Brinker M, Hokken-Koelega AC, Hazelzet JA, et al. One single dose of etomidate negatively influences adrenocortical performance for at least 24h in children with meningococcal sepsis. Intensive Care Med 2008;34(1):163–8.

53. Jabre P, Combes X, Lapostolle F, et al. Etomidate versus ketamine for rapid sequence intubation in acutely ill patients: a multicentre randomised controlled trial. Lancet 2009;374(9686):293–300.

54. Marino BS, Tabbutt S, MacLaren G, et al. Cardiopulmonary resuscitation in infants and children with cardiac disease: a scientific statement from the American Heart Association. Circulation 2018;137(22):e691–782.

55. Part 5: management of respiratory distress and failure. In: Chameides L, Samson RA, Schexnayder SM, et al, editors. Pediatric advanced life support provider manual. Dallas (TX): American Heart Association; 2011. p. 49–58.

56. Herzenberg JE, Hensinger RN, Dedrick DK, et al. Emergency transport and positioning of young children who have an injury of the cervical spine. The standard backboard may be hazardous. J Bone Joint Surg Am 1989;71(1):15–22.

57. Skippen P, Seear M, Poskitt K, et al. Effect of hyperventilation on regional cerebral blood flow in head-injured children. Crit Care Med 1997;25(8):1402–9.

58. Rothenberg SS, Moore EE, Moore FA, et al. Emergency department thoracotomy in children–a critical analysis. J Trauma 1989;29(10):1322–5.

59. Gitman M, Fettiplace MR, Weinberg GL, et al. Local anesthetic systemic toxicity: a narrative literature review and clinical update on prevention, diagnosis and management. Plast Reconstr Surg 2019;144(3):783–95.

60. Bartlett JW, Walker PL. Management of calcium channel blocker toxicity in the pediatric patient. J Pediatr Pharmacol Ther 2019;24(5):378–89.

61. Hegenbarth MA. Preparing for pediatric emergencies: drugs to consider. Pediatrics 2008;121(2):433–43.

62. Stewart SA. Parents experience during a child's resuscitation: getting through it. J Pediatr Nurs 2019;47:58.

63. McAlvin SS, Carew-Lyons A. Family presence during resuscitation and invasive procedures in pediatric critical care: a systematic review. Am J Crit Care 2014; 23(6):477–84 [quiz: 485].

64. Moler FW, Donaldson AE, Meert K, et al. Multicenter cohort study of out-of-hospital pediatric cardiac arrest. Crit Care Med 2011;39(1):141–9.

65. López-Herce J, Del Castillo J, Matamoros M, et al. Factors associated with mortality in pediatric in-hospital cardiac arrest: a prospective multicenter multinational observational study. Intensive Care Med 2013;39(2):309–18.

The Crashing Toxicology Patient

Aaron Skolnik, MD[a,b],*, Jessica Monas, MD[b]

KEYWORDS

- Toxicology • Poisoning • Overdose • Critical care • Intensive care • ECMO
- Kidney injury • Hemodialysis

KEY POINTS

- Conventional antiepileptics are typically ineffective at terminating drug-induced seizures or status epilepticus.
- Drug-induced cardiogenic shock treatment differs from conventional shock therapy in the use of antidotes, such as hyperinsulinemic-euglycemic therapy for calcium-channel blocker or beta-blocker toxicity, among first-line treatments.
- Poisoned patients who require extracorporeal life support (ECLS) for refractory drug-induced acute respiratory distress syndrome, cardiogenic shock, or cardiac arrest may have improved survival compared with those with other indications and should be considered for emergent ECLS.
- Drugs are the leading cause of acute liver failure in the United States and Europe. Treatment with N-acetylcysteine should be started for all patients with suspected drug-induced liver failure and such patients should be referred to a transplant-capable center.
- Many critically poisoned patients have a conventional indication for renal replacement therapy. If drug or toxin removal is desired, intermittent hemodialysis provides superior clearance to continuous therapies.

INTRODUCTION

Emergency physicians are well equipped to deal with routine drug- and toxin-related visits to the emergency department (ED). Recently, poisoning-related ED visits have been increasing, and with them, lengths of stay, patient complexity, resource utilization, and likelihood of hospital admission.[1] In 2017, the Centers for Disease Control and Prevention reported 75,354 poisoning deaths in the United States.[2] Patients are often sickest in the first few hours of their illness. Therefore, emergency physicians

[a] Department of Critical Care Medicine, Mayo Clinic Hospital, 5777 East Mayo Boulevard, Phoenix, AZ 85054, USA; [b] Department of Emergency Medicine, Mayo Clinic Alix School of Medicine, Mayo Clinic Hospital, 5777 East Mayo Boulevard, Phoenix, AZ 85054, USA
* Corresponding author. Department of Critical Care Medicine, Mayo Clinic Hospital, 5777 East Mayo Boulevard, Phoenix, AZ 85054, USA.
E-mail address: Skolnik.aaron@mayo.edu
Twitter: @ToxCCM (A.S.)

Emerg Med Clin N Am 38 (2020) 841–856
https://doi.org/10.1016/j.emc.2020.06.014
0733-8627/20/© 2020 Elsevier Inc. All rights reserved.
emed.theclinics.com

and intensivists bear the primary responsibility for the diagnosis and management of the crashing toxicology patient. Diagnostic testing and specific antidotes are secondary to the immediate resuscitation and stabilization of these patients with multiple organ failure.

NEUROLOGIC TOXICITY
Seizures and Status Epilepticus

Drug-induced seizures are common, responsible for up to 9% of status epilepticus cases and 6% of new-onset seizures in some series.[3] Status epilepticus may develop more frequently in drug-induced seizures, complicating up to 10% of cases.[3] Compared with non–drug-induced seizures, seizures due to drug ingestion have a higher rate of complications, including hypoxia, hypercapnia, rhabdomyolysis, metabolic acidosis, elevated lactate, and brain injury from excessive metabolic demand,[4] as well as mortality. Unlike most epilepsy, drug-induced seizures begin as a generalized brain process, often resulting from an acute imbalance in inhibitory (gamma aminobutyric acid [GABA]) and excitatory (acetylcholine, glutamate, dopamine, norepinephrine, and serotonin) transmission. This may be related to $GABA_A$ receptor antagonism or modulation, withdrawal from chronic use of $GABA_A$ or $GABA_B$ agonists, or excessive excitatory transmission (**Table 1**). For this reason, conventional antiepileptic drugs, notably phenytoin, are typically ineffective in terminating them.[5]

Treatment of drug-induced seizures is focused on immediate stabilization and restoration of inhibitory neurotransmission. Although assessing and managing the patient's airway, point-of-care (POC) glucose and sodium should be tested or empirical dextrose administered if testing is unavailable. Hypotension may be treated with empirical administration of balanced crystalloid solution or vasopressors if fluid-nonresponsive. Core temperature should be measured and hyperthermia treated with active cooling measures. The first-line agents in the treatment of drug-induced seizures are the $GABA_A$ agonists and benzodiazepines, listed in **Table 2**.[6] If isoniazid or hydrazine (ie, *Gyromitra esculenta* [false morel] mushroom poisoning) is suspected, pyridoxine should be administered.[7] If the patient remains in status epilepticus, second-line agents should be used. Second-line agents include phenobarbital, high-dose midazolam infusion, and propofol. The dose of propofol required to achieve burst suppression is higher than typically used for intensive care unit (ICU) sedation.[8] Ketamine shows promise, but a lack of randomized controlled trials prohibits its recommendation as part of algorithmic treatment.[9]

Table 1
Seizures related to poisonings

Mechanism	Common Agents
$GABA_A$ receptor antagonism or modulation	Flumazenil, ciprofloxacin, clozapine, cicutoxin
Withdrawal from chronic use of $GABA_A$ or $GABA_B$ agonists	Ethanol, benzodiazepines, barbiturates, baclofen, gamma hydroxybutyrate (GHB), gamma butyrolactone (GBL)
Excessive excitatory transmission	Sympathomimetics, serotonin syndrome, monoamine oxidase inhibitors
Inhibition of GABA generation	Isoniazid, hydrazines, *Gyromitra* mushrooms
Adenosine antagonism	Carbamazepine, caffeine, theophylline

Table 2 Treatment of drug-induced seizures	

Initial Stabilization	• Provide supportive care
	  ○ Assess and manage the airway
	  ○ Manage hypotension
	    ■ Give balanced crystalloid solution
	    ■ Give vasopressors if fluid-unresponsive
	  ○ Check for and manage hyperthermia
	• Check point-of-care laboratories (glucose, basic metabolic panel)
	  ○ Give empirical dextrose, 25 grams, IV if unable to assess

First-line Treatment	• Give first-line medication
	  ○ Benzodiazepines
	    ■ Lorazepam, 4 mg, IV q4–5 min or
	    ■ Midazolam, 5 mg, IM
	  ○ If isoniazid or hydrazine suspected
	    ■ Pyridoxine
	      • Gram-for-gram based on ingested isoniazid amount or
	      • 25 mg/kg IV over 15–30 min up to 5 g

Second-line Treatment	• Secure the airway if not already done
	• Give second-line medication
	  ○ Phenobarbital IV or
	  ○ High-dose midazolam or
	  ○ Propofol, 80 mcg/kg/min

Diagnostic Considerations	• Send urine drug screen, acetaminophen, and salicylate levels
	• Send antiepileptic drug levels as indicated
	• Obtain head CT scan
	  ○ If status epilepticus, head trauma, or prolonged postictal state
	• Obtain continuous EEG monitoring
	  ○ If status epilepticus

Disposition	• Admit to ICU

Diagnostic Considerations: Neurotoxicity

Patients with underlying epilepsy may experience drug-induced seizures, even while taking medications as prescribed. In addition, some antiepileptic drugs, such as carbamazepine, may induce seizures at supratherapeutic concentrations.[10] Patients with antiepileptic drug exposure should have drug levels tested. A urine or serum drugs of abuse screen is of limited utility, but a positive result may be helpful if subsequent workup is otherwise negative. Blood levels of common poisons, including acetaminophen and salicylate, should be tested, as salicylates may cause fatal neurotoxicity. Patients with status epilepticus, a prolonged postictal period, or signs or history concerning for head trauma should undergo noncontrast computed tomography (CT) scan of the head. Regardless of the use of neuromuscular blockers for intubation, patients who presented with status epilepticus should undergo continuous electroencephalography monitoring, as 14% of treated generalized convulsive status epilepticus may evolve into nonconvulsive status epilepticus.[11] All patients with drug-induced status epilepticus or complicated seizures should be admitted to the ICU.

RESPIRATORY FAILURE

A large number of drugs are capable of causing acute respiratory failure through multiple mechanisms. Numerous central nervous system depressants cause central hypoventilation. In the current era, opioids are one of the most commonly encountered causes of drug-induced respiratory failure by the emergency physician.[12] If opioid intoxication is on the differential in a patient with hypoventilation, trial administration of naloxone is warranted. Naloxone has proved to be relatively safe but can rarely cause serious pulmonary and cardiac complications.[13] These may be due to a rapid increase in catecholamine levels associated with acute opioid antagonism and seem to increase in incidence with higher initial (>0.4 mg) and total (>4.4 mg) doses of naloxone.[14] Unfortunately, multiple administrations and higher initial doses of naloxone may be required to reverse overdoses of fentanyl analogues or other novel synthetics.[15] Many sedating agents can also cause or exacerbate hypercapnic respiratory failure or lead to loss of airway protective reflexes.

Toxins that cause neuromuscular weakness, such as organophosphate pesticides or nerve agents, can cause hypoventilation, failure of secretion clearance, and respiratory arrest. Many drugs can cause acute respiratory distress syndrome (ARDS) in overdose (ie, salicylate, calcium channel blockers).[16] Cardiogenic (ie, beta blockers, cocaine) and neurogenic (ie, naloxone) pulmonary edema are also well described.

All causes of respiratory failure are initially managed supportively with endotracheal intubation and lung-protective mechanical ventilation strategies. Toxicology patients may have suffered prolonged immobilization, and acute kidney injury is common, so nondepolarizing neuromuscular blockers are recommended for rapid sequence intubation. For refractory hypoxic or hypercapnic respiratory failure, venovenous extracorporeal membrane oxygenation (V-V ECMO) has also been used with relatively high survival rates (see the later discussion *Mechanical Circulatory Support*).[17]

CARDIOVASCULAR TOXICITY
Drug-Induced Tachycardia and Malignant Dysrhythmias

Sympathomimetic or anticholinergic poisoning may produce sinus tachycardia. Classically, these entities are distinguished by dry mucous membranes and axillary skin in the anticholinergic patient.[18] Reflex tachycardia in response to peripheral vasodilation can occur but is relatively rare, with the exception of dihydropyridine calcium channel blocker poisoning. Many drugs are associated with increased risk for malignant tachydysrhythmias. Common mechanisms include sodium channel blockade resulting in QRS widening, potassium efflux blockade resulting in QTc prolongation and torsades de pointes, sympathomimesis leading to increased myocardial irritability, and sensitization of the myocardium to endogenous catecholamines.[19] The agents associated with tachydysrhythmias in a retrospective review of poison control data are listed in **Table 3**.[20] Initial treatment of pulseless dysrhythmias of unknown cause should follow Advanced Cardiac Life Support (ACLS) guidelines, in an attempt to restore spontaneous circulation.

Drug-Induced Bradycardia

Drug-induced bradycardia, including atrioventricular conduction blocks of varying degree, can be attributed to several drug classes. Most notorious are calcium channel antagonists and beta-adrenergic antagonists, the 2 classes responsible for most of the fatalities among cardiac drug poisoning. In nondiabetic patients, a markedly elevated glucose in the presence of hypotension and bradycardia or conduction blocks directs suspicion to calcium channel blocker poisoning.[21] **Table 3** lists agents known to cause significant bradycardia.[22] Drug-induced symptomatic bradycardia is treated according to ACLS and may respond to atropine. Calcium administered via IV bolus or infusion may improve inotropy and blood pressure but fails to improve

Table 3
Dysrhythmias related to poisonings

Cardiac Disturbance	Common Agents
Sinus tachycardia	Sympathomimetics, anticholinergics
Wide-complex tachycardia	Tricyclic antidepressants, stimulants (cocaine), diphenhydramine, citalopram, propoxyphene, bupropion, lithium, lamotrigine, and antiarrhythmic drugs
Torsades de pointes	Cyclic antidepressants, methadone, antipsychotics, and antiarrhythmics
Bradycardia/heart block	Calcium channel antagonists, beta adrenergic antagonists, cardiac glycosides (ie, digoxin), organophosphorous or carbamate compounds (ie, nerve agents, malathion, pyridostigmine, central alpha-2 agonists (ie, clonidine, guanfacine)

bradycardia in animal models; effects in human case reports have been mixed.[23] Treatment of toxicologic bradycardia has included transcutaneous and transvenous cardiac pacing, but electrical capture may not occur reliably.[23] For patients with significant dysrhythmia, hyperkalemia (>6 mmol/L), or hemodynamic instability following known or suspected cardiac glycoside poisoning, digoxin Fab fragments may be administered as described in **Table 4**.[24]

Sodium Bicarbonate

Drug-induced sodium channel blockade and resulting wide complex tachycardia have been reported across a wide variety of drugs (see **Table 3**). The first-line antidote of choice is sodium bicarbonate, although the exact mechanism by which sodium bicarbonate reverses blockade is incompletely understood. Traditional treatment thresholds for sodium bicarbonate administration have been based on QRS duration, although there is variability on when to begin treatment.[25] Because a normal QRS duration varies from 80 to 100 msec, in wide complex tachycardia suspected to be drug related, it is reasonable to administer a trial dose of sodium bicarbonate if QRS duration is greater than 120 msec and promptly reexamine the ECG for QRS narrowing. If the QRS narrows, an infusion of sodium bicarbonate should be administered to maintain a target blood pH of 7.45 to 7.55. Patients should be monitored with serial arterial blood gases to control pH and serial electrolyte testing because of the risk of hypokalemia due to transcellular potassium shifts.[26]

Lipid Emulsion

Antidotal intravenous lipid emulsion (ILE) first emerged as a treatment of local anesthetic toxicity. Administration of large amounts of concentrated lipid (typically a 20% solution) reversed cardiovascular toxicity of local anesthetics in animal models and human case reports.[27] Thereafter, rescue use of ILE was reported across a wide variety of overdoses including cyclic antidepressants, calcium channel blockers, and beta blockers. Several mechanisms have been proposed for lipid emulsion's reported salutary effects on hemodynamics: a "lipid sink" into which soluble drugs preferentially distribute, supply of free fatty acids for cardiac metabolism in the stunned heart, and inhibition of endothelial nitric oxide synthase.[28] Use of ILE to treat overdose patients has expanded to include non–life-threatening overdoses, but a recent systematic review found the effects in these cases to be heterogeneous.[28] Multiple complications have been reported including lipemic laboratory interference, acute kidney

Table 4
Dosing for common antidotes

Antidote	Indications	Bolus	Infusion
Intravenous NAC	Acetaminophen poisoning (based on >4-h level and nomogram) Acute liver failure	150 mg/kg loading dose over 1 h, followed by:	12.5 mg/kg/h for 4 h, followed by 6.25 mg/kg/h at least 16 h (see text for termination criteria)
Glucagon	Beta blocker overdose with myocardial dysfunction	50–150 µg/kg, up to 10 mg IV	Start infusion at same dose in mg required for response. For example, 5 mg effective bolus dose followed by a 5 mg/h infusion
Insulin	Calcium channel or beta blocker overdose with myocardial dysfunction	1 U/kg IV bolus, followed by:	1–2 U/kg/h titrated every 15 min, up to a maximum rate of 10 U/kg/h
Sodium bicarbonate	Wide QRS dysrhythmia (QRS duration >120 msec) Urine alkalization	1–2 mEq/kg of 8.4% sodium bicarbonate IV	150 mEq/L of sodium bicarbonate in 1 L of dextrose 5% water or 8.4% sodium bicarbonate solution (1mEq/mL)
Digoxin fab fragments	Life-threatening dysrhythmia, hemodynamic instability, or hyperkalemia >5 mEq/L associated with digoxin or cardiac glycoside poisoning	May be administered at an initial empirical dose of 400 mg (10 vials) in cases of imminent cardiac arrest or 80 mg (2 vials) otherwise	Can consider half-molar reversal in patients at risk of cardiac deterioration due to underlying heart disease
Lorazepam	Drug-induced status epilepticus (first-line agent)	4 mg IV every 4–5 min until seizures abate	
Pyridoxine	Isoniazid poisoning Hydrazine or *Gyromitra mushroom poisoning* Intractable drug-induced seizures	Administer on a gram-for-gram basis to the amount of isoniazid ingested OR 25 mg/kg IV over 15–30 min, up to 5 g in adult patients	
Propofol	Drug-induced status epilepticus		Propofol titration is required to achieve EEG burst suppression (typically >80 mcg/kg/min).
Naloxone	Opioid poisoning	In hospital settings where oxygenation and ventilation are supported, titration of 0.04 mg IV every 1–2 min until respiratory rate is >10 may avoid rapidly precipitated	For patients with recurrent respiratory depression or resedation after naloxone, start IV infusion at 2/3 of the dose required

	withdrawal	Can also be given 0.4–2 mg IM OR 4 mg intranasal if no IV access. Initial dosing may be repeated if fails to respond. Higher doses (>10 mg) may be required for novel or highly potent opioids	for reversal, given hourly (ie, if 1 mg reversed, start infusion at 0.66 mg/h)
Hydroxo-cobalamin	Cyanide poisoning Refractory vasoplegia	5 g IV over 15 min	5 g dose may be repeated, infused intravenously over 15 min to 2 h, based on clinical status, for a total dose of 10 g

injury, cardiac arrest, ventilation/perfusion mismatch, ARDS, venous thromboembolism, hypersensitivity, fat embolism or overload syndrome, pancreatitis, allergic reaction, and increased susceptibility to infection.[29] In patients on venoarterial extracorporeal membrane oxygenation (VA-ECMO), fat emulsion has been reported to cause agglutination in the circuit, cracking of stopcocks, oxygenator dysfunction, and an increase in circuit thrombosis.[30]

The American Academy of Clinical Toxicology's evidence-based recommendations support ILE use for cardiac arrest resulting from bupivacaine toxicity but recommend *against* using ILE as first-line therapy for most other poisonings. If other therapies fail, they recommend ILE for bupivacaine toxicity and suggest ILE for toxicity due to other local anesthetics, amitriptyline, and bupropion, but their recommendations are neutral for all other toxins.[31] Lipid emulsion may be considered for drug-induced cardiac arrest when other antidotes have failed, and advanced therapies such as mechanical circulatory support are not immediately available.

CARDIOGENIC AND VASODILATORY SHOCK
Vasopressors and Inotropes

Emergency physicians commonly use intravenous fluids and vasopressors in the initial resuscitation of patients with hypotension or shock of unknown cause, including patients with drug-induced shock. With the advent of ED POC ultrasonography, distinguishing between vasodilatory, cardiogenic, and mixed shock should guide empirical therapy with respect to fluid tolerance, vasopressors, and inotropes. For example, dihydropyridine calcium channel antagonists may initially produce vasodilatory shock that may respond to calcium and vasopressors alone. Other calcium channel antagonists, or dihydropyridines taken in sufficient quantity such that receptor specificity is lost, may produce cardiogenic shock with myocardial depression, favoring the use of inotropes.

Concerns around the use of vasopressors to treat drug-induced shock have centered around ischemic complications and adverse effects on cardiac metabolism and cardiac output, primarily based on animal models.[32] A single-center retrospective review of verapamil and diltiazem overdoses managed with high doses of vasopressors and inotropes reported high survival with a low rate of ischemic complications.[33] In a systematic review of vasopressors in the treatment of toxin-induced cardiogenic shock, the investigators reported a lack of detrimental effects of vasopressors and high survival among the patients included in their study.[32] Although the investigators note that treatment failures of vasopressors are likely underreported, it is also likely that treatment successes are underreported, as the reversal of hypotension with vasopressors is not a case-reportable event. A systematic review of the treatment of calcium channel blocker poisoning found that dopamine and norepinephrine improved hemodynamic parameters and survival without documented severe side effects, although evidence quality was very low.[34] It is therefore reasonable, after optimizing volume status, to administer vasopressors or inotropes to support hemodynamic parameters in patients with cardiovascular drug toxicity. Ideally, this should be guided by invasive (pulmonary artery catheterization) or noninvasive (echocardiography, pulse contour analysis) hemodynamic monitoring.

Hyperinsulinemic-Euglycemic Therapy

Hyperinsulinemic-euglycemic therapy (HIET), primarily used for calcium channel blocker and beta blocker poisoning, consists of administration of very high doses of insulin, often coadministered with concentrated dextrose infusions to maintain euglycemia. Cardiac myocytes stunned by drug toxicity alter their metabolism from primarily free fatty acid utilization to favor carbohydrate metabolism.[35] In animal models of drug-induced cardiogenic shock, insulin administration has been shown to improve both systolic and diastolic cardiac function[36] and seems to have independent positive inotropic effects on failing human myocardium.[37] Calcium channel blocker poisoning causes insulin resistance, and antagonism of pancreatic L-type calcium channels inhibits calcium-mediated insulin release.[3] These effects, combined with the physiologic stress response, lead to hyperglycemia and relative hypoinsulinemia.[38] In one retrospective study of verapamil and diltiazem overdose, the degree of hyperglycemia was a better predictor of illness severity than hemodynamics.[21] The mechanism of HIET as an antidote relies on meeting altered cardiac metabolic demands, improving inotropy, and peripheral vasodilation, improving organ perfusion. Therefore, HIET is best used in cases of calcium channel blocker– or beta blocker–induced cardiogenic shock with impaired myocardial contractility.

Recent consensus guidelines on treatment of calcium channel blocker poisoning recommend HIET as part of first-line therapies.[39] Once initiated, insulin infusion rates can be titrated to clinical effect.[40,41] A concentrated dextrose infusion, often dextrose 50% at 25 g/h, is used to maintain euglycemia. All infusions should be concentrated to avoid pulmonary edema resulting from drug effect, volume overload, or acute left ventricular dysfunction. Hypokalemia, hyponatremia, and hypoglycemia are common, even with poison center or toxicologist oversight, and must be carefully monitored during treatment.[42]

Glucagon

The pancreatic hormone glucagon circumvents poisoning of the β1 adrenergic receptor via agonism at the G-protein coupled glucagon receptor. The downstream result is similar to stimulation of adenylate cyclase and increase in cellular cyclic AMP. Pharmacologic effects include increased inotropy and chronotropy, supported by animal models of beta blocker poisoning.[43] Use of glucagon in the treatment of human beta blocker overdose has shown mixed results, however.[23] In animal models of propranolol and verapamil toxicity, glucagon was inferior to HIET as an antidote.[44] The side effect profile of glucagon is favorable, with dose-dependent nausea, vomiting, and hyperglycemia. In patients with appropriate level of consciousness and intact airway protective reflexes, or a protected airway, glucagon may be used for known or suspected beta antagonist poisoning with myocardial dysfunction or cardiogenic shock. If a favorable clinical response is observed after a bolus, an infusion can then be started at the same dose in milligram required for response per hour.[23]

Methylene Blue

Methylene blue is proposed to treat refractory vasodilatory shock through inhibition of soluble guanylyl cyclase and nitric oxide synthase in the nitric oxide pathway, with a downstream decrease in vasodilation and concomitant increase in systemic vascular resistance.[45] A systematic review of methylene blue for drug-induced shock found only case reports and abstracts, with variable effects on hemodynamics. These data being subject to lack of randomization, publication bias, confounding by other therapies, and incomplete reporting, the investigators concluded there is insufficient evidence to recommend methylene blue for drug-induced shock.[46] Methylene blue is contraindicated in patients with glucose-6-phosphate dehydrogenase deficiency due to risk of hemolysis.[47] Although no serious adverse effects were reported in any of the cases reviewed earlier, it should be noted that methylene blue has been reported to precipitate serotonin syndrome in patients taking other serotonergic medications.[48]

Hydroxocobalamin

Hydroxocobalamin is well established as a cyanide antidote. In cases of severe cyanide exposure, defined by unconsciousness, seizure, and cardiac or respiratory compromise, there is little downside to empirical treatment with hydroxocobalamin. For patients with smoke inhalation and possible cyanide exposure, one evidence-based algorithm for cyanide treatment based on ED POC testing recommends immediate empirical treatment of any severe exposure.[49]

Hydroxocobalamin has also been used as a rescue therapy for refractory vasodilatory shock, based on its ability to scavenge nitric oxide (NO) and reverse NO-mediated vasoplegia.[50] This effect was noted as a hypertensive response in volunteer studies of the drug and later followed by its successful use in cardiac surgery to reverse postcardiopulmonary bypass vasoplegic syndrome.[51] There are no reports of hydroxocobalamin treatment of shock resulting from noncyanide overdoses. In a large (greater than 5-fold) iatrogenic overdose of hydroxocobalamin, the only clinically significant effect was erythroderma, which resolved.[52] Hydroxocobalamin, administered at the cyanide treatment dose, has a favorable side-effect profile and can be considered a last-line treatment of refractory drug-induced vasoplegia, although evidence is limited.[53]

Mechanical Circulatory Support in Toxicology Patients

Critically poisoned patients may be ideal candidates for extracorporeal life support (ECLS). Overdose patients tend to be younger and have fewer comorbid conditions than those with cardiac indications. If these patients can be supported until toxicity wanes, excellent recovery is anticipated. Despite this, the use of ECLS in poisoned patients remains rare.[54] The use of mechanical circulatory supports including the intra-aortic balloon pump and the Impella (Abiomed, Danvers, MA, USA) percutaneous left ventricular assist device has been reported in poisoned patients, but the evidence for these devices is sparse.

Although still uncommon, ECMO is the most reported mechanical support modality for poisoned patients. In a series of patients undergoing emergent percutaneous ECMO, outcomes were superior in the poisoned cohort to those with primary cardiac indications.[55] Another series compared 12 patients treated with ECMO for poisoning-related shock with 5 patients with cardiovascular indications. All patients required continuous CPR for greater than 45 minutes at the time of cannulation for VA-ECMO. Three of 12 poisoned patients survived, whereas none of the nonpoisoned patients survived.[56] Masson and colleagues[57] examined 62 poisoned patients in persistent shock or cardiac arrest, of whom 14 were treated with VA-ECMO. In the ECMO cohort, 86% survived compared with 48% of the conventionally treated cohort. Notably, the number of included patients is small and the results fragile. An analysis of the Extracorporeal Life Support Organization registry showed that use of ECMO for poisoned patients continues to increase dramatically, and survival was 59% overall and 89% for the subgroup undergoing V-V ECMO for inhalational or aspiration injury.[17] Poisoned patients with severe refractory hypoxia failing conventional treatment, persistent cardiogenic shock, or cardiac arrest should be evaluated for ECMO, if available. If an ECMO retrieval service is available at a non-ECMO capable center, they should be consulted urgently for the critically ill poisoned patients described earlier, based on high predicted mortality with conventional treatment and high rates of ECLS survival in this population.

Drug-Induced Liver Failure

Acute liver failure (ALF), also referred to as acute fulminant hepatic failure, is defined by an acute (<26 weeks) insult with liver injury, encephalopathy, and synthetic dysfunction (elevated international normalized ratio >1.5), in a patient without underlying liver disease.[58] Drugs are the leading cause of ALF in the United States and Europe, with acetaminophen (APAP) comprising most of the cases and nonacetaminophen–induced ALF (11%) of all cases in the United States Acute Liver Failure Study Group registry.[59] Patients who present with ALF from APAP are already late in the course of their illness because of the time required to develop liver injury from its toxic metabolite, N-acetyl-p-benzoquinone imine (NAPQI). Patients who present in ALF with marked transaminitis, low bilirubin, and elevated INR are most likely to have APAP-induced ALF.

N-acetylcysteine (NAC), which works by replenishing hepatic glutathione stores, detoxification of NAPQI, and antiinflammatory properties, has been shown to improve survival from APAP overdose.[60] NAC has a favorable safety profile when dosed correctly. All adult patients with ALF should be started on NAC according to the acetaminophen antidote dosing, until APAP level is undetectable, with improving aminotransferases and improving clinical biomarkers such as creatinine, lactate, pH, prothrombin time/INR, and phosphate. Pre-bolusing NAC or infusions at higher rates may be warranted in some cases and should be guided by toxicology consultation.[61] Reversal of coagulopathy is not recommended unless clinically significant bleeding occurs or it is required for invasive procedures, as degree of coagulopathy influences all predictive models for liver transplantation.

Hyperammonemia can cause cerebral edema and elevated intracranial pressure (ICP) via its conversion to glutamine in astrocytes. There is no evidence for the utility of lactulose or rifaximin to lower ammonia in ALF. For refractory hyperammonemia (>100 μmol/L) or high-grade encephalopathy in which the prevalence of intracranial hypertension is high, continuous renal replacement therapy can be used to reduce ammonia levels, although outcomes-based evidence is limited.[58] There is no accepted consensus on the risks versus benefits of invasive ICP monitoring in patients with ALF, and institutional practice varies.[62,63]

The only other treatment proved to improve survival for ALF is emergency liver transplantation, although survival is lower than in those undergoing elective liver transplant.[64] Multiple prognostic criteria exist for both APAP and all-cause ALF. Two of the most widely used are the King's College Criteria (composed of one set of criteria for APAP and another for non-APAP patients) and the Model for End-Stage Liver Disease (MELD) score.[65,66] King's College Criteria are more specific and MELD score more sensitive with respect to the need for liver transplant in cases of drug-induced ALF.[67] In cases of suspected drug-induced ALF, urgent hepatology consultation and transfer to a liver transplant center are recommended.

Enhanced Elimination

Although many drugs' elimination can be enhanced by urinary alkalization, the most clinically relevant are salicylate, methotrexate, and phenobarbital.[18] By using sodium bicarbonate and targeting a urinary pH of 8, renal elimination of these toxins can be enhanced. In the case of salicylate, alkalization of blood and urine also helps to minimize the volume of distribution of salicylate and central nervous system toxicity.[68]

Extracorporeal Toxin Removal

Many crashing toxicology patients will have acute kidney injury with conventional indications for hemodialysis, such as metabolic acidosis, electrolyte derangements, volume overload, or uremia. In those cases, nephrology should be consulted early, and toxin removal is a secondary consideration. Extracorporeal toxin removal (ECTR) can be achieved via hemodialysis or continuous renal replacement therapy (CRRT).[69] Technical advances in renal replacement therapy and an enhanced understanding of toxicokinetics have changed the classic criteria for ECTR.[18] High-efficiency, high-flux dialysis membranes allow for enhanced clearance of substances up to 15,000 Da. Larger hemodialysis catheters and improved hemodialysis machines permit higher blood flows during dialysis.[70] Several drugs with high protein binding, such as salicylate, valproic acid, phenytoin, and carbamazepine, are amenable to ECTR in overdose, as protein binding becomes saturated, and free drug is then removed by hemodialysis.

Extracorporeal clearance of a poison must also comprise a significant portion of total clearance to render ECTR effective treatment, and there must not be an effective antidote for the poison that renders the risk/benefit ratio of ECTR unfavorable.[69] For example, insulin is dialyzable via high-flux membranes, but concentrated dextrose therapy is easily instituted.

CRRT is often used in ICU patients too hemodynamically unstable to undergo hemodialysis, but clearance of drugs and toxins by these methods is too low for effective toxin removal.[71] CRRT may be helpful, however, in permitting greater net fluid removal over time and preserving cerebral perfusion pressure in patients with ALF.[72] In general, the decision to perform ECTR should not be based on a single drug level, as this is often a poor surrogate measure of drug concentration at the target organ of toxicity. Rather, patients with severe organ dysfunction or life-threatening poisoning by toxins amenable to ECTR should have urgent nephrology consultation and consideration of hemodialysis.

SUMMARY

The crashing toxicology patient presents a unique critical care challenge for the emergency physician. Patients may present in extremis, requiring a unique set of antidotes and treatments for clinical entities associated with poisoning with which emergency physicians are otherwise familiar, such as status epilepticus, cardiogenic shock, kidney injury, or liver failure. The brunt of resuscitation of the crashing poisoned patient falls to the ED, although all of these patients will ultimately require ICU management. Frequently, critical decisions regarding emergent mechanical circulatory support, consideration for organ transplant, or extracorporeal toxin removal and renal replacement therapy will be made in the ED, by emergency physicians. Rapid diagnostic evaluation, hemodynamic stabilization, and application of drug- and class-specific antidotes as outlined earlier are therefore crucial for improved patient survival and clinical outcomes.

DISCLOSURE

The authors have nothing to disclose.

REFERENCES

1. Mazer-Amirshahi M, Sun C, Mullins P, et al. Trends in emergency department resource utilization for poisoning-related visits, 2003-2011. J Med Toxicol 2016; 12(3):248–54.
2. Prevention CfDCa. Available at: https://www.cdc.gov/nchs/fastats/injury.htm. Accessed November 28, 2019.

3. Chen HY, Albertson TE, Olson KR. Treatment of drug-induced seizures. Br J Clin Pharmacol 2016;81(3):412–9.
4. Hocker SE, Britton JW, Mandrekar JN, et al. Predictors of outcome in refractory status epilepticus. JAMA Neurol 2013;70(1):72–7.
5. Shah AS, Eddleston M. Should phenytoin or barbiturates be used as second-line anticonvulsant therapy for toxicological seizures? Clin Toxicol (Phila) 2010;48(8): 800–5.
6. Silbergleit R, Durkalski V, Lowenstein D, et al. Intramuscular versus intravenous therapy for prehospital status epilepticus. N Engl J Med 2012;366(7):591–600.
7. Lheureux P, Penaloza A, Gris M. Pyridoxine in clinical toxicology: a review. Eur J Emerg Med 2005;12(2):78–85.
8. Rossetti AO, Reichhart MD, Schaller MD, et al. Propofol treatment of refractory status epilepticus: a study of 31 episodes. Epilepsia 2004;45(7):757–63.
9. Rosati A, De Masi S, Guerrini R. Ketamine for refractory status epilepticus: a systematic review. CNS Drugs 2018;32(11):997–1009.
10. Schmidt S, Schmitz-Buhl M. Signs and symptoms of carbamazepine overdose. J Neurol 1995;242(3):169–73.
11. DeLorenzo RJ, Waterhouse EJ, Towne AR, et al. Persistent nonconvulsive status epilepticus after the control of convulsive status epilepticus. Epilepsia 1998; 39(8):833–40.
12. Beauchamp GA, Hendrickson RG, Hatten BW. Endotracheal intubation for toxicologic exposures: a retrospective review of toxicology investigators consortium (ToxIC) cases. J Emerg Med 2016;51(4):382–8.e1.
13. van Dorp E, Yassen A, Dahan A. Naloxone treatment in opioid addiction: the risks and benefits. Expert Opin Drug Saf 2007;6(2):125–32.
14. Farkas A, Lynch MJ, Westover R, et al. Pulmonary complications of opioid overdose treated with naloxone. Ann Emerg Med 2020;75(1):39–48.
15. Somerville NJ, O'Donnell J, Gladden RM, et al. Characteristics of fentanyl overdose - Massachusetts, 2014-2016. MMWR Morb Mortal Wkly Rep 2017;66(14): 382–6.
16. Otani Y, Kanno K, Toh Yoon EW, et al. Acute respiratory distress syndrome caused by salicylate intoxication. Clin Case Rep 2018;6(9):1905–6.
17. Ramanathan K, Tan CS, Rycus P, et al. Extracorporeal membrane oxygenation for poisoning in adult patients: outcomes and predictors of mortality. Intensive Care Med 2017;43(10):1538–9.
18. Levine M, Brooks DE, Truitt CA, et al. Toxicology in the ICU: Part 1: general overview and approach to treatment. Chest 2011;140(3):795–806.
19. Bass M. Sudden sniffing death. JAMA 1970;212(12):2075–9.
20. Al-Abri SA, Woodburn C, Olson KR, et al. Ventricular dysrhythmias associated with poisoning and drug overdose: a 10-year review of statewide poison control center data from California. Am J Cardiovasc Drugs 2015;15(1):43–50.
21. Levine M, Boyer EW, Pozner CN, et al. Assessment of hyperglycemia after calcium channel blocker overdoses involving diltiazem or verapamil. Crit Care Med 2007;35(9):2071–5.
22. Delk C, Holstege CP, Brady WJ. Electrocardiographic abnormalities associated with poisoning. Am J Emerg Med 2007;25(6):672–87.
23. Kerns W 2nd. Management of beta-adrenergic blocker and calcium channel antagonist toxicity. Emerg Med Clin North Am 2007;25(2):309–31 [abstract: viii].
24. Chan BS, Buckley NA. Digoxin-specific antibody fragments in the treatment of digoxin toxicity. Clin Toxicol (Phila) 2014;52(8):824–36.

25. Seger DL, Hantsch C, Zavoral T, et al. Variability of recommendations for serum alkalinization in tricyclic antidepressant overdose: a survey of U.S. Poison Center medical directors. J Toxicol Clin Toxicol 2003;41(4):331–8.

26. Bruccoleri RE, Burns MM. A literature review of the use of sodium bicarbonate for the treatment of QRS widening. J Med Toxicol 2016;12(1):121–9.

27. Litz RJ, Popp M, Stehr SN, et al. Successful resuscitation of a patient with ropivacaine-induced asystole after axillary plexus block using lipid infusion. Anaesthesia 2006;61(8):800–1.

28. Levine M, Hoffman RS, Lavergne V, et al. Systematic review of the effect of intravenous lipid emulsion therapy for non-local anesthetics toxicity. Clin Toxicol (Phila) 2016;54(3):194–221.

29. Hayes BD, Gosselin S, Calello DP, et al. Systematic review of clinical adverse events reported after acute intravenous lipid emulsion administration. Clin Toxicol (Phila) 2016;54(5):365–404.

30. Lee HM, Archer JR, Dargan PI, et al. What are the adverse effects associated with the combined use of intravenous lipid emulsion and extracorporeal membrane oxygenation in the poisoned patient? Clin Toxicol (Phila) 2015;53(3):145–50.

31. Gosselin S, Hoegberg LC, Hoffman RS, et al. Evidence-based recommendations on the use of intravenous lipid emulsion therapy in poisoning. Clin Toxicol (Phila) 2016;54(10):899–923.

32. Skoog CA, Engebretsen KM. Are vasopressors useful in toxin-induced cardiogenic shock? Clin Toxicol (Phila) 2017;55(4):285–304.

33. Levine M, Curry SC, Padilla-Jones A, et al. Critical care management of verapamil and diltiazem overdose with a focus on vasopressors: a 25-year experience at a single center. Ann Emerg Med 2013;62(3):252–8.

34. St-Onge M, Dube PA, Gosselin S, et al. Treatment for calcium channel blocker poisoning: a systematic review. Clin Toxicol (Phila) 2014;52(9):926–44.

35. Kline JA, Leonova E, Raymond RM. Beneficial myocardial metabolic effects of insulin during verapamil toxicity in the anesthetized canine. Crit Care Med 1995; 23(7):1251–63.

36. Kline JA, Raymond RM, Leonova ED, et al. Insulin improves heart function and metabolism during non-ischemic cardiogenic shock in awake canines. Cardiovasc Res 1997;34(2):289–98.

37. von Lewinski D, Bruns S, Walther S, et al. Insulin causes [Ca2+]i-dependent and [Ca2+]i-independent positive inotropic effects in failing human myocardium. Circulation 2005;111(20):2588–95.

38. Kline JA, Raymond RM, Schroeder JD, et al. The diabetogenic effects of acute verapamil poisoning. Toxicol Appl Pharmacol 1997;145(2):357–62.

39. St-Onge M, Anseeuw K, Cantrell FL, et al. Experts consensus recommendations for the management of calcium channel blocker poisoning in adults. Crit Care Med 2017;45(3):e306–15.

40. Cole JB, Arens AM, Laes JR, et al. High dose insulin for beta-blocker and calcium channel-blocker poisoning. Am J Emerg Med 2018;36(10):1817–24.

41. Krenz JR, Kaakeh Y. An overview of hyperinsulinemic-euglycemic therapy in calcium channel blocker and beta-blocker overdose. Pharmacotherapy 2018; 38(11):1130–42.

42. Beavers JR, Stollings JL, Rice TW. Hyponatremia induced by hyperinsulinemia-euglycemia therapy. Am J Health Syst Pharm 2017;74(14):1062–6.

43. Love JN, Leasure JA, Mundt DJ, et al. A comparison of amrinone and glucagon therapy for cardiovascular depression associated with propranolol toxicity in a canine model. J Toxicol Clin Toxicol 1992;30(3):399–412.

44. Kerns W 2nd, Schroeder D, Williams C, et al. Insulin improves survival in a canine model of acute beta-blocker toxicity. Ann Emerg Med 1997;29(6):748–57.

45. Mayer B, Brunner F, Schmidt K. Inhibition of nitric oxide synthesis by methylene blue. Biochem Pharmacol 1993;45(2):367–74.

46. Warrick BJ, Tataru AP, Smolinske S. A systematic analysis of methylene blue for drug-induced shock. Clin Toxicol (Phila) 2016;54(7):547–55.

47. SAS P. Prescribing Information. 2016. Available at: https://www.americanregent. com/media/1802/provayblue-prescribing-information.pdf. Accessed November 27, 2019.

48. Lo JC, Darracq MA, Clark RF. A review of methylene blue treatment for cardiovascular collapse. J Emerg Med 2014;46(5):670–9.

49. Hamad E, Babu K, Bebarta VS. Case files of the university of massachusetts toxicology fellowship: does this smoke inhalation victim require treatment with cyanide antidote? J Med Toxicol 2016;12(2):192–8.

50. Jentzer JC, Vallabhajosyula S, Khanna AK, et al. Management of refractory vasodilatory shock. Chest 2018;154(2):416–26.

51. Burnes ML, Boettcher BT, Woehlck HJ, et al. Hydroxocobalamin as a rescue treatment for refractory vasoplegic syndrome after prolonged cardiopulmonary bypass. J Cardiothorac Vasc Anesth 2017;31(3):1012–4.

52. Friedman BT, Chen BC, Latimer AJ, et al. Iatrogenic pediatric hydroxocobalamin overdose. Am J Emerg Med 2019;37(7):1394.e1-2.

53. SAS MS. Cyanokit administration guide. Available at: https://www.cyanokit.com/ sites/default/files/CYANOKIT_Administration_Guide_PP-CYA-USA-0091.pdf. Accessed January 29, 2020.

54. Wang GS, Levitan R, Wiegand TJ, et al. Extracorporeal membrane oxygenation (ECMO) for severe toxicological exposures: review of the toxicology investigators consortium (ToxIC). J Med Toxicol 2016;12(1):95–9.

55. Vanzetto G, Akret C, Bach V, et al. [Percutaneous extracorporeal life support in acute severe hemodynamic collapses: single centre experience in 100 consecutive patients]. Can J Cardiol 2009;25(6):e179–86.

56. Megarbane B, Leprince P, Deye N, et al. Emergency feasibility in medical intensive care unit of extracorporeal life support for refractory cardiac arrest. Intensive Care Med 2007;33(5):758–64.

57. Masson R, Colas V, Parienti JJ, et al. A comparison of survival with and without extracorporeal life support treatment for severe poisoning due to drug intoxication. Resuscitation 2012;83(11):1413–7.

58. Khan R, Koppe S. Modern management of acute liver failure. Gastroenterol Clin North Am 2018;47(2):313–26.

59. Thomas AM, Lewis JH. Nonacetaminophen drug-induced acute liver failure. Clin Liver Dis 2018;22(2):301–24.

60. McPhail MJ, Kriese S, Heneghan MA. Current management of acute liver failure. Curr Opin Gastroenterol 2015;31(3):209–14.

61. ACMT position statement: duration of intravenous acetylcysteine therapy following acetaminophen overdose. J Med Toxicol 2017;13(1):126–7.

62. Rajajee V, Fontana RJ, Courey AJ, et al. Protocol based invasive intracranial pressure monitoring in acute liver failure: feasibility, safety and impact on management. Crit Care 2017;21(1):178.

63. Porteous J, Cioccari L, Ancona P, et al. Outcome of acetaminophen-induced acute liver failure managed without intracranial pressure monitoring or transplantation. Liver Transpl 2019;25(1):35–44.

64. Germani G, Theocharidou E, Adam R, et al. Liver transplantation for acute liver failure in Europe: outcomes over 20 years from the ELTR database. J Hepatol 2012;57(2):288–96.
65. O'Grady JG, Alexander GJ, Hayllar KM, et al. Early indicators of prognosis in fulminant hepatic failure. Gastroenterology 1989;97(2):439–45.
66. Kamath PS, Wiesner RH, Malinchoc M, et al. A model to predict survival in patients with end-stage liver disease. Hepatology 2001;33(2):464–70.
67. Mishra A, Rustgi V. Prognostic models in acute liver failure. Clin Liver Dis 2018; 22(2):375–88.
68. Klig JE, Sharma A, Skolnik AB. Case records of the Massachusetts General Hospital. Case 26-2014. A 21-month-old boy with lethargy, respiratory distress, and abdominal distention. N Engl J Med 2014;371(8):767–73.
69. Ghannoum M, Nolin TD, Lavergne V, et al. Blood purification in toxicology: nephrology's ugly duckling. Adv Chronic Kidney Dis 2011;18(3):160–6.
70. Garlich FM, Goldfarb DS. Have advances in extracorporeal removal techniques changed the indications for their use in poisonings? Adv Chronic Kidney Dis 2011;18(3):172–9.
71. Fertel BS, Nelson LS, Goldfarb DS. Extracorporeal removal techniques for the poisoned patient: a review for the intensivist. J Intensive Care Med 2010;25(3): 139–48.
72. Tandukar S, Palevsky PM. Continuous renal replacement therapy: who, when, why, and how. Chest 2019;155(3):626–38.

The Crashing Obese Patient

Sara Manning, MD

KEYWORDS

- Obesity • Airway • Pharmacology • Sepsis • Trauma

KEY POINTS

- Obesity imparts anatomic and physiologic changes that have an impact on resuscitative treatments in critical illness, including airway and ventilator management, pharmacology, and fluid management.
- Obesity is a risk factor for difficult bag-valve mask ventilation and may predict difficult intubation.
- Obese patients are at risk for inaccurate medication dosing, including underdosing and overdosing of resuscitative medications, such as sedatives, paralytics, and antibiotics.
- Obese patients are at risk for under-resuscitation in the setting of critical illness and injury.

INTRODUCTION

Obesity is defined as a body mass index (BMI) greater than or equal to 30 kg/m² and can be subdivided into 3 classes (**Table 1**). In the past 3 decades, obesity rates have increased dramatically worldwide.[1] Current obesity rates in the United States are approaching 40%, with increases in rates across ages, races, and social demographics.[1,2] As rates of obesity continue to climb, emergency physicians will increasingly resuscitate critically ill obese patients. Obesity imparts important anatomic and physiologic changes, including alterations to airway anatomy, respiratory mechanics, cardiovascular function, and drug metabolism. The emergency physician should be well acquainted with the challenges faced in the resuscitation of the critically ill or injured obese patient and be equipped with strategies to overcome them.

ACCESS AND MONITORING

Obesity poses challenges in the most basic aspects of patient care, including venous access and cardiovascular monitoring. A BMI greater than 30 mg/kg² has been shown to predict difficult intravenous (IV) access.[3] Obscured landmarks and increased tissue depth can complicate both central venous and intraosseous access in obese patients.[4,5] Ultrasound guidance can improve the likelihood of successful placement

Department of Emergency Medicine, University of Maryland School of Medicine, 110 South Paca Street, 6th Floor, Suite 200, Baltimore, MD 21201, USA
E-mail address: smanning@som.umaryland.edu
Twitter: @EM_SaraM (S.M.)

Emerg Med Clin N Am 38 (2020) 857–869
https://doi.org/10.1016/j.emc.2020.06.013
0733-8627/20/© 2020 Elsevier Inc. All rights reserved.
emed.theclinics.com

Table 1	
Body mass index categorization	
Category	**Body Mass Index (kg/m^2)**
Underweight	<18.5
Normal weight	18.5 to <25
Overweight	25 to <30
Obesity class I	30 to <35
Obesity class II	35 to <40
Obesity class III	40 and above

of a peripheral IV in patients with difficult access.[6] Ultrasound guidance also can improve successful cannulation and complication rates in central venous access in the obese.[7] If available, ultrasound guidance for central venous access placement is recommended.[8]

Accurate blood pressure monitoring can be difficult in obese patients in part due to an increase in arm circumference and an exaggerated conical shape of the upper arm that limit the fit of noninvasive blood pressure cuffs.[9,10] An inappropriately fitting noninvasive blood pressure cuff can provide inaccurate blood pressure readings—an effect that is exaggerated in the critically ill obese patient.[10] When available, a properly fitted upper arm cuff provides the most accurate noninvasive blood pressure measurements followed by a properly fitting wrist cuff.[11] In the critically ill obese patient requiring close and accurate blood pressure monitoring, early arterial access should be considered.

AIRWAY ANATOMY

Obesity is associated with several important anatomic changes that influence emergent airway management. Neck extension may be limited due to dorsocervical fat deposition and increased circumference. Redundant soft tissues in the oropharynx can lead to airway obstruction, and excess thoracoabdominal fat can limit lung expansion.[12] These changes contribute to the demonstrated association between obesity and difficult bag-valve mask ventilation.[13] The influence of BMI on the rates of difficult intubation is less clear, with studies yielding conflicting results.[14,15] Obesity and obesity-related anatomic changes frequently are included in various difficult airway prediction tools.[16–18] Although it remains unclear whether obesity is an independent risk factor for a difficult airway, the emergency physician should consider this possibility and approach these airways with caution.

RESPIRATORY PATHOPHYSIOLOGY

Alterations to respiratory physiology also are observed in obese patients. Lung volumes are significantly reduced, including functional residual capacity (FRC), respiratory reserve volume, vital capacity, total lung capacity, and residual capacity.[19] Volume loss increases with BMI, with reductions of 0.5% to 5% observed for each unit increase in BMI.[19] Reductions in FRC are associated with closure of small airways and increased airway resistance.[20] Premature airway closure results in under-ventilated lung space, producing a shunt phenomenon and contributing to rapid desaturation.[21] Additionally, compliance can be limited by decreased lung volumes and excess chest wall adipose. Supine positioning exacerbates reductions in lung volumes.

Obese patients demonstrate higher rates of oxygen consumption and carbon dioxide production that contribute to the adoption of a resting rapid shallow breathing pattern with baseline respiratory rates of 15 to 21 breaths per minute observed in the severely obese.[19,22,23] Obesity also is linked to several distinct respiratory disease states, including obstructive sleep apnea (OSA) and obesity hypoventilation syndrome (OHS).

The cumulative result of these anatomic and physiologic changes in the obese patient is a dramatic reduction in pulmonary reserve with risk for rapid desaturation during intubation and challenges with mechanical ventilator support.

APPROACH TO THE OBESE AIRWAY

Airway management of the obese patient should begin with effective preoxygenation. Traditional methods of preoxygenation, including face mask oxygen with 100% fractional inspired oxygen concentration and bag-valve mask ventilation, often are insufficient.[22] Noninvasive positive pressure ventilation (NIPPV) can improve preoxygenation and prolong time to desaturation.[22,24] To avoid premature airway closure observed in the supine position, obese patients should be preoxygenated in a seated or semiupright position.[25]

Safe apnea time may be prolonged further through the use of apneic oxygenation, although the utility and best means of delivery are yet to be determined.[26,27] Alterations to routine intubation techniques should be employed to maximize safety in airway management of the obese. A ramped or head-up position during intubation technique can improve laryngoscopic view compared with supine positioning.[28] Ramping consists of supporting a patient's upper back and head with towels, pillows, or specifically designed devices to achieve alignment of the external auditory meatus and the sternal notch. Head-up positioning aims to achieve the same alignment by raising the head of the bed to approximately 25° and supporting the head with additional pillows or towels as needed (**Fig. 1**).

An obese neck can make surgical airway management difficult. Some experts advocate making a partial-thickness, vertical incision to facilitate palpation of deeper structures.[29] If a tracheostomy device is used, care should be taken to choose a device with sufficient length to securely enter the trachea.

RESPIRATORY SUPPORT

NIPPV is commonly used in the outpatient and perioperative treatment of OSA and OHS.[30,31] Although it is less well studied in the treatment of acute respiratory failure, it is used widely with good success.[32–34] Treatment protocols relying on bilevel

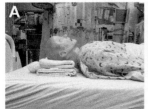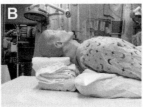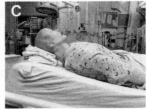

Fig. 1. Comparison of 3 intubation positions. (*A*) Sniffing position—patient flat with head elevated. (*B*) Ramped position —patient's head and shoulders elevated. (*C*) Semirecumbent position—head of bed elevated to approximately 25° with further head elevation with towels or pillows.

positive pressure ventilation emphasizing relatively high inspiratory (12–25 cm H_2O) and expiratory (5–9 cm H_2O) pressures have been described, with success rates approaching those of similar protocols for chronic obstructive pulmonary disease.[33,34] Predictors of failure of NIPPV treatment include pneumonia and mutiorgan dysfunction, whereas idiopathic hypercarbic respiratory failure has been shown to be predictive of success.[32]

Mechanical ventilation support strategies should take into account the altered respiratory physiology of obese patients. Muscle paralysis and sedation can further impair lung function, compliance, and gas exchange through worsened lung volume loss and atelectasis.[35] Improper ventilation strategies can result in significant respiratory or hemodynamic instability.

Obese patients can be supported successfully with both volume-controlled and pressure-controlled ventilation modes, with no single mode demonstrating superiority.[22] Increased airway resistance and decreased compliance can produce inadequate ventilation and resultant respiratory acidosis in pressure-controlled ventilation. Conversely, volume-controlled ventilation carries the risk of barotrauma because high pressures may be required to deliver the specified volume.

The use of low-tidal-volume (6–8 mL/kg) ventilation strategies in patients with acute respiratory distress syndrome (ARDS) is well supported and its use in patients without ARDS is gaining support.[36–38] In volume-controlled modes, tidal volume should be calculated based on ideal body weight (IBW). Use of total body weight (TBW) may result in significant ventilator-associated lung injury from barotrauma.

Obese patients can experience significant alveolar derecruitment and expiratory flow limitation during mechanical ventilation.[22,25,35] Application of positive end-expiratory pressure (PEEP) can improve respiratory mechanics and atelectasis. Obese patients may require higher PEEP than nonobese patients (eg, 10 cm H_2O).[22] Obese patients also can demonstrate expiratory flow limitation with resultant air-trapping and auto-PEEP, also referred to as intrinsic PEEP.[35] In this instance, it is important to monitor for the development of auto-PEEP using an expiratory hold maneuver on the ventilator. The application of extrinsic PEEP should be limited to two-thirds of the intrinsic PEEP.[22,25] High PEEP also can precipitate hemodynamic compromise through limitations of venous return, right ventricular output, and pulmonary perfusion.[25]

The increased work of breathing, CO_2 production, and oxygen consumption observed in the obese results in a rapid, shallow breathing pattern.[22,23] This resting rate should be mirrored in ventilator settings and monitored for adequate expiration.[22,35]

As with preoxygenation and intubation, positioning is an important component of successful mechanical ventilation of the obese patient. Patients should be kept in a head-elevated position (ie, reverse Trendelenburg) so as to lessen the volume loss observed in supine positioning.[35]

PHARMACOLOGY

Changes in body composition, cardiac output, and renal and hepatic function can have important impacts on pharmacokinetics and pharmacodynamics of many important medications (**Fig. 2**). The use of weight-based dosing scalars can lead to incorrect dosing of medications through the use of an inappropriate dosing weight. Obese patients often are excluded from pharmaceutical dosing studies, limiting understanding of effective dosing in this population.[25,39,40] At increasing weights, adipose tissue contributes disproportionately to TBW, resulting in larger than expected volumes of

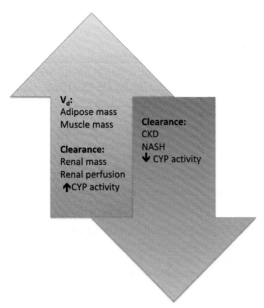

Fig. 2. Impacts of obesity on drug pharmacokinetics and pharmacodynamics. CKD, chronic kidney disease; CYP, cytochrome P450; NASH, nonalcoholic steatohepatitis.

distribution (V_d) of lipophilic compounds (**Fig. 3**).[39] Alterations in V_d are particularly relevant to emergency physicians, because they have significant impacts on loading doses. Drug clearance has a more significant impact on maintenance doses and dosing intervals.[40] Drug clearance is determined primarily by hepatic and renal functions, both of which can be variably affected by obesity, with an overall trend toward more rapid drug clearance.[41] Several different dosing weights are commonly used in obese patients (**Table 2**). The appropriate dosing weight takes into consideration drug

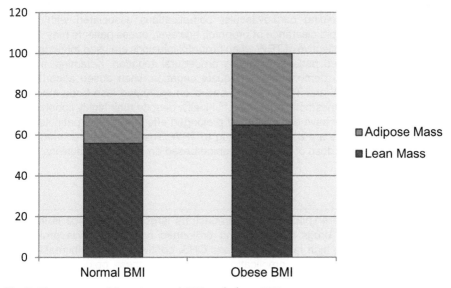

Fig. 3. Tissue composition at normal BMI and obese BMI.

Table 2 Dosing weight definitions		
Weight	**Abbreviation**	**Definition**
Ideal body weight	IBW	The weight at a given height that is associated with the lowest mortality
Total body weight	TBW	Measured weight without adjustment
Adjusted body weight	AdjBW ABW	IBW + cf(TBW − IBW)
Lean body mass	LBM	Estimated mass of nonfat tissues, including muscle, bone, and so forth, with various calculations available.

Abbreviation: cf, correction factor, most commonly 0.4.

lipophilicity, protein binding characteristics, and risk of toxicity. In general, more lipophilic compounds are best dosed according to TBW, whereas more hydrophilic compounds are best dosed according to IBW or adjusted body weight (ABW). The following sections highlight particularly relevant resuscitative medications and special cases in obese pharmacology.

Sedatives and Paralytics

Incorrect dosing of sedatives and paralytics in rapid sequence intubation (RSI) can affect intubation conditions adversely. Obese patients frequently experience underdosing of common RSI medications, such as etomidate and succinylcholine.[42] In general, medications used for RSI should be dosed according to TBW or IBW, depending on drug lipophilicity, with some notable exceptions (**Table 3**). Rocuronium, although weakly lipophilic, has been demonstrated to cause prolonged neuromuscular blockade in obese patients when dosed at TBW and, therefore, should be dosed according IBW.[39] Propofol is highly lipophilic and dosing studies have demonstrated that dosing according to IBW during RSI achieves similar sedation goals and intubating conditions, while avoiding cardiovascular complications associated with higher doses.[39] Given the rapid clearance of propofol, however, obese patients may require higher dosing more reflective of TBW when propofol infusions are used for sedation in mechanically ventilated patients or during procedural sedation. Ketamine, another highly lipophilic drug, demonstrates adequate sedation when dosed according to weights between IBW and TBW. Dosing based on estimated lean body mass has demonstrated good anesthetic outcomes.[43] Finally, despite their highly lipophilic nature, benzodiazepines have demonstrated prolonged effects in obese patients when maintenance infusions are dosed according to TBW. Therefore, it is recommended to calculate the initial dose of a benzodiazepine based on TBW, with infusions dosed according to IBW.[44]

Analgesics

Opioid medications are lipophilic and demonstrate large V_d. Clearance is variably affected, with some drugs demonstrating prolonged half-lives.[44] This prolonged half-life, coupled with high rates of OSA and OHS, contributes to an increased risk of opiate-related respiratory complications.[39] Dosing of these opioid medications should consider the intended effect and clinical scenario. When used in the peri-intubation time period, consideration should be given to the rapid dispersal to tissues;

				Lean Body	Adjusted
	High	**Total Body**	**Ideal Body**	**Lean Body**	**Adjusted**
Drug Class	**Standard**	**Weight**	**Weight**	**Mass**	**Body Weight**
RSI Medications		Etomidate Succinylcholine Midazolam Fentanyl	Propofol Rocuronium Vecuronium	Ketamine	
Antibiotics	Cephalosporins Carbapenems Fluoroquinolones	Vancomycin			Aminoglycosides
Cariovascular Medications		Calcium channel blockers Epinephrine Norepinephrine	β-Blockers Lidocaine Procainamide Digoxin		

Table 3
Weight-based dosing for selected medications

dosing based on TBW likely is beneficial.[25] When dosed for analgesia, dosing should reflect IBW so as to minimize risk for respiratory complications.[39,44,45]

Antibiotics

Early, appropriate antibiotic administration is a critical component of sepsis care.[46] It is incumbent on emergency physicians to accurately dose antibiotics to expediently achieve therapeutic levels. As with other drug classes, drug-specific dosing recommendations for antibiotics in obese patients are sparse. Vancomycin is among the best-studied antibiotics in obese patients. Generally, the initial dose of vancomycin is best dosed according to TBW, owing to relatively large V_d; however, increases in V_d do not scale proportionally with BMI; therefore, patients with very large BMIs may require lower doses.[47] Subsequent doses are best determined via therapeutic drug monitoring, because Cl can be significantly altered by both obesity and sepsis-related organ dysfunction.[47] Although evidence of improved therapeutic drug levels with this dosing strategy have been reported for decades, underdosing is still observed among many obese patients.[48] A study of more than 2500 ED patients demonstrated an 8-fold increase in the likelihood of underdosing of vancomycin for every 10 kg increase in body weight.[48]

Aminoglycosides have also been relatively well studied in the obese population. The most commonly recommended dosing strategy is based on an ABW, in which a correction factor, typically 0.4, is used for excess weight above IBW.[47]

Penicillins, cephalosporins, carbapenems, and fluoroquinolones require relatively little dosing adjustment and should be dosed at the higher end of the standard recommended range.[47]

Antibiotic therapy for the critically ill obese patient can be challenging, because multiple patient and disease factors can alter the pharmacokinetics and pharmacodynamics of commonly used medications. Where available, therapeutic drug monitoring can play a crucial role in treatment.[40,47]

Cardiovascular Medications

Unlike many of the medications discussed previously, cardiovascular drugs like β-adrenergic receptor blockers, lidocaine, procainamide, and digoxin are relatively hydrophilic and have little alteration in their V_d with increasing BMI. Because their V_d are relatively unchanged, dosing according to IBW is recommended.[25,41] Conversely, calcium channel blockers are more lipophilic and should be dosed according to TBW.[25]

Both weight-based and non–weight-based dosing strategies for vasoactive medications like norepinephrine have demonstrated similar efficacy in achieving clinically meaningful outcomes like mean arterial blood pressure goal and mortality.[49,50] When weight-based dosing strategies are used, TBW should be used for dosing calculations.

CONDITION-SPECIFIC CONSIDERATIONS
Cardiovascular Disease and Cardiac Arrest

Obesity is a significant contributor to cardiovascular disease mortality.[1] Even in the absence of common congestive heart failure risk factors, obesity can lead directly to the development of heart failure. This often is termed, *obesity cardiomyopathy*. In this condition, hypertension, OSA, and OHS lead to alterations in cardiac structure and function, ultimately producing a reduction in ejection fraction. Despite the well-documented association with cardiovascular disease and cardiovascular death, the impact of obesity on outcome after cardiac arrest is less clear.[51,52] Obesity does have measurable impacts on the delivery of high-quality cardiopulmonary resuscitation. Increased abdominal girth may shift the optimal location for chest compressions to a more cephalad position than advanced cardiac life support guidelines would suggest.[53] Additionally, the force required to generate appropriate chest compression depth may lead to more rapid compressor fatigue.[54]

Trauma

In addition to increased rates of illness, obese patients also demonstrate higher rates of traumatic injury. When compared with patients with normal BMI, overweight individuals have an increased rate of injury of approximately 10%, whereas the risk of obese individuals can be as high as 48%[55] Obese patients demonstrate altered patterns of injury, particularly in blunt trauma, with fewer liver and head injuries but increased rates of extremity and thoracic injury.[56] Although increased abdominal adipose tissue may protect from intra-abdominal injury, increased inertia from excess weight may contribute to more severe extremity injury and the increased frequency of severe extremity injury from relatively low mechanism trauma.[57]

Many studies have demonstrated worsened morbidity in obese trauma patients.[58–61] Mortality results are mixed, with the overall trend favoring worsened mortality with high BMI.[58–61] Increased morbidity is driven largely by posttrauma complications, including infection, respiratory failure, venous thromboembolism, and multiorgan failure.[58–61] Increased incidence of respiratory disease, airway obstruction, chronic inflammation, and poor glycemic control may contribute to these complications.[57,61] The poor reliability of traditional resuscitation endpoints like central venous pressure monitoring can result in under-resuscitation of obese trauma patients.[61] Other contributors to worsened outcomes span the spectrum of care of the trauma patient, including challenges with prehospital care (limitations of routine equipment, prolonged extrication times),[57] limitations of diagnostic imaging,[62] and challenges in operative management with intraoperative patient positioning, table size, and tissue depth at operative sites.[57]

Care of the injured obese patient should focus on aggressive supportive care, including respiratory support, appropriate perioperative antibiotic dosing, and aggressive early resuscitative care.

Sepsis

The link between obesity and chronic disease, morbidity, and decreased life expectance has been well established.[1] The effects of obesity in critical illness, however, including sepsis, remain unclear. A systematic review noted significant heterogeneity in the available literature and demonstrated no clear effect of obesity on mortality risk in sepsis.[63] Adipose produces a variety of inflammatory mediators leading to a state chronic inflammatory state.[64] It has been suggested that this may lead to an altered host response during infection, conferring a protective effect.[65]

Despite inconsistent effects on mortality, obesity has a well-demonstrated impact on morbidity. Hospital and ICU lengths of stay, cost of care, and ventilator dependence frequently are increased in the obese.[64,66–68] Additionally, several studies note that the average age of obese cohorts are younger than those of normal BMI or underweight BMI, suggesting a potential increased risk of developing sepsis in this group.[66,67] Obese patients also have altered patterns of infection compared with their normal and underweight counterparts, with fewer incidents of pulmonary infections and increased rates of skin and soft tissue infections and of gram-positive infections.[64–66]

The Surviving Sepsis Campaign recommends a weight-based fluid resuscitation strategy but does not specify a dosing weight.[46] Obese patients are frequently under-resuscitated compared with normal weight and underweight patients.[64,68,69] ABW with a correction factor of 40% for body weight in excess of IBW has been associated with improved morbidity and mortality.[68] Prospective studies are needed in order to determine the best fluid resuscitation strategy in the obese patient with sepsis-induced hypotension. Early administration of appropriately dosed antibiotics remains critically important in the care of the septic obese patient.

SUMMARY

Obesity imparts important anatomic and physiologic changes that have an impact on resuscitative measures in critical illness. Obesity poses significant challenges to the most basic aspects of resuscitative care, including IV access and cardiovascular monitoring. Invasive procedures like central venous and arterial access may be necessary to provide appropriate monitoring and treatment. Altered airway anatomy and respiratory mechanics contribute to a decrease in respiratory reserve and can contribute to rapid desaturation during RSI. Although it remains unclear if obesity is an independent risk factor for difficult intubation, preparing for a potentially difficult intubation is prudent because obesity and obesity-associated conditions frequently are considered in difficult airway scoring systems. Emergency physicians should be cognizant of altered pharmacokinetics in the obese and choose appropriate dosing weights based on drug and patient characteristics and therapeutic intent.

DISCLOSURE

No financial disclosures.

REFERENCES

1. Afshin A, Forouzanfar MH, Reitsma MB, et al. Health effects of overweight and obesity in 195 countries over 25 years. N Engl J Med 2017;377(1):13–27.

2. Flegal KM, Kruszon-Moran D, Carroll MD, et al. Trends in obesity among adults in the United States, 2005 to 2014. JAMA 2016;315(21):2284–91.

3. Sebbane M, Claret PG, Lefebvre S, et al. Predicting peripheral venous access difficulty in the Emergency Department using body mass index and a clinical evaluation of venous accessibility. J Emerg Med 2013;44(2):299–305.

4. Helwani M, Saied N, Ikeda S. Accuracy of anatomical landmarks in locating the internal jugular vein cannulation site among different levels of anesthesia trainees. J Educ Perioper Med 2008;10(2):E050.

5. Kehrl T, Becker BA, Simmons DE, et al. Intraosseous access in the obese patient: assessing the need for extended needle length. Am J Emerg Med 2016;34(9): 1831–4.

6. Costantino TG, Parikh AK, Satz WA, et al. Ultrasonography-guided peripheral intravenous access versus traditional approaches in patients with difficult intravenous access. Ann Emerg Med 2005;46(5):456–61.

7. Brusasco C, Corradi F, Zattoni PL, et al. Ultrasound-guided central venous cannulation in bariatric patients. Obes Surg 2009;19(10):1365–70.

8. Brass P, Hellmich M, Kolodziej L, et al. Ultrasound guidance versus anatomical landmarks for internal jugular vein catheterization. Cochrane Database Syst Rev 2015;(1):CD006962.

9. Anast N, Olejniczak M, Ingrande J, et al. The impact of blood pressure cuff location on the accuracy of noninvasive blood pressure measurements in obese patients: an observational study. Can J Anaesth 2016;63(3):298–306.

10. Araghi A, Bander JJ, Guzman JA. Arterial blood pressure monitoring in overweight critically ill patients: invasive or noninvasive? Crit Care 2006;10(2):R64.

11. Irving G, Holden J, Stevens R, et al. Which cuff should I use? Indirect blood pressure measurement for the diagnosis of hypertension in patients with obesity: A diagnostic accuracy review. BMJ Open 2016;6(11):1–9.

12. Isono S. Obesity and obstructive sleep apnoea: Mechanisms for increased collapsibility of the passive pharyngeal airway. Respirology 2012;17(1):32–42.

13. Langeron O, Masso E, Huraux C, et al. Prediction of difficult mask ventilation. Anesthesiology 2000;92(5):1229–36.

14. Wang T, Sun S, Huang S. The association of body mass index with difficult tracheal intubation management by direct laryngoscopy: A meta-analysis. BMC Anesthesiol 2018;18(1):1–13.

15. Moon TS, Fox PE, Somasundaram A, et al. The influence of morbid obesity on difficult intubation and difficult mask ventilation. J Anesth 2019;33(1):96–102.

16. Wilson ME, Spiegelhalter D, Robertson JA, et al. Predicting difficult intubation. Br J Anaesth 1988;61(2):211–6.

17. Kuzmack E, Inglis T, Olvera D, et al. A novel difficult-airway prediction tool for emergency airway management: validation of the HEAVEN criteria in a large air medical cohort. J Emerg Med 2018;54(4):395–401.

18. Reed MJ, Dunn MJG, McKeown DW. Can an airway assessment score predict difficulty at intubation in the emergency department? Emerg Med J 2005;22(2): 99–102.

19. Salome CM, King GG, Berend N. Physiology of obesity and effects on lung function. J Appl Physiol 2010;108(1):206–11.

20. Sebastian JC. Respiratory physiology and pulmonary complications in obesity. Best Pract Res Clin Endocrinol Metab 2013;27(2):157–61.

21. Benumof J, Dagg RBR. Critical hemoglobin desaturation will occur before return to an unparalyzed state following 1 mg/kg intravenous succinylcholine. Anesthesiology 1997;97(4):979–82.

22. De Jong A, Chanques G, Jaber S. Mechanical ventilation in obese ICU patients: From intubation to extubation. Crit Care 2017;21(1):1–8.

23. Chlif M, Keochkerian D, Choquet D, et al. Effects of obesity on breathing pattern, ventilatory neural drive and mechanics. Respir Physiol Neurobiol 2009;168(3): 198–202.

24. Baillard C, Fosse JP, Sebbane M, et al. Noninvasive ventilation improves preoxygenation before intubation of hypoxic patients. Am J Respir Crit Care Med 2006;174(2):171–7.
25. Parker BK, Manning S, Winters ME. The crashing obese patient. West J Emerg Med 2019;20(2):323–30.
26. Heard A, Toner AJ, Evans JR, et al. Apneic oxygenation during prolonged laryngoscopy in obese patients: A randomized, controlled trial of buccal RAE tube oxygen administration. Anesth Analg 2017;124(4):1162–7.
27. Ramachandran SK, Cosnowski A, Shanks A, et al. Apneic oxygenation during prolonged laryngoscopy in obese patients: a randomized, controlled trial of nasal oxygen administration. J Clin Anesth 2010;22(3):164–8.
28. Collins JS, Lemmens HJM, Brodsky JB, et al. Laryngoscopy and morbid obesity: A comparison of the "sniff" and "ramped" positions. Obes Surg 2004;14(9): 1171–5.
29. Freeman BD. Tracheostomy update: when and how. Crit Care Clin 2017;33(2): 311–22.
30. Pierce AM, Brown LK. Obesity hypoventilation syndrome: Current theories of pathogenesis. Curr Opin Pulm Med 2015;21(6):557–62.
31. Chau EHL, Lam D, Wong J, et al. Obesity hypoventilation syndrome: a review of epidemiology, pathophysiology, and perioperative considerations. Anesthesiology 2012;117(1):188–205.
32. Lemyze M, Taufour P, Duhamel A, et al. Determinants of noninvasive ventilation success or failure in morbidly obese patients in acute respiratory failure. PLoS One 2014;9(5):5–11.
33. Carrillo A, Ferrer M, Gonzalez-Diaz G, et al. Noninvasive ventilation in acute hypercapnic respiratory failure caused by obesity hypoventilation syndrome and chronic obstructive pulmonary disease. Am J Respir Crit Care Med 2012; 186(12):1279–85.
34. Masa JF, Utrabo I, Gomez de Terreros J, et al. Noninvasive ventilation for severely acidotic patients in respiratory intermediate care units: Precision medicine in intermediate care units. BMC Pulm Med 2016;16(1):1–13.
35. Junhasavasdikul D, Telias I, Grieco DL, et al. Expiratory Flow Limitation During Mechanical Ventilation. Chest 2018;154(4):948–62.
36. Petrucci N, De Feo C. Lung protective ventilation strategy for the acute respiratory distress syndrome. Cochrane Database Syst Rev 2013;2013(2):CD003844.
37. De Jong A, Verzilli D, Jaber S. ARDS in obese patients: specificities and management. Crit Care 2019;23(1):74.
38. Fuller BM, Mohr NM, Drewry AM, et al. Lower tidal volume at initiation of mechanical ventilation may reduce progression to acute respiratory distress syndrome: A systematic review. Crit Care 2013;17(1):R11.
39. Ingrande J, Lemmens HJ. Dose adjustment of anaesthetics in the morbidly obese. Br J Anaesth 2010;105(Suppl):16–23.
40. Barras M, Legg A. Drug dosing in obese adults. Aust Prescr 2017;40(5):189–93.
41. Blouin RA, Warren GW. Pharmacokinetic considerations in obesity. J Pharm Sci 1999;88(1):1–7.
42. Bhat R, Mazer-Amirshahi M, Sun C, et al. Accuracy of rapid sequence intubation medication dosing in obese patients intubated in the ED. Am J Emerg Med 2016; 34(12):2423–5.
43. Wulfsohn NL. Ketamine dosage for induction based on lean body mass. Anesth Analg 1972;51(2):299–305.

44. De Baerdemaeker LEC, Mortier EP, Struys MMRF. Pharmacokinetics in obese patients. Contin Educ Anaesthesia, Crit Care Pain 2004;4(5):152–5.

45. Nelson JA, Loredo JS, Acosta JA. The obesity-hypoventilation syndrome and respiratory failure in the acute trauma patient. J Emerg Med 2011;40(4):e67–9.

46. Rhodes A, Evans LE, Alhazzani W, et al. Surviving sepsis campaign: international guidelines for management of sepsis and septic shock: 2016. Intensive Care Med 2017;43(3):304–77.

47. Meng L, Mui E, Holubar MK, et al. Comprehensive Guidance for Antibiotic Dosing in Obese Adults. Pharmacotherapy 2017;37(11):1415–31.

48. Fuller BM, Mohr N, Skrupky L, et al. Emergency Department vancomycin use: dosing practices and associated outcomes. J Emerg Med 2013;44(5):910–8.

49. Adams C, Tucker C, Allen B, et al. Disparities in hemodynamic resuscitation of the obese critically ill septic shock patient. J Crit Care 2017;37:219–23.

50. Radosevich JJ, Patanwala AE, Erstad BL. Norepinephrine dosing in obese and nonobese patients with septic shock. Am J Crit Care 2016;25(1):27–32.

51. Shahreyar M, Dang G, Waqas Bashir M, et al. Outcomes of In-hospital cardiopulmonary resuscitation in morbidly obese patients. JACC Clin Electrophysiol 2017; 3(2):174–83.

52. Geri G, Savary G, Legriel S, et al. Influence of body mass index on the prognosis of patients successfully resuscitated from out-of-hospital cardiac arrest treated by therapeutic hypothermia. Resuscitation 2016;109:49–55.

53. Lee J, Oh J, Lim TH, et al. Comparison of optimal point on the sternum for chest compression between obese and normal weight individuals with respect to body mass index, using computer tomography: A retrospective study. Resuscitation 2018;128:1–5.

54. Secombe PJ, Sutherland R, Johnson R. Morbid obesity impairs adequacy of thoracic compressions in a simulation-based model. Anaesth Intensive Care 2018;46(2):171–7.

55. Finkelstein EA, Chen H, Prabhu M, et al. The relationship between obesity and injuries among U.S. adults. Am J Health Promot 2007;21(5):460–8.

56. Stroud T, Bagnall NM, Pucher PH. Effect of obesity on patterns and mechanisms of injury: Systematic review and meta analysis. Int J Surg 2018;56:148–54.

57. Spitler CA, Hulick RM, Graves ML, et al. Obesity in the Polytrauma Patient. Orthop Clin North Am 2018;49(3):307–15.

58. Newell MA, Bard MR, Goettler CE, et al. Body mass index and outcomes in critically injured blunt trauma patients: weighing the impact. J Am Coll Surg 2007; 204(5):1056–61.

59. Byrnes MC, McDaniel MD, Moore MB, et al. The effect of obesity on outcomes among injured patients. J Trauma 2005;58(2):232–7.

60. Bochicchio GV, Joshi M, Bochicchio K, et al. Impact of obesity in the critically ill trauma patient: a prospective study. J Am Coll Surg 2006;203(4):533–8.

61. Winfield RD, Delano MJ, Lottenberg L, et al. Traditional resuscitative practices fail to resolve metabolic acidosis in morbidly obese patients after severe blunt trauma. J Trauma 2010;68(2):317–30.

62. Modica MJ, Kanal KM, Gunn ML. The obese emergency patient: imaging challenges and solutions. Radiographics 2011;31(3):811–23.

63. Trivedi V, Bavishi C, Jean R. Impact of obesity on sepsis mortality: A systematic review. J Crit Care 2015;30(3):518–24.

64. Wacharasint P, Boyd JH, Russell JA, et al. One size does not fit all in severe infection: Obesity alters outcome, susceptibility, treatment, and inflammatory response. Crit Care 2013;17(3):R122.

65. Falagas ME, Kompoti M. Obesity and infection. Lancet Infect Dis 2006;6(7): 438–46.
66. Arabi YM, Dara SI, Tamim HM, et al. Clinical characteristics, sepsis interventions and outcomes in the obese patients with septic shock: An international multi-center cohort study. Crit Care 2013;17(2):R72.
67. Nguyen AT, Tsai CL, Hwang LY, et al. Obesity and mortality, length of stay and hospital cost among patients with sepsis: A nationwide inpatient retrospective cohort study. PLoS One 2016;11(4):1–12.
68. Taylor SP, Karvetski CH, Templin MA, et al. Initial fluid resuscitation following adjusted body weight dosing is associated with improved mortality in obese patients with suspected septic shock. J Crit Care 2018;43:7–12.
69. Kuttab HI, Lykins JD, Hughes MD, et al. Evaluation and Predictors of Fluid Resuscitation in Patients With Severe Sepsis and Septic Shock. Crit Care Med 2019; 47(11):1.

Massive Gastrointestinal Hemorrhage

Katrina D'Amore, DO, MPH[a],*, Anand Swaminathan, MD, MPH[b]

KEYWORDS

- Gastrointestinal hemorrhage • Resuscitation • Massive hemorrhage
- Massive transfusion • Thromboelastography • Anticoagulant reversal

KEY POINTS

- Massive gastrointestinal hemorrhage requires aggressive resuscitation with prompt transfusion of blood products and initiation of a massive transfusion protocol if clinical instability does not improve.
- Successful resuscitation begins with the placement of reliable, large-bore, peripheral intravenous or intraosseous access.
- Reversal of anticoagulant medications is a critical component in the management of patients with massive gastrointestinal hemorrhage. Using thromboelastography or rotational thromboelastometry can guide transfusion strategies specific to the patient's unique needs.
- Consider delayed sequence intubation; bed-up head-elevated positioning; reduced dose of the sedative; increased dose of the paralytic; and the SALAD (suction-assisted laryngoscopy for airway decontamination) technique to intubate the patient and minimize aspiration.
- Consult gastroenterology, interventional radiology, and acute care emergency surgery early in the patient's resuscitation for definitive source control.

INTRODUCTION

Massive gastrointestinal (GI) hemorrhage is a life-threatening condition that requires prompt recognition and skilled resuscitation to increase the chance of good outcomes. Although no consensus definition exists, any gastrointestinal bleeding (GIB) that results in hemodynamic instability, signs of poor perfusion (eg, altered mental status, syncope, pallor), transfusion of more than 2 units of packed red blood cells (pRBCs) during the initial resuscitation, or the presence of bleeding that is overt and rapid can be considered massive.[1] Although the mortality of all patients with a GIB ranges from 3% to 14%, the mortality from massive hemorrhage is much higher.[2] Successful resuscitation of massive GIB (MGIB) involves prompt establishment of reliable

[a] Department of Emergency Medicine, Good Samaritan Hospital Medical Center, 1000 Montauk Highway, West Islip, NY 11795, USA; [b] St. Joseph's University Medical Center, 703 Main Street, Paterson, NJ 07503, USA
* Corresponding author.
E-mail address: damoreka@gmail.com

Emerg Med Clin N Am 38 (2020) 871–889
https://doi.org/10.1016/j.emc.2020.06.008
0733-8627/20/© 2020 Elsevier Inc. All rights reserved.

emed.theclinics.com

vascular access, transfusion of appropriate blood products, reversal of coagulopathies, early involvement of consultants, and, in many cases, definitive airway management.

DOES THIS PATIENT HAVE A MASSIVE GASTROINTESTINAL HEMORRHAGE?

MGIB describes patients with severe bleeding who require emergency intervention in order to prevent mortality and limit morbidity.[3] Patients with clinically obvious MGIB include those with overt hematemesis, brisk hematochezia, or hemodynamic instability (eg, hypotension) in the setting of bleeding. When significant hemorrhage leads to poor perfusion, organs such as the skin and distal extremities manifest distinct signs and symptoms. Physical examination signs of poorly perfused organs are markers of circulatory shock and impending organ failure. These signs are listed in **Box 1**.[4]

Several findings from the history and physical examination have been shown to predict the need for immediate intervention in patients with an upper GI bleed (UGIB). MGIB is more likely if the patient reports a history of cirrhosis or malignancy (Likelihood Ratio (LR), 3.7; 95% confidence interval [CI], 1.6–8.8) or syncope (LR, 3.0; 95% CI, 1.7–5.4).[3] Clinical signs of MGIB include tachycardia (LR, 4.9; 95% CI, 3.2–7.6) and a nasogastric lavage that shows red blood (LR, 3.1; 95% CI, 1.2–14.0).[3] A normal heart rate (LR, 0.34; 95% CI, 0.22–0.53) was the most predictive clinical factor of a nonsevere UGIB.[3] However, tachycardia may not be present if the patient is taking a β-blocker or calcium channel blocker medication. β-Blocker medication use is particularly common in patients with advanced cirrhosis, because they are first-line therapy in the treatment of portal hypertension. Similar factors (tachycardia, syncope, hemodynamic instability) have also been shown to predict MGIB in the setting of a lower GI bleed (LGIB).[5] Additional characteristics of severe LGIB include active bleeding per rectum during the initial evaluation, a nontender abdominal examination, history of aspirin use, and more than 2 comorbid conditions.[6,7] Comorbidities such as renal failure, liver failure, and malignancy are considered higher risk. Regardless of the patient's initial presentation and vital sign measurements, all patients with signs and

---

Box 1
Signs of poor perfusion

- Altered or decreased mental status
- Decreased peripheral pulses
- Delayed capillary refill
- Skin pallor or mottling, most commonly around the knees and fingers (limited utility in darker complexions)
- Cold skin
- Low peripheral oxygen saturation
- Decreased mean arterial pressure
- Increased lactate level

Data from Hasanin A, Mukhtar A, Nassar H. Perfusion indices revisited. *Journal of Intensive Care.* 2017;5(1). https://doi.org/10.1186/s40560-017-0220-5.

symptoms of GIB should be taken seriously and prompt treatment initiated. The potential for rapid decompensation among GIB patients is high.

Shock index (SI) is defined as the heart rate divided by systolic blood pressure and can be used as an indicator of impending hemodynamic instability or collapse.[8] An SI greater than 0.7 is considered abnormal. An abnormal SI in the presence of bleeding indicates considerable hypovolemia and, possibly, occult shock. An SI greater than 0.9 portends a poorer prognosis, and an SI greater than 1.0 indicates the need for a massive transfusion (MT).[8,9] Calculation of the SI can aid in the recognition of critical illness before a patient becomes overtly hypotensive and can prompt more aggressive evaluation and treatment.[10,11]

IDENTIFYING THE LOCATION OF HEMORRHAGE

MGIB can result from both upper and lower GI sources (**Tables 1** and **2**).[12] It is important to differentiate between upper and lower sources of GIB, because this affects the type of diagnostic studies and consultants needed for definitive source control. In hemodynamically unstable patients, an UGIB is more likely. Although UGIB carries a higher mortality, recent data show that the prevalence of hospitalizations and inpatient death from LGIB are approaching those seen in UGIB.[13]

UGIB occurs at locations proximal to the ligament of Treitz, a suspensory ligament located at the duodenojejunal flexure (**Fig. 1**). Massive UGIB can present in several ways: hematemesis, melena, or hematochezia. Hematemesis can occur as either bright red blood or so-called coffee-ground emesis, which gains its appearance from gastric acids converting hemoglobin to the brown-pigmented hematin. Melena occurs when hemoglobin undergoes digestion by intestinal enzymes and endogenous gastrointestinal flora. UGIB that presents as hematochezia results from a brisk bleed that passes rapidly through the small and large intestines and encounters little digestion. One in 10 patients presenting with hematochezia are bleeding from an upper GI source.[14]

LGIB originates anywhere distal to the ligament of Treitz and typically presents with hematochezia, with or without associated clots. LGIB rarely presents with melena, although it can occur with very proximal lower sources that undergo some intestinal digestion. Up to 80% of LGIB stops spontaneously.[15]

Table 1	
Common causes of massive upper gastrointestinal bleed	
Cause	**Frequency (%)**
Peptic ulcer disease	55–74

Varices
  Esophageal and gastric
  Portal hypertensive
    gastropathy
	5–14

Hemorrhagic gastritis	11–15
Vascular lesions	2–3
Malignancy	2–5
Aortoenteric fistula	<1

Data from Lee E, Laberge J. Differential Diagnosis of Gastrointestinal Bleeding. Techniques in vascular and interventional radiology. 2004;7: 112-22. https://doi.org/10.1053/j.tvir.2004.12.001.

Table 2
Common causes of massive lower gastrointestinal bleed

Cause	Prevalence (%)
Diverticular disease	5–42
Colitis	
Ischemic	6–18
Infectious	3–29
Radiation related	1–3
Vascular lesions	0–3
Malignancy	3–11
Rectal varices	1–8
Inflammatory bowel disease	2–4

Data from Lee E, Laberge J. Differential Diagnosis of Gastrointestinal Bleeding. Techniques in vascular and interventional radiology. 2004;7: 112-22. https://doi.org/10.1053/j.tvir.2004.12.001.

EMERGENCY DEPARTMENT RESUSCITATION OF THE PATIENT WITH MASSIVE GASTROINTESTINAL BLEED
Vascular Access

Effective resuscitation of a patient with MGIB begins with the urgent placement of reliable and appropriate intravenous (IV) or intraosseous (IO) access, so that additional therapies can be given rapidly and safely. The rate of flow through IV or IO catheters can be described by Poiseuille's law, which states that the larger the diameter and the shorter the length, the faster the flow through the catheter will be. Maximal flow rates have been determined for a variety of IV and IO catheters.[16] **Table 3** summarizes the gravity and pressure bag flow rates of commonly used catheters. Application of a pressure bag, a decrease in the length or an increase in the diameter of the catheter, increases the flow rate.[16] Two large-bore (14-gauge to 18-gauge) peripheral IV catheters are ideal for resuscitating patients with MGIB, because these patients often require large-volume transfusions.[17] Importantly, the largest port of a central venous

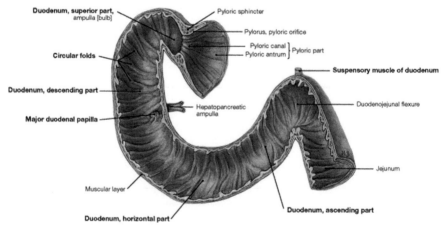

Fig. 1. Suspensory muscle of the duodenum/ligament of Treitz at the duodenojejunal flexure.

Table 3
Flow rates of commonly used intravenous and intraosseous catheters

Catheter Size	Gravity Flow Rate[a] (mL/min)	Pressure Bag Flow Rate[a] (mL/min)	Time[b] to Infuse 1 L of 0.9% NS (min)	Time[b] to Infuse 1 L of 0.9% NS Under Pressure (min)
14 G, 50 mm	236	384	4	3
16 G, 50 mm	154	334	7	3
18 G, 45 mm	98	153	10	7
Humeral IO	82	148	12	7
16 G port, central line 34 cm	69	116	15	9
Tibial IO	68	204	15	5
20 G, 33 mm	64	105	16	10
22 G, 25 mm	35	71	29	14
18 G port, central line 35 cm	30	79	33	13

Abbreviations: IO, intraosseous; NS, normal saline.
[a] Rounded to the nearest 1 mL/min.
[b] Rounded to the nearest minute.
Data from Reddick AD, Ronald J, Morrison WG. Intravenous fluid resuscitation: was Poiseuille right? Emergency Medicine Journal. 2010;28(3):201-202. https://doi.org/10.1136/emj.2009. 083485; and Ngo AS, Oh JJ, Chen Y, Yong D, Ong ME. Intraosseous vascular access in adults using the EZ-IO in an emergency department. Int J Emerg Med. 2009;2(3):155–160. Published 2009 Aug 11. https://doi.org/10.1007/s12245-009-0116-9

catheter has a slow flow rate caused mostly by its long length (>33 cm). Therefore, these are often inadequate for efficient resuscitation of patients with MGIB. Patients with a history of diabetes mellitus, IV drug abuse, sickle cell disease, end-stage renal disease, and obesity have been shown to be challenging to obtain emergent peripheral vascular access.[18] Ultrasonography guidance may aid in placement of IV catheters in these patients.

If reliable IV access proves difficult to quickly obtain, a humeral or tibial IO catheter should be inserted.[19] Modern IO devices allow rapid insertion (average insertion time of 4 seconds) and are safe options for infusing blood products and most medications.[19,20] IO marrow aspirate can also be used to obtain point-of-care hemoglobin, hematocrit, blood urea nitrogen, creatinine, and glucose values. IO values for these laboratory studies have all shown good correlation with serum samples.[21]

Although a humeral IO catheter can infuse 1 L of 0.9% normal saline (NS) faster than a tibial IO catheter (12 vs 14 minutes), the application of a pressure bag has been shown to produce the opposite result, with 1 L of 0.9% NS administered in 5 minutes via the tibial route compared with 7 minutes via the humeral route.[19] A tibial IO catheter should be placed 2 finger widths below the patella and 1 to 2 cm medial to the tibial tuberosity (**Fig. 2**). A humeral IO catheter is placed on the most prominent aspect of the greater tuberosity with the patient's hand on the abdomen or the humerus in an internally rotated position (**Fig. 3**).

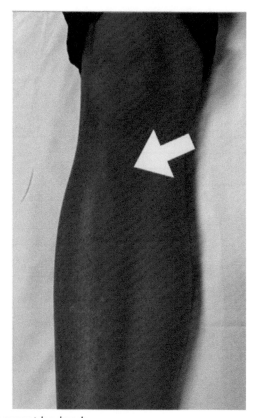

Fig. 2. Tibial IO placement landmark.

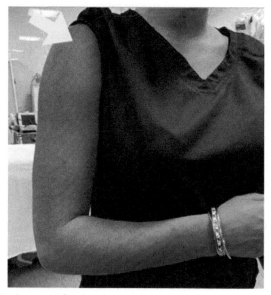

Fig. 3. Humeral IO placement landmark.

Transfusion Strategies

The harms of massive bleeding center on end-organ ischemia secondary to decreased perfusion through a lack of oxygen-carrying red blood cells. Transfusing pRBCs sustains hemoglobin levels and oxygen delivery to tissues. Because patients with MGIB can rapidly deteriorate, exsanguination from hematemesis or hematochezia is a real and feared outcome. Early administration of blood products is a cornerstone of management. Although restrictive transfusion strategies that target a hemoglobin level of 7 g/dL are recommended for patients with an acute UGIB, patients with MGIB should be transfused as soon as possible.[22–24]

Excessive crystalloid infusion should be avoided. Fluid administration may worsen anemia and coagulation through further dilution. Large volumes of 0.9% NS can result in a hyperchloremic acidosis and, if not warmed, decrease body temperature as well.[25] Both hypothermia and acidosis have been shown to increase the time to clot formation and impair hemostasis.[26,27] Administration of small volumes of warmed balanced solutions (eg, Ringer's lactate, Plasma-lyte) is reasonable to support mean arterial pressure while waiting for emergency blood products to be available.

It is important to recall that hemoglobin measurement lags behind the true serum concentrations and is not reliable in the face of brisk bleeding.[28] Initial transfusion of 2 to 4 units of type-O pRBCs should be initiated as soon as MGIB is recognized. All persons less than the age of 16 years and women of childbearing age should receive Rh-negative type-O blood. Men and women past childbearing age may receive initial resuscitation with Rh-positive type-O blood. If there is no significant improvement after initial pRBC administration, initiate a massive transfusion protocol (MTP). Clinical stability and signs of end-organ perfusion should guide transfusion.[4,29] Avoid hypertension and over-resuscitation, because this can disrupt nascent clots at sites of bleeding, especially in the setting of variceal bleeding. Permissive hypotension with a target systolic blood pressure of 90 mm Hg is acceptable.

Platelets are the component of blood responsible for initiating blood clot formation at sites of endothelial injury. There are no clear guidelines for transfusion of platelets in patients with MGIB. Expert opinion recommends transfusion of platelets in the face of thrombocytopenia to a goal of at least 50,000.[30–32]

Massive Transfusion Protocols

Unstable patients with GIB may require large transfusion volumes. Solely transfusing erythrocytes can lead to a dilutional coagulopathy and worse outcomes. MTPs have been designed to mimic replacement of whole blood, providing an equal ratio of red blood cells, plasma, and platelets.[33,34] MT has been defined as administration of greater than 10 units of pRBC in 24 hours or transfusion of 4 units of pRBC in the first 30 minutes of resuscitation.[17,35] The latter definition is more useful to the emergency department resuscitation of MGIB. Although these protocols have largely been developed for patients with trauma, the authors believe they can reasonably be extrapolated to the management of other forms of hemorrhagic shock, such as MGIB.

In patients with hemorrhagic trauma, MTPs that use a 1:1:1 ratio of blood products, compared with isolated erythrocyte transfusion, have shown a decrease in mortality and total pRBC transfusions.[35,36] A combination of MT with thromboelastography (TEG) or rotational thromboelastometry (ROTEM) further improves survival while decreasing overall amounts of blood product given in trauma.[37] Evidence of benefit of MTP and TEG/ROTEM in patients with MGIB does not exist, but the benefit can be extrapolated from the trauma research.[35–39] If the initial transfusion of 2 to 4 units of pRBC is not effective in improving hemodynamic stability, perfusion, or hemostasis, consider activating an MTP.

Known complications of MT are hypothermia, hypocalcemia, and hyperkalemia.[17] Warming blood through a rapid transfuser and keeping the patient covered in warm blankets can combat hypothermia. Because fractionated blood products are preserved with citrate, their administration can cause precipitation with calcium and resultant hypocalcemia. Monitor calcium levels closely throughout the resuscitation or consider empiric calcium administration. Potassium levels should be monitored as well and hyperkalemia treated accordingly. Familiarity and anticipation of these complications are important during resuscitation.

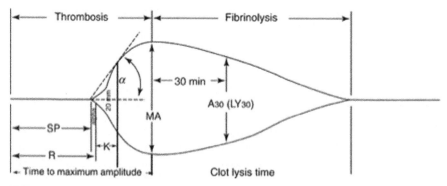

Parameter	Description	Function Measured	Treatment when abnormal
Reaction ("R") time	Time from start of test to initial fibrin formation	Coagulation factors	FFP
Kinetic ("K") time	Time to achieve a clot strength of 20 mm	Fibrinogen & Platelets	Cryoprecipitate
α angle	Angle that represents the rate of clot formation	Fibrinogen & Platelets	Cryoprecipitate +/- Platelets
Maximum amplitude (MA)	Highest amplitude measures the overall strength of the clot	Platelets	Platelets and/or Desmopressin
Lysis time at 30 minutes ("LY 30")	Amount of clot dissolution 30 minutes after MA is reach	Amount of Fibrinolysis	Tranexamic acid (TXA)

Fig. 4. Normal thromboelastogram. MA, maximum amplitude (mm); SP, initial fibrin formation; R, reaction time (seconds); K, kinetics (seconds); A30/LY30, amplitude/lysis at 30 minutes after MA (percentage decrease).

Assessing Coagulation Status

Although traditional coagulation tests such as prothrombin time and activated partial thromboplastin time evaluate a portion of the coagulation cascade, they do not give clinicians the entire picture of in vivo coagulation in patients with massive hemorrhage. Although frequently ordered, the ability of these tests to inform transfusion strategy is limited. Importantly, an International Normalized Ratio (INR) value should not be interpreted as a degree of anticoagulation or bleeding risk unless the patient is taking warfarin. In patients not taking warfarin, the INR indicates the synthetic function of the liver, which is responsible for both procoagulant and anticoagulant (AC) protein production.[40]

TEG and ROTEM are laboratory blood assays that measure the efficiency of blood coagulation, clot strength, and fibrinolysis. Through TEG/ROTEM, platelet mapping displays real-time platelet function and shows the degree to which platelets are inhibited by aspirin and clopidogrel. **Fig. 4** shows a normal thromboelastogram. Each part of the curve correlates to a specific aspect of either clot formation or dissolution. Characteristic changes to the thromboelastogram signal the need for specific product transfusion, such as cryoprecipitate, platelets, or fresh frozen plasma.[41]

Much of the literature on the role of TEG/ROTEM in transfusions has been published in cardiac surgery and trauma. However, its clinical use is expanding and it may be applicable to patients with MGIB. A Cochrane Review in 2018 evaluated a total of 17 studies of adults and children with bleeding. Despite the totality of evidence being categorized as lower quality, the use of TEG/ROTEM reduced overall blood product transfusion with a trend toward improved mortality and reduced hemodialysis-dependent renal failure.[42] There was no significant difference between the need for surgical reintervention and MT.[42] A 2019 randomized controlled trial evaluating the effect of TEG on outcomes in cirrhotic patients with nonvariceal UGIB similarly found that patients in the TEG-guided transfusion group received fewer blood product transfusions.[43] There was no significant difference in rates of hemorrhage control, rebleeding, or mortality.[43] Although more high-quality evidence is needed, there are emerging data that the use of TEG/ROTEM decreases the amount of blood products transfused with no resultant increase in mortality.[42–44] Because transfusion and overtransfusion can have deleterious effects and complications, using TEG/ROTEM when available is advised.

If TEG or ROTEM is not available, a fibrinogen level may be informative and help guide transfusion. Fibrinogen is a protein abundant in the human body and is converted to fibrin by the enzyme thrombin. Fibrin molecules then polymerize to aid in forming hemostatic clots. Fibrinogen also actively aids in platelet aggregation. Normal fibrinogen levels range from 150 to 400 mg/dL. A low fibrinogen level results from decreased production (liver disease), hemodilution, or consumption.[45–47] Cryoprecipitate is a blood product that contains fibrinogen, factor VIII, von Willebrand factor (vWF), factor XIII, and platelet microparticles. Fibrinogen concentrate is also available at some institutions. In patients with MGIB and fibrinogen levels less than 100 mg/dL, consider administration of cryoprecipitate (1 unit/5 kg body weight up to 10 units).

Reversing Anticoagulant and Antiplatelet Medications

A thorough medication history can provide valuable information in controlling hemorrhage. An increase in cardiovascular disease coupled with the advent of newer oral ACs has seen an increase in the overall prevalence of outpatient antiplatelet and AC (AC) medication use. These medications impair hemostasis and may contribute to worsening hemorrhage in patients with GIB. The most commonly used oral ACs are

Table 4
Oral anticoagulants and suggested reversal agents

Oral AC	Mechanism of Action	Reversal and Suggested Dosing
Warfarin	Inhibits the production of vitamin K–dependent factors (II, VII, IX, X)	50 U/kg PCC plus vitamin K 5–10 mg IV Or 15 mL/kg FFP plus vitamin K 5–10 mg IV
Rivaroxaban Apixaban Edoxaban Betrixaban	Factor Xa inhibitor	50 U/kg PCC Or Andexanet alfa[a]
Dabigatran	Direct thrombin inhibitor	Idarucizumab 5 mg IV with option to repeat the dose once Or 50 U/kg PCC

Abbreviations: FFP, fresh frozen plasma; PCC, prothrombin complex concentrate (3 or 4 factor).
  [a] Recommended dosing varies depending on which Xa inhibitor is being reversed as well as the time since the last dose.
  Data from Tomaselli GF, Mahaffey KW, Cuker A, et al. 2017 ACC Expert Consensus Decision Pathway on Management of Bleeding in Patients on Oral Anticoagulants. *Journal of the American College of Cardiology.* 2017;70(24):3042-3067. https://doi.org/10.1016/j.jacc.2017.09.1085; and Cuker A, Burnett A, Triller D, et al. Reversal of direct oral anticoagulants: Guidance from the Anti-coagulation Forum. *American Journal of Hematology.* 2019;94(6):697-709. https://doi.org/10.1002/ajh.25475

warfarin, dabigatran, and direct oral ACs (DOACs), such as rivaroxaban, apixaban, and edoxaban.[48,49] Importantly, patients with renal dysfunction have decreased excretion of DOACs and therefore can be expected to have longer half-lives and higher levels of active drug.[50] Dabigatran is the only oral AC amenable to hemodialysis; however, gaining access and initiating dialysis may not be feasible during the initial resuscitation of patients with MGIB.[50]

In a recent meta-analysis, DOACs were noted to have significantly lower mortalities caused by major bleeding compared with warfarin (7% v 11%).[51] However, once bleeding has occurred, the presence of an AC increases morbidity and mortality and clinicians should consider reversal to aid in achieving hemostasis. **Table 4** outlines the common oral ACs, their mechanism of action, and recommended reversal strategies.[50,52,53] Although there is no strong clinical evidence to support its routine use for factor Xa inhibitor reversal, andexanet alfa is recommended when available.[52]

Antiplatelet agents such as aspirin, clopidogrel, and ticagrelor decrease platelet function, but they do not affect the overall number of platelets. There are no clear guidelines for transfusion of platelets in patients with MGIB taking these medications. Platelet transfusion is not recommended in patients on antiplatelet therapy with normal platelet counts.[32,54] Platelet mapping through a viscoelastic assay, such as TEG, can provide more information regarding platelet activity and contribution to clot integrity, thus better informing the need for platelet transfusion.

Patients with MGIB on antiplatelet therapy may benefit from IV desmopressin.[55] Desmopressin is thought to increase the levels of factor VIII and vWF and has been shown to expedite thrombus formation in animal models and decrease pRBC transfusion in cardiac surgery patients.[55,56] An IV desmopressin bolus of 0.4 µg/kg is recommended in patients taking antiplatelet therapy and presenting with MGIB.

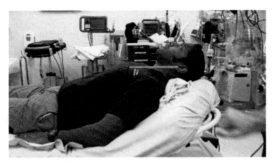

Fig. 5. Bed-up head-elevated positioning.

Airway Management

Intubation in the setting of massive UGIB is a critical and challenging task. Although real-world scenarios are likely to have multiple resuscitative efforts occurring simultaneously, securing a definitive airway in the face of massive hematemesis is a high priority and may be indicated to limit aspiration of blood and other GI contents, protect the airway in patients with altered mentation, and anticipate the need for emergent intervention such as endoscopy. Patients with MGIB are often hemodynamically unstable and at risk of peri-intubation cardiovascular collapse. Resuscitation should be initiated before intubation in order to maximize the patient's physiology and, it is hoped, prevent peri-intubation cardiovascular collapse.

All of the basic strategies of effective emergency airway management hold true in the case of MGIB. The following recommendations should be considered when time, resources, and clinical scenario allow:

1. Preoxygenate the patient: a nonrebreather mask in additional to high-flow nasal cannula is recommended.[57,58] Avoid ventilating with a bag-valve-mask (BVM) device, because this may lead to further stomach insufflation, vomiting, airway contamination, and aspiration. If BVM ventilation is necessary, use in conjunction with a positive end expiratory pressure (PEEP) valve. Aim for a PEEP of less than 20 cm H_2O, because this level is unlikely to cause gastric insufflation.[59]
2. Properly position the patient: elevate the head of the bed to 45° to aid in reducing the risk of gastric contents filling the hypopharynx and mouth. Keeping the patient semiupright may also improve preoxygenation by decreasing the collapse of both upper airway soft tissues and lower airway alveoli. Although the bed-up head-elevated positioning (**Fig. 5**) has been shown to improve safe apnea times and first-pass success and decrease intubation-related complications in the anesthesia literature, no difference has been found in first-pass success among ED intubations in limited studies.[60–63]
3. Consider placement of a nasogastric tube (NGT) before intubation. NGT placement can empty the stomach and decrease the risk of large-volume aspiration and airway contamination. If the patient is unable to tolerate NGT placement but it is determined to be of benefit, ketamine can be used to facilitate placement followed by intubation (ie, delayed sequence intubation).[64]
4. Provide proper medication doses: all sedative medications decrease the patient's release of catecholamines and decrease sympathetic tone. In hemodynamically unstable patients, sedative doses should be reduced to minimize this issue. Although lower doses of sedatives are recommended to facilitate intubation, higher

---

Box 2
Suction-assisted laryngoscopy for airway decontamination technique

1. Lead with a rigid suction catheter (held in the right hand) and suction any proximal airway contaminant.

2. Insert the laryngoscope into the midline of the mouth (with left hand).

3. Continue to advance the suction catheter followed by the laryngoscope. The suction catheter not only clears the airway of any blood, vomitus, or other secretions but also helps to lift the tongue.

4. Place the laryngoscope in the vallecula and visualize the vocal cords.

5. Move and park the suction catheter at the left corner of the mouth, with the tip of the catheter in the proximal esophagus. The catheter can then be pinned in place by the laryngoscope in the left hand, resulting in continuous esophageal suctioning with endotracheal tube insertion on the right.

6. Advance the endotracheal tube through the vocal cords. Secure and suction the tube.

Data from Suction Assisted Laryngoscopy and Airway Decontamination (SALAD). https://www.sscor.com/suction-assisted-laryngoscopy-and-airway-decontamination-salad. Accessed November 30, 2019.

---

doses of paralytics are needed because the hypotensive state leads to longer circulation time for the paralytic.

5. Use suction-assisted laryngoscopy for airway decontamination (SALAD): SALAD is a set of actions developed by Dr Jim Ducanto in order to manage grossly contaminated airways, and, if used prophylactically, may decrease the risk of contamination.[65] Please refer to the following video for a demonstration of the technique: https://spaces.hightail.com/receive/V0YyRzYPqP. The steps are summarized in **Box 2**.

Balloon Tamponade Devices

Consider placement of a Sengstaken-Blakemore or Minnesota tube if massive UGIB continues despite aggressive resuscitation and establishment of a definitive airway. These devices work by applying direct pressure to the mucosal surfaces and, theoretically, the bleeding vessels of the esophagus and stomach through inflation of balloons located on the device. There are risks of gastric and esophageal perforation or necrosis; however, these devices are potentially lifesaving efforts to tamponade ongoing hemorrhage in the upper GI tract.[66,67] Because the insertion procedure is infrequently performed, it is recommended to review the steps and equipment before placement (EM:RAP Productions, Placement of a Blakemore Tube for Bleeding Varices: https://www.youtube.com/watch?v=NHeICd5Jtp4&t=10s).

Medications

In the management of GIB, there are several medications that can be considered after the initial resuscitation and stabilization. These medications should not be a routine part of the resuscitative phase of care, because they can be safely administered after patient stabilization. With the exception of antibiotics for variceal UGIB, none of the pharmacologic agents have been shown to improve mortality.

Antibiotics

Antibiotics are a crucial medication to administer to patients with massive UGIB with either variceal bleeding or a history of cirrhosis.[68] In these patients, those who survive the initial bleeding episode are at risk of developing subsequent bacterial infections and sepsis. A third-generation cephalosporin, such as ceftriaxone (1 g IV every 24 hours) or cefotaxime (2 g IV every 8 hours), has been shown to decrease the incidence of subsequent infection with a number needed to treat (NNT) of 4 and decrease mortality with an NNT of 22.[68,69] In patients who cannot receive cephalosporins because of an anaphylactic allergy, a fluoroquinolone can be used (eg, ciprofloxacin 400 mg IV every 12 hours). The increasing prevalence of multidrug-resistant bacteria, particularly to quinolones, should be noted. The antibiotic should possess activity against pathogens such as *Escherichia coli*, *Klebsiella* species, *Pseudomonas* species, and *Enterococcus*.[70]

Octreotide
Octreotide is a somatostatin analogue that acts as a vasoconstrictor on the splanchnic circulation. This action reduces portal hypertension and, thus, decreases the circulation to esophageal and gastric varices. Decreasing cardiac output to the splanchnic circulation also shunts blood away from those vessels supplying gastric and duodenal ulcers. In undifferentiated GIB, octreotide has been shown to decrease initial bleeding, total transfusion requirements, and the need for surgery. However, it has not been shown to decrease mortality in undifferentiated patients with GIB.[71] Consider a 50-μg bolus followed by 50-μg/h infusion.

Proton pump inhibitors
Proton pump inhibitors (PPIs) are frequently administered to patients with GIB but have limited utility in patients with MGIB. PPIs have not shown a significant benefit in terms of mortality, rebleeding, or need for surgery.[72,73] Although PPIs may decrease the presence of high-risk stigmata (active bleeding, visible vessel, overlying clot) in peptic ulcer disease, they have little other use in the resuscitation setting.

Tranexamic acid
Tranexamic acid (TXA) acts as a competitive inhibitor and prevents the activation of plasminogen to plasmin.[74] At high concentrations, TXA also directly inhibits plasmin. This relative decrease in active plasmin reduces the degradation of fibrin clots, fibrinogen, and other plasma proteins. TXA has been widely used in several hemorrhagic conditions and is often also included in MTPs.[75] TXA is inexpensive and generally well tolerated, with nausea or diarrhea among the commonly reported adverse effects.[75] Studies on the use of TXA in GIB have had inconsistent outcomes with regard to mortality benefit; however there was no evidence that the use of TXA in patients with GIB increased the incidence of thromboembolic events and so it has been used for MGIB.[76] The recently published HALT-IT trial has provided more conclusive evidence of its possible impact on mortality.[77] This multicenter, randomized, placebo-controlled trial demonstrated no difference in five-day mortality due to bleeding in those patients receiving TXA versus those receiving placebo.[77] Additionally, there was a significant increase in venous thromboembolic events in the TXA treatment group.[77] Until further strong evidence is produced, administering TXA to all-comers with MGIB is not recommended. However, if TEG/ROTEM is available and demonstrates excessive fibrinolysis, then TXA may be indicated.

Source Control
Early consultation with an endoscopist, interventional radiologist, and acute care surgeon is paramount to the care of patients with MGIB after initiating the resuscitation and stabilization.

Upper gastrointestinal source

MGIB is more commonly a result of an upper GI source. Many upper GI sources of bleeding, such as varices and ulcers, are amenable to endoscopic interventions such as injection (of a vasoconstricting or sclerosing agent), thermal (through electro-coagulation), or mechanical therapies (endoscopic clipping or band ligation).[78] Endos-copy within the first 24 hours of hemorrhage has been shown to decrease resource use and transfusion requirements.[79] A recent cohort study showed that patients who presented with hemodynamic instability from bleeding peptic ulcers experienced lower in-hospital mortality if they received endoscopic intervention within the first 24 hours.[80] With regard to variceal bleeding, the combination of octreotide and endos-copy was associated with significantly improved initial and 5-day hemostasis rates, although mortality was not affected.[81] The endoscopist ultimately decides on the timing of endoscopy. Surgical involvement for resection may be necessary when endoscopic therapies fail to control hemorrhage.

Lower gastrointestinal source

Much of acute massive LGIB is self-limiting with proper medical resuscitation. After initial stabilization, many patients require computed tomography angiography in or-der to localize the source of bleeding. Pending this information, interventional radi-ologists (IRs) should be consulted for possible embolization of amenable vessels. General surgeons should be consulted as well. In the case of massive LGIB that is either not amenable to IR intervention or that is continuing in the face of appro-priate resuscitation, surgical resection may be indicated. With regard to direct visu-alization, the evidence supporting early colonoscopy for LGIB is mixed and generally of lower quality; however, a colonoscopy in the first 24 hours is recom-mended in patients with high-risk features (eg, hemodynamic compromise, older age, syncope, bright red rectal bleeding) who can undergo appropriate bowel preparation.[82,83] Patients with hemodynamic instability and hematochezia should prompt suspicion of an upper GI source and thus esophagogastroduodenoscopy would be warranted.

SUMMARY

MGIB is a condition with high morbidity and mortality that must be recognized promptly and resuscitated aggressively. The cornerstones of management include the establishment of large-bore IV access, early transfusion of blood products, reversal of coagulopathies, as well as the consideration of technology such as TEG/ROTEM when available. Definitive airway management and early involvement of con-sultants are also essential to a successful resuscitation.

DISCLOSURE

Dr A. Swaminathan is a deputy editor for EM:RAP and the managing editor of EM Ab-stracts. Dr K. D'Amore has nothing to disclose.

REFERENCES

1. Nagata N, Sakurai T, Shimbo T, et al. Acute severe gastrointestinal tract bleeding is associated with an increased risk of thromboembolism and death. Clin Gastro-enterol Hepatol 2017;15(12):1882–9.

2. Leerdam MV. Epidemiology of acute upper gastrointestinal bleeding. Best Pract Res Clin Gastroenterol 2008;22(2):209–24.

3. Srygley FD, Gerardo CJ, Tran T, et al. Does this patient have a severe upper gastrointestinal bleed? JAMA 2012;307(10):1072–9.
4. Hasanin A, Mukhtar A, Nassar H. Perfusion indices revisited. J Intensive Care 2017;5(1). https://doi.org/10.1186/s40560-017-0220-5.
5. Barnert J, Messmann H. Management of lower gastrointestinal tract bleeding. Best Pract Res Clin Gastroenterol 2008;22(2):295–312.
6. Velayos FS, Williamson A, Sousa KH, et al. Early predictors of severe lower gastrointestinal bleeding and adverse outcomes: a prospective study. Clin Gastroenterol Hepatol 2004;2:485–90.
7. Strate LL, Ayanian JZ, Kotler G, et al. Risk factors for mortality in lower intestinal bleeding. Clin Gastroenterol Hepatol 2008;6(9):1004–955.
8. Montoya KF, Charry JD, Calle-Toro JS, et al. Shock index as a mortality predictor in patients with acute polytrauma. Journal of Acute Disease 2015;4(3):202–4.
9. Rau C-S, Wu S-C, Kuo S, et al. Prediction of massive transfusion in trauma patients with shock index, modified shock index, and age shock index. Int J Environ Res Public Health 2016;13(7):683.
10. Cannon CM, Braxton CC, Kling-Smith M, et al. Utility of the shock index in predicting mortality in traumatically injured patients. J Trauma 2009;67(6):1426–30.
11. Vandromme MJ, Griffin RL, Kerby JD, et al. Identifying risk for massive transfusion in the relatively normotensive patient: utility of the prehospital shock index. J Trauma 2011;70(2):384–90.
12. Lee E, Laberge J. Differential diagnosis of gastrointestinal bleeding. Tech Vasc Interv Radiol 2004;7:112–22.
13. El-Tawil AM. Trends on gastrointestinal bleeding and mortality: Where are we standing? World J Gastroenterol 2012;18(11):1154.
14. Jensen DM, Machicado GA. Diagnosis and treatment of severe hematochezia. Gastroenterology 1988;95(6):1569–74.
15. Zuckerman GR, Prakash C. Acute lower intestinal bleeding. Part I: Clinical presentation and diagnosis. Gastrointest Endosc 1998;48(6):606–16.
16. Reddick AD, Ronald J, Morrison WG. Intravenous fluid resuscitation: was Poiseuille right? Emerg Med J 2010;28(3):201–2.
17. Jennings LK, Watson S. Massive transfusion. Treasure Island (FL): StatPearls Publishing; 2019. Available at: https://www.ncbi.nlm.nih.gov/books/NBK499929/.
18. Fields JM, Piela NE, Au AK, et al. Risk factors associated with difficult venous access in adult ED patients. Am J Emerg Med 2014;32(10):1179–82.
19. Ngo AS, Oh JJ, Chen Y, et al. Intraosseous vascular access in adults using the EZ-IO in an emergency department. Int J Emerg Med 2009;2(3):155–60.
20. Burgert J. Intraosseous infusion of blood products and epinephrine in an adult patient in hemorrhagic shock. AANA J 2009;77:359–63.
21. Miller LJ, Philbeck TE, Montez D, et al. A new study of intraosseous blood for laboratory analysis. Arch Pathol Lab Med 2010;134(9):1253–60.
22. Villanueva C, Colomo A, Bosch A, et al. Transfusion strategies for acute upper gastrointestinal bleeding. N Engl J Med 2013;368:11–21.
23. Jairath V, Kahan BC, Gray A, et al. Restrictive versus liberal blood transfusion for acute upper gastrointestinal bleeding (TRIGGER): a pragmatic, open-label, cluster randomised feasibility trial. Lancet 2015;386(9989):137–44.
24. Ley EJ, Clond MA, Srour MK, et al. Emergency department crystalloid resuscitation of 1.5 l or more is associated with increased mortality in elderly and nonelderly trauma patients. J Trauma 2011;70(2):398–400.

25. Kaczynski J, Wilczynska M, Hilton J, et al. Impact of crystalloids and colloids on coagulation cascade during trauma resuscitation-a literature review. Emerg Med Health Care 2013;1(1):1.

26. Kettner SC, Kozek SA, Groetzner JP, et al. Effects of hypothermia on thrombelastography in patients undergoing cardiopulmonary bypass. Br J Anaesth 1998; 80(3):313–7.

27. Engström M, Schött U, Romner B, et al. Acidosis impairs the coagulation: a thromboelastographic study. J Trauma 2006;61(3):624–8.

28. American College of Surgeons, Committee on Trauma. Advanced trauma life support for doctors. 6th edition. Chicago: American College of Surgeons; 1997.

29. van Genderen ME, Engels N, Ralf J, et al. Early peripheral perfusion–guided fluid therapy in patients with septic shock. Am J Respir Crit Care Med 2015;191(4): 477–80.

30. Maltz GS, Siegel JE, Carson JL. Hematologic management of gastrointestinal bleeding. Gastroenterol Clin North Am 2000;29(1):169–87.

31. Hunt BJ, Allard S, Keeling D, et al. A practical guideline for the haematological management of major haemorrhage. Br J Haematol 2015;170(6):788–803.

32. Razzaghi A, Barkun AN. Platelet transfusion threshold in patients with upper gastrointestinal bleeding. J Clin Gastroenterol 2012;46(6):482–6.

33. Bolliger D, Görlinger K, Tanaka KA. Pathophysiology and treatment of coagulopathy in massive hemorrhage and hemodilution. Anesthesiology 2010;113(5): 1205–19.

34. Holcomb JB, Tilley BC, Baraniuk S, et al. Transfusion of plasma, platelets, and red blood cells in a 1:1:1 vs a 1:1:2 ratio and mortality in patients with severe trauma: the PROPPR randomized clinical trial. JAMA 2015;313(5):471–82.

35. O'Keeffe T. A massive transfusion protocol to decrease blood component use and costs. Arch Surg 2008;143(7):686.

36. Cole E, Weaver A, Gall L, et al. A decade of damage control resuscitation. Ann Surg 2019;1. https://doi.org/10.1097/sla.0000000000003657.

37. Gonzalez E, Moore EE, Moore HB, et al. Goal-directed hemostatic resuscitation of trauma-induced coagulopathy. Ann Surg 2016;263(6):1051–9.

38. Johansson PI, Stensballe J. REVIEWS: Hemostatic resuscitation for massive bleeding: the paradigm of plasma and platelets-a review of the current literature. Transfusion 2009;50(3):701–10.

39. Johansson PI, Sørensen AMM, Larsen CF, et al. Low hemorrhage-related mortality in trauma patients in a Level I trauma center employing transfusion packages and early thromboelastography-directed hemostatic resuscitation with plasma and platelets. Transfusion 2013;53(12):3088–99.

40. Harrison MF. The misunderstood coagulopathy of liver disease: a review for the acute setting. West J Emerg Med 2018;19(5):863–71.

41. Hans GA, Besser MW. The place of viscoelastic testing in clinical practice. Br J Haematol 2016;173(1):37–48.

42. Wikkelsø A, Wetterslev J, Møller AM, et al. Thromboelastography (TEG) or thromboelastometry (ROTEM) to monitor haemostatic treatment versus usual care in adults or children with bleeding. Cochrane Database Syst Rev 2018. https://doi.org/10.1002/14651858.cd007871.pub3.

43. Kumar M, Ahmad J, Maiwall R, et al. Thromboelastography-guided blood component use in patients with cirrhosis with nonvariceal bleeding: a randomized controlled trial. Hepatology 2019. https://doi.org/10.1002/hep.30794.

44. Spiezia L, Mazza A, Pelizzaro E, et al. Thromboelastometry-guided therapy of massive gastrointestinal bleeding in a 12-year old boy with severe Graft-versus-Host Disease. Blood Transfus 2014;13:1–3.
45. Besser M, Macdonald S. Acquired hypofibrinogenemia: current perspectives. J Blood Med 2016;7:217–25.
46. Leal-Noval SR, Casado M, Arellano-Orden V, et al. Administration of fibrinogen concentrate for refractory bleeding in massively transfused, non-trauma patients with coagulopathy: a retrospective study with comparator group. BMC Anesthesiol 2014;14(1). https://doi.org/10.1186/1471-2253-14-109.
47. Harr JN, Moore EE, Ghasabyan A, et al. Functional fibrinogen assay indicates that fibrinogen is critical in correcting abnormal clot strength following trauma. Shock 2013;1. https://doi.org/10.1097/shk.0b013e3182787122.
48. Barnes GD, Lucas E, Alexander GC, et al. National trends in ambulatory oral anticoagulant use. Am J Med 2015;128(12). https://doi.org/10.1016/j.amjmed.2015.05.044.
49. Kirley K, Qato DM, Kornfield R, et al. National Trends in oral anticoagulant use in the United States, 2007 to 2011. Circ Cardiovasc Qual Outcomes 2012;5(5): 615–21.
50. Tomaselli GF, Mahaffey KW, Cuker A, et al. 2017 ACC expert consensus decision pathway on management of bleeding in patients on oral anticoagulants. J Am Coll Cardiol 2017;70(24):3042–67.
51. Chai-Adisaksopha C, Hillis C, Isayama T, et al. Mortality outcomes in patients receiving direct oral anticoagulants: a systematic review and meta-analysis of randomized controlled trials. J Thromb Haemost 2015;13(11):2012–20.
52. Cuker A, Burnett A, Triller D, et al. Reversal of direct oral anticoagulants: Guidance from the Anticoagulation Forum. Am J Hematol 2019;94(6):697–709.
53. Hussain SS, Tyroch AH, Mukherjee D. Reversal of newer direct oral anticoagulant drugs (DOACs). Cardiovasc Hematol Agents Med Chem 2016;14:76.
54. Zakko L, Rustagi T, Douglas M, et al. No benefit from platelet transfusion for gastrointestinal bleeding in patients taking antiplatelet agents. Clin Gastroenterol Hepatol 2017;15(1):46–52.
55. Desborough MJR, Oakland KA, Landoni G, et al. Desmopressin for treatment of platelet dysfunction and reversal of antiplatelet agents: a systematic review and meta-analysis of randomized controlled trials. J Thromb Haemost 2017;15(2): 263–72.
56. Peter FW, Benkovic C, Muehlberger T, et al. Effects of desmopressin on thrombogenesis in aspirin-induced platelet dysfunction. Br J Haematol 2002;117(3): 658–63.
57. Weingart SD, Levitan RM. Preoxygenation and prevention of desaturation during emergency airway management. Ann Emerg Med 2012;59(3). https://doi.org/10.1016/j.annemergmed.2011.10.002.
58. Weingart SD. Preoxygenation, reoxygenation, and delayed sequence intubation in the emergency department. J Emerg Med 2011;40(6):661–7.
59. Bucher JT, Cooper JS. Bag mask ventilation (bag valve mask, BVM). Treasure Island (FL): StatPearls Publishing; 2019. Available at: https://www.ncbi.nlm.nih.gov/books/NBK441924/.
60. Lane S, Saunders D, Schofield A, et al. A prospective, randomised controlled trial comparing the efficacy of pre-oxygenation in the 20° head-up vs supine position. Anaesthesia 2005;60(11):1064–7.

61. Dixon BJ, Dixon JB, Carden JR, et al. Preoxygenation is more effective in the 25° head-up position than in the supine position in severely obese patients. Anesthesiology 2005;102(6):1110–5.

62. Khandelwal N, Khorsand S, Mitchell SH, et al. Head-elevated patient positioning decreases complications of emergent tracheal intubation in the ward and intensive care unit. Anesth Analg 2016;122(4):1101–7.

63. Stoecklein HH, Kelly C, Kaji AH, et al. Multicenter comparison of nonsupine versus supine positioning during intubation in the emergency department: a national emergency airway registry (NEAR) study. Acad Emerg Med 2019;26(10):1144–51.

64. Weingart SD, Trueger NS, Wong N, et al. Delayed sequence intubation: a prospective observational study. Ann Emerg Med 2015;65(4):349–55.

65. Suction Assisted Laryngoscopy and Airway Decontamination (SALAD). Available at: https://www.sscor.com/suction-assisted-laryngoscopy-and-airway-decontamination-salad. Accessed November 30, 2019.

66. Vlavianos P, Gimson AE, Westaby D, et al. Balloon tamponade in variceal bleeding: use and misuse. BMJ 1989;298(6681):1158.

67. Chong C-F. Esophageal rupture due to Sengstaken-Blakemore tube misplacement. World J Gastroenterol 2005;11(41):6563.

68. Chavez-Tapia NC, Barrientos-Gutierrez T, Tellez-Avila F, et al. Meta-analysis: antibiotic prophylaxis for cirrhotic patients with upper gastrointestinal bleeding - an updated Cochrane review. Aliment Pharmacol Ther 2011;34(5):509–18.

69. Jun C-H, Park C-H, Lee W-S, et al. Antibiotic prophylaxis using third generation cephalosporins can reduce the risk of early rebleeding in the first acute gastroesophageal variceal hemorrhage: a prospective randomized study. J Korean Med Sci 2006;21(5):883.

70. Lee YY. Role of prophylactic antibiotics in cirrhotic patients with variceal bleeding. World J Gastroenterol 2014;20(7):1790.

71. Gøtzsche P. Somatostatin analogues for acute bleeding oesophageal varices. Cochrane Database Syst Rev 2002. https://doi.org/10.1002/14651858.cd000193.

72. Sreedharan A, Martin J, Leontiadis GI, et al. Proton pump inhibitor treatment initiated prior to endoscopic diagnosis in upper gastrointestinal bleeding. Cochrane Database Syst Rev 2010. https://doi.org/10.1002/14651858.cd005415.pub3.

73. Leontiadis GI, Mcintyre L, Sharma VK, et al. Proton pump inhibitor treatment for acute peptic ulcer bleeding. Cochrane Database Syst Rev 2004. https://doi.org/10.1002/14651858.cd002094.pub2.

74. Chauncey JM, Wieters JS. Tranexamic acid. Treasure Island (FL): StatPearls Publishing; 2019. Available at: https://www.ncbi.nlm.nih.gov/books/NBK532909/.

75. Dunn CJ, Goa KL. Tranexamic acid: a review of its use in surgery and other indications. Drugs 1999;57:1005.

76. Bennett C, Klingenberg SL, Langholz E, et al. Tranexamic acid for upper gastrointestinal bleeding. Cochrane Database Syst Rev 2014. https://doi.org/10.1002/14651858.cd006640.pub3.

77. Roberts I, Shakur-Still H, Afolabi A, et al. Effects of a high-dose 24-h infusion of tranexamic acid on death and thromboembolic events in patients with acute gastrointestinal bleeding (HALT-IT): an international randomised, double-blind, placebo-controlled trial. The Lancet 2020;395(10241). https://doi.org/10.1016/S0140-6736(20)30848-5 NCT01713101.

78. Jung K, Moon W. Role of endoscopy in acute gastrointestinal bleeding in real clinical practice: An evidence-based review. World J Gastrointest Endosc 2019;11(2):68–83.

79. Spiegel BMR, Vakil NB, Ofman JJ. Endoscopy for acute nonvariceal upper gastrointestinal tract hemorrhage: is sooner better? Arch Intern Med 2001; 161(11):1393.
80. Laursen SB, Leontiadis GI, Stanley AJ, et al. Relationship between timing of endoscopy and mortality in patients with peptic ulcer bleeding: a nationwide cohort study. Gastrointest Endosc 2017;85(5). https://doi.org/10.1016/j.gie.2016.08.049.
81. Banares R, Albillos A, Rincon D, et al. Endoscopic treatment versus endoscopic plus pharmacologic treatment for variceal bleeding. J Hepatol 2002;36:44.
82. Jang BI. Lower gastrointestinal bleeding: is urgent colonoscopy necessary for all hematochezia? Clin Endosc 2013;46(5):476.
83. Strate LL, Gralnek IM. ACG clinical guideline: management of patients with acute lower gastrointestinal bleeding. Am J Gastroenterol 2016;111(4):459–74.

Updates in Traumatic Cardiac Arrest

William Teeter, MD, MS*, Daniel Haase, MD

KEYWORDS

- Cardiac arrest • Traumatic cardiac arrest • Pediatric trauma
- Cardiopulmonary resuscitation
- Resuscitative endovascular balloon occlusion of the aorta • Thoracotomy

KEY POINTS

- Traumatic cardiac arrest has persistently poor outcomes despite decades of research and refinement of treatment guidelines.
- Factors that predict survival in traumatic arrest include penetrating injury, short length of prehospital cardiopulmonary resuscitation, signs of life with emergency medical services or on arrival, cardiac motion on ultrasound, and pediatric patients.
- Emergency department thoracotomy can be performed in select situations that include pericardial tamponade, tension pneumothorax, and for external aortic cross-clamping to improve proximal tissue perfusion.
- Open chest compressions or cardiac massage may not be superior to closed chest compressions for traumatic arrest.
- Pediatric traumatic arrest patients remain poorly studied and represent a distinct clinical challenge.

INTRODUCTION

Trauma is among the leading causes of mortality and morbidity in industrialized nations.[1] Cardiac arrest caused by trauma historically carries a low likelihood of survival, with a high rate of permanent neurologic disability in survivors.[2,3] Approximately one-third of patients who sustain a traumatic cardiac arrest (TCA) die before arrival to a hospital.[4] Early studies suggested that patients with a TCA who had more than a few minutes of cardiopulmonary resuscitation (CPR) rarely survived.[5–7] As a result, some clinicians have advocated no resuscitation in most cases of TCA.[5–7] More recent studies have consistently reported that survival for TCA can be as high as 7%.[8–10] Pickens and colleagues reported that prehospital assessment of TCA was not reliable

Department of Emergency Medicine, University of Maryland, 22 South Greene Street, T1R51, Baltimore, MD 21201, USA
* Corresponding author.
E-mail address: william.teeter@som.umaryland.edu

Emerg Med Clin N Am 38 (2020) 891–901
https://doi.org/10.1016/j.emc.2020.06.009
0733-8627/20/© 2020 Elsevier Inc. All rights reserved.

emed.theclinics.com

and recommended that all patients with TCA should be transported to the emergency department (ED) for further assessment and intervention. This and additional studies have demonstrated survival in patients despite receiving treatment and CPR outside of the time window currently recommended in guidelines for TCA.[9,10] Furthermore, survival from TCA may be higher with select etiologies that are rapidly reversible, including tension pneumothorax and cardiac tamponade.[11] Unfortunately, there has been relatively little improvement in patients outcomes despite evidence that neurologic outcomes may be higher than previously thought.[1,12] TCA is a complex disease and presents unique challenges to the ED physician for evaluation and treatment. This article focuses on a review of criteria for termination of resuscitation, important etiologies of TCA, and important components of the ED resuscitation of patients with TCA.

WITHHOLDING AND TERMINATION OF RESUSCITATION

TCA is a distinct disease process from patients who present to the ED with out-of-hospital cardiac arrest (OHCA) from medical causes. Predictors of survival following TCA include the mechanism of TCA, location of injury, and signs of life (SOLs) on arrival.[9] Although it is important to recognize that TCA can be a survivable disease, it is equally important to identify predictors of mortality when resuscitative efforts should be discontinued, or even withheld. Various guidelines exist for withholding or terminating resuscitation in TCA.[13–15]

In 2003, The National Association of EMS Physicians and the American College of Surgeons Committee on Trauma (NAEMSP/ASCOT) consensus guidelines stated "termination of resuscitation (TOR) may be considered when there are no SOL and there is no return of spontaneous circulation despite appropriate field EMS treatment that includes minimally interrupted cardiopulmonary resuscitation (CPR)."[14] Similarly, The Eastern Association for the Surgery of Trauma recommends thoracotomy for penetrating injury to thorax, but favors using SOLs as a measure of futility in resuscitative efforts.[16] The Western Trauma Association recommends time-based criteria based on the mechanism of injury (blunt trauma with >10 minutes of prehospital CPR and penetrating trauma with >15 minutes of prehospital CPR) that cessation of resuscitation and withholding ED thoracotomy should be considered.[15]

In 2012, NAEMSP/ASCOT updated their recommendations and marked a difference between criteria for withholding resuscitation and termination of resuscitation (**Boxes 1** and **2**). They concluded "In the setting of cardiopulmonary arrest secondary to trauma from both blunt and penetrating mechanisms, an evidence guided protocol for withholding resuscitation includes clear evidence that the patient is dead, and a protocol for TOR should include the following elements: no evidence of SOL including no pulse, no respirations, no blood pressure; and no ROSC after initiation of resuscitation by the EMS providers, which should include minimally interrupted chest compressions."[13]

ETIOLOGY OF TRAUMATIC CARDIAC ARREST

The etiology of TCA is due to many causes, but can be categorized largely due to penetrating or blunt injury.[10] TCA patients can be further categorized according to location of injury (**Boxes 3**and **4**) with several injuries that are potentially life-saving, correctable causes of TCA, amenable to immediate treatment by the ED physician.

Although subject to large regional variation, especially in North America where penetrating injury is much more common than in other countries, hemorrhage remains a leading cause of traumatic death.[4] The mechanism and location of hemorrhage are both important predictors of outcome following TCA. The literature has shown that

---

Box 1
The National Association of EMS Physicians and the American College of Surgeons Committee on Trauma 2012 position on withholding resuscitation in traumatic cardiopulmonary arrest

- It is appropriate to withhold resuscitative efforts for certain trauma patients for whom death is the predictable outcome.
- Resuscitative efforts should be withheld for trauma patients with injuries that are obviously incompatible with life, such as decapitation or hemicorporectomy.
- Resuscitative efforts should be withheld for patients of either blunt or penetrating trauma when there is evidence of prolonged cardiac arrest, including rigor mortis or dependent lividity.
- Resuscitative efforts may be withheld for a blunt trauma patient who, on the arrival of EMS personnel, is found to be apneic, pulseless, and without organized electrocardiographic activity.
- Resuscitative efforts may be withheld for a penetrating trauma patient who, on arrival of EMS personnel, is found to be pulseless and apneic and there are no other SOLs, including spontaneous movement, electrocardiographic activity, and papillary response.
- When the mechanism of injury does not correlate with the clinical condition, suggesting a nontraumatic cause of cardiac arrest, standard resuscitative measures should be followed.

From Millin MG, Galvagno SM, Khandker SR, et al. Withholding and termination of resuscitation of adult cardiopulmonary arrest secondary to trauma: resource document to the joint NAEMSP-ACSCOT position statements. J Trauma Acute Care Surg 2013;75:459-67.

---

penetrating trauma is associated with better outcome than blunt mechanisms, but the location of the injury greatly affects survival.[16] In 2015, Seamon and colleagues published an evidence-based approach to TCA following a systematic review of the literature. In their analysis, the authors report that patients who sustained a penetrating injury had an overall survival of 10.6%, with approximately 90% of survivors neurologically intact. However, only 15.8% of stab wounds survived, and just 7.2% of gunshot wounds survived. This contrasts sharply with blunt injuries, where only 2.3% of patients survived. Of these patients with blunt injuries, only 59.4% remained neurologically intact.

Tension pneumothorax (tPTX) accounts for approximately 6% to 13% of cases of TCA[8,17] and must be quickly evaluated and treated. Tube thoracostomy can be lifesaving, as tPTX is a potentially correctable cause of TCA. A robust urban emergency medical services (EMS) system in Berlin identified that approximately half of TCAs required a chest tube (one-third for tPTX), but only approximately 13% received a chest tube prior to hospital arrival.[17] Huber-Wagner and colleagues[8] found that early, prehospital thoracostomy was associated with increased survival. Identifying and releasing tension pneumothorax as soon as possible should be among the highest priorities in TCA.

Pericardial tamponade is a potentially reversible cause of TCA. Rapid identification and treatment with thoracotomy, or needle decompression if thoracotomy is unavailable, is important for patient survival and is a priority in treatment of TCA. Davies and Lockey[18] of the London Air Ambulance found that by utilizing early thoracotomy by prehospital physicians, the etiology of all survivors (13) of 71 patients in TCA was pericardial tamponade. Eleven of these patients were discharged with good neurologic outcome. The rapid identification and evacuation of pericardial tamponade should be a high priority for emergency physicians.

Box 2

The National Association of EMS Physicians and the American College of Surgeons Committee on Trauma 2012 position on termination of resuscitation of traumatic cardiopulmonary arrest

- A principle focus of EMS treatment of trauma patients is efficient evacuation to definitive care, where major blood loss can be corrected. Resuscitative efforts should not prolong on-scene time.

- EMS systems should have protocols that allow EMS providers to terminate resuscitative efforts for certain adult patients in traumatic cardiopulmonary arrest.

- Termination of resuscitation (TOR) may be considered when there are no SOLs, and there is no ROSC despite appropriate field EMS treatment that includes minimally interrupted CPR.

- Protocols should require a specific interval of CPR that accompanies other resuscitative interventions. Past guidance has indicated that up to 15 minutes of CPR should be provided before resuscitative efforts are terminated, but the science in this regard remains unclear.

- TOR protocols should be accompanied by standard procedures to ensure appropriate management of the deceased patient in the field and adequate support services for the patient's family.

- Implementation of TOR protocols mandates active physician oversight.

- TOR protocols should include any locally specific clinical, environmental, or population-based situations for which the protocol is not applicable. TOR may be impractical after transport has been initiated.

- Further research is appropriate to determine the optimal duration of CPR before terminating resuscitative efforts.

From Millin MG, Galvagno SM, Khandker SR, et al. Withholding and termination of resuscitation of adult cardiopulmonary arrest secondary to trauma: resource document to the joint NAEMSP-ACSCOT position statements. J Trauma Acute Care Surg 2013;75:459-67.

KEY COMPONENTS OF EMERGENCY MEDICAL MANAGEMENT OF TRAUMATIC CARDIAC ARREST

Ultrasound

The use of ultrasound in the primary survey of trauma has been a mainstay for decades.[19,20] It continues to be a valuable adjunct for the initial assessment of a trauma patient, both for the identification of reversible causes of arrest and the assessment of cardiac function when considering whether to withhold or terminate resuscitation efforts.[21] Ultrasound examination of the heart in the setting of cardiac arrest is part of the focused abdominal sonography for trauma (FAST) examination, specifically to identify

---

Box 3

Injury patterns in traumatic cardiac arrest

Polytrauma

Exsanguination

Isolated traumatic brain injury

Thoracic trauma

Abdominal trauma

Other causes

Box 4	
Correctable causes of traumatic cardiac arrest and treatments	
Injury	**Treatment**
Pericardial tamponade	Thoracotomy/needle pericardiocentesis
Tension pneumothorax	Thoracostomy
Thoracic hemorrhage	Thoracotomy
Abdominal hemorrhage	Thoracotomy/REBOA
Extremity hemorrhage	Tourniquet application
Hypoxia	Definitive airway management

hemopericardium leading to cardiac tamponade, which accounts for 10% of TCA cases.[17]

Cardiac ultrasound can also help predict survival in patients with TCA. In a single-center study of 162 patients with TCA who received cardiac ultrasound and electrocardiogram (EKG) tracing found a 4.3% survival to hospital admission.[22] "Survival was higher for those with cardiac motion on ultrasound than for those without cardiac." Ultrasound cardiac motion predicted survival to hospital admission with 86% sensitivity, 91% specificity, 30% positive predictive value, and 99% negative predictive value.[22] Sensitivity was 100% for penetrating trauma and 75% for blunt trauma. The authors concluded that "cardiac ultrasound had a negative predictive value approaching 100% for survival to hospital admission. For patients with prolonged prehospital cardiopulmonary resuscitation, ultrasound evaluation of cardiac motion in pulseless patients with trauma may be a rapid way to help determine which patients have no chance of survival in the setting of lethal injuries, so that futile resuscitations can be stopped."[22]

As discussed previously, the rapid assessment for pneumothorax in TCA is a high priority. The eFAST examination (**Box 5**) has become standard practice in trauma, with a higher sensitivity than chest radiograph for identifying pneumothorax. The authors recommend that the eFAST examination start with the subxiphoid or parasternal views, quickly followed by intercostal views to identify tPTX, which must be quickly evaluated and treated. Although needle decompression is classically the first-line treatment for tPTX, problems with catheter depth[23] and insertion[24] limit its effectiveness and should always be followed by finger or tube thoracostomy.

Emergency Department Thoracotomy

A patient with TCA who arrives to the ED should immediately be assessed for SOLs, as well as a determination of the length of CPR, as these data points inform the decision whether to proceed with an ED thoracotomy (EDT). Early studies on EDT suggested that only 4% of patients with TCA who received an EDT survived neurologically intact. Importantly, survival was found to be higher for patients with a stab wound to the thorax with SOLs (23%) and 38% among moribund patients who showed some SOLs.[25–27] Guidelines have been developed to guide clinicians on the critical decision to perform an EDT.

Importantly, current guidelines differ slightly by organization on whether EDT may be beneficial (**Boxes 6** and **7**) The Eastern Association for the Surgery of Trauma strongly recommends that EDT be performed in any patient with SOLs after penetrating thoracic injury, but make weaker conditional recommendations for patients with SOLs after penetrating extrathoracic and blunt injuries, as well as those without SOLs after penetrating thoracic and extrathoracic injuries.[16] The Western Association

---

Box 5
Components of an extended focused abdominal sonography for trauma examination

Subcostal

Inferior vena cava

Right upper quadrant

Left upper quadrant

Pelvis
   Sagittal view
   Transverse view

Intercostal views (bilateral)

---

for the Surgery of Trauma currently recommends EDT for patients undergoing less than 10 minutes of prehospital CPR after blunt injury, less than 15 minutes of prehospital CPR following penetrating injury to the thorax, less than 5 minutes of prehospital CPR in patients following penetrating injury to the neck or extremity, and patients in profound refractory shock. The Eastern Guidelines also recommend against EDT in those without SOLs following blunt injury.[28] These guidelines have remained relatively constant, with most experts agreeing that EDT should be performed in those with SOLs, especially following penetrating injury, during prehospital transport or on arrival to the hospital.

Closed Chest Compressions Versus Open Cardiac Compression

During the initial phases of resuscitation following TCA, closed chest compressions are the most expedient means to provide some degree of circulation to the body and perfuse the myocardium and brain. However, EDT allows the clinician the option to perform open chest cardiac massage (OCCM). OCCM is hand-assisted cardiac

---

Box 6
Eastern Association for the surgery of trauma guidelines for resuscitative thoracotomy

Strong Recommendation:
   Pulseless patient presenting to ED with SOLs after penetrating thoracic injury

Conditional Recommendations:
   Pulseless patient presenting to ED without SOLs after penetrating thoracic injury (consider time without SOL in decision making)
   Pulseless patient presenting to ED with SOL after penetrating nonthoracic injury (consider location of injury in decision making)
   Pulseless patient presenting to ED without SOLs after penetrating nonthoracic injury (few patients may benefit, low quality evidence, and excludes isolated intracranial injury)
   Pulseless patient presenting to ED with SOLs after blunt injury (some patients may not wish to undergo EDT considering concomitant severe traumatic brain injury)

Recommendation Against:
   Pulseless patient presenting to ED without SOLs after blunt injury (most patients would not wish to undergo EDT considering concomitant severe traumatic brain injury and dismal outcomes)

From Seamon MJ, Haut ER, Van Arendonk K, et al. An evidence-based approach to patient selection for emergency department thoracotomy: A practice management guideline from the Eastern Association for the Surgery of Trauma. J Trauma Acute Care Surg 2015;79:159-73.

Box 7
Western Trauma Association guidelines for resuscitative thoracotomy

Penetrating injury with CPR less than 15 minutes

Profound refractory shock (CPR with SOLs or systolic blood pressure <60 mm Hg)

Blunt injury with CPR <10 minutes

Data from Burlew CC, Moore EE, Moore FA, et al. Western Trauma Association critical decisions in trauma: resuscitative thoracotomy. J Trauma Acute Care Surg 2012;73:1359-63.

---

compression and is thought to augment or stimulate cardiac compression, improve filling of the heart, and improve perfusion to distal tissues. Some animal data suggest OCCM may be superior to closed chest compression (CCC) following nontraumatic cardiac arrest.[29] However, recent clinical data in TCA patients showed no difference in patient-oriented outcomes or end-tidal CO_2 ($EtCO_2$) in those who received CCC compared with those who received OCCM.[30] Although $EtCO_2$ has been shown to predict survival in patients with OHCA, it has been studied relatively little in the trauma population.[31,32] A recent study found that combining CCC with resuscitative endovascular balloon occlusion of the aorta (REBOA) in the setting of TCA resulted in "higher EtCO2 and cardiac compression fraction before and after aortic occlusion (AO) compared with patients who receive OCCM."[33] These data suggest that cardiac compressions following TCA utilizing endovascular adjuncts may benefit from more aggressive study.

Resuscitative Balloon Occlusion of the Aorta

The terms EDT and resuscitative thoracotomy (RT) are often used interchangeably. This can lead to confusion when discussing the use of REBOA in TCA. These are distinct procedures with similar, but not identical, indications. EDT is the term used for a thoracotomy performed for the reasons previously described. RT is a thoracotomy performed for the purpose of external cross-clamping of the aorta. Regardless of the method, the use of aortic cross-clamping in the setting of TCA is for the temporization of distal hemorrhage, supplementing cerebral and coronary perfusion by reduction of the vascular bed that requires perfusion by CPR or native cardiac output.

Recent small studies have suggested a benefit in the use of REBOA in TCA. One study found that mean cardiac compression fraction was significantly improved in TCA patients who received REBOA compared with patients who underwent RT. REBOA was also associated with shorter pauses in cardiac compression.[34] However, this study was not powered for patient-oriented outcomes. A follow-up study found that $EtCO_2$ was significantly improved among a similar population of patients who received REBOA.[33] This suggests that although chest compressions in a hypovolemic patient may be of limited benefit, CCC with or without aortic occlusion may carry some patient benefit versus OCCM.

In 2013, the American Association for the Surgery of Trauma (AAST) created the Aortic Occlusion in Resuscitation for Trauma and Acute Care Surgery (AORTA) multi-institutional registry to more rigorously study REBOA and RT. A recent interim analysis of the database has shown an improvement in survival beyond the ED and improved survival to discharge in patients who receive REBOA compared with RT. Eighty-five percent of those discharged had a Glasgow Coma Scale score of 15. Although the survival benefit in those who did not require CPR before aortic occlusion was more pronounced, there was no survival benefit in those who arrived after prehospital arrest or in arrest. Patients who did not require CPR but presented with a systolic blood pressure less than 90 mm Hg had a significantly higher survival beyond the ED and to discharge with REBOA. The authors concluded "overall, REBOA can confer a survival benefit over RT, particularly in patients not requiring CPR. Considerable additional study is required to definitively recommend REBOA for specific subsets of injured patients." These preliminary data suggest a potential benefit of REBOA in the setting of TCA, but outside of a few high-volume centers, the data do not support widespread adoption of REBOA for this indication. It remains an active area of discussion and investigation at the time of publication of this article.[35]

PEDIATRIC PATIENTS

Pediatric TCA is a difficult issue for the emergency physician. This is further complicated by the lack of clear guidelines for this population. Zwingmann and colleagues[1] showed that children with TCA have a higher survival rate compared with adults, but suffered from worse neurologic outcomes. In this systematic review, it was unclear why blunt injury predicted better outcomes for pediatric patients with TCA, or why children suffer worse neurologic outcomes. Some have suggested that the etiology of TCA in children is respiratory compromise rather than exsanguination, and this may represent different pathology from adult patients.[36] There is no clear consensus on the resuscitation of pediatric populations in TCA. Most guidelines and recommendations are derived from data from primarily adult populations,[13,16,28] limiting their use in the pediatric TCA patient.

NOVEL ADVANCES

Extracorporeal resuscitation is an active area of research in TCA. Selective aortic arch perfusion (SAAP) has been shown to salvage a TCA swine model in 90% of animals. This technique has been studied for decades and is close to active clinical trials, but remains an investigative technique.[37] Extracorporeal preservation and resuscitation is currently being evaluated in clinical trials and has shown a survival benefit in dogs compared with a standard treatment model of TCA. However, this technique requires substantial resources to implement and will likely be outside the capabilities of most centers.[38] Extracorporeal life support is becoming more frequent in the setting of trauma, but is primarily using venovenous support for complications following trauma, including TCA. Use of ECLS as a primary adjunct for TCA remains exceedingly rare.[39] Extracorporeal membrane oxygenation (ECMO) is discussed in a separate article, "ECMO in the Emergency Department," in this issue.

SUMMARY

The evaluation and treatment of traumatic cardiac arrest remains a challenge to the emergency medicine provider. Guidelines have establish criteria for the patients who can benefit from treatment and resuscitation versus those who will likely not survive. Patient factors that predict survival are penetrating injury, SOLs with EMS or on arrival to the Emergency Department, short length of prehospital CPR, cardiac motion on ultrasound, pediatric patients, and those with reversible causes including pericardial tamponade and tension pneumothorax. Newer technologies such as REBOA, SAAP, and ECMO may improve outcomes, but remain primarily investigational.

DISCLOSURE

The authors have nothing to disclose.

REFERENCES

1. Zwingmann J, Mehlhorn AT, Hammer T, et al. Survival and neurologic outcome after traumatic out-of-hospital cardiopulmonary arrest in a pediatric and adult population: a systematic review. Crit Care 2012;16:R117.
2. Martin SK, Shatney CH, Sherck JP, et al. Blunt trauma patients with prehospital pulseless electrical activity (PEA): poor ending assured. J Trauma 2002;53: 876–80 [discussion: 880–1].
3. Battistella FD, Nugent W, Owings JT, et al. Field triage of the pulseless trauma patient. Arch Surg 1999;134:742–5 [discussion: 745–6].
4. Sauaia A, Moore FA, Moore EE, et al. Epidemiology of trauma deaths: a reassessment. J Trauma 1995;38:185–93.
5. Rosemurgy AS, Norris PA, Olson SM, et al. Prehospital traumatic cardiac arrest: the cost of futility. J Trauma 1993;35:468–73 [discussion: 473–4].
6. Mattox KL, Feliciano DV. Role of external cardiac compression in truncal trauma. J Trauma 1982;22:934–6.
7. Stockinger ZT, McSwain NE Jr. Additional evidence in support of withholding or terminating cardiopulmonary resuscitation for trauma patients in the field. J Am Coll Surg 2004;198:227–31.
8. Huber-Wagner S, Lefering R, Qvick M, et al. Outcome in 757 severely injured patients with traumatic cardiorespiratory arrest. Resuscitation 2007;75:276–85.
9. Lockey D, Crewdson K, Davies G. Traumatic cardiac arrest: who are the survivors? Ann Emerg Med 2006;48:240–4.
10. Pickens JJ, Copass MK, Bulger EM. Trauma patients receiving CPR: predictors of survival. J Trauma 2005;58:951–8.
11. Sherren PB, Reid C, Habig K, et al. Algorithm for the resuscitation of traumatic cardiac arrest patients in a physician-staffed helicopter emergency medical service. Crit Care 2013;17:308.
12. Barnard EBG, Sandbach DD, Nicholls TL, et al. Prehospital determinants of successful resuscitation after traumatic and non-traumatic out-of-hospital cardiac arrest. Emerg Med J 2019;36:333–9.
13. Millin MG, Galvagno SM, Khandker SR, et al. Withholding and termination of resuscitation of adult cardiopulmonary arrest secondary to trauma: resource document to the joint NAEMSP-ACSCOT position statements. J Trauma Acute Care Surg 2013;75:459–67.
14. National Association of EMSP, American College of Surgeons Committee on Trauma. Termination of resuscitation for adult traumatic cardiopulmonary arrest. Prehosp Emerg Care 2012;16:571.
15. Moore EE, Knudson MM, Burlew CC, et al. Defining the limits of resuscitative emergency department thoracotomy: a contemporary Western Trauma Association perspective. J Trauma 2011;70:334–9.
16. Seamon MJ, Haut ER, Van Arendonk K, et al. An evidence-based approach to patient selection for emergency department thoracotomy: a practice management guideline from the Eastern Association for the Surgery of Trauma. J Trauma Acute Care Surg 2015;79:159–73.
17. Kleber C, Giesecke MT, Lindner T, et al. Requirement for a structured algorithm in cardiac arrest following major trauma: epidemiology, management errors, and preventability of traumatic deaths in Berlin. Resuscitation 2014;85:405–10.

18. Davies GE, Lockey DJ. Thirteen survivors of prehospital thoracotomy for penetrating trauma: a prehospital physician-performed resuscitation procedure that can yield good results. J Trauma 2011;70:E75–8.

19. Asher WM, Parvin S, Virgillo RW, et al. Echographic evaluation of splenic injury after blunt trauma. Radiology 1976;118:411–5.

20. Rozycki GS, Ochsner MG, Schmidt JA, et al. A prospective study of surgeon-performed ultrasound as the primary adjuvant modality for injured patient assessment. J Trauma 1995;39:492–8 [discussion: 498–500].

21. Truhlar A, Deakin CD, Soar J, et al. European Resuscitation Council Guidelines for Resuscitation 2015: Section 4. Cardiac arrest in special circumstances. Resuscitation 2015;95:148–201.

22. Cureton EL, Yeung LY, Kwan RO, et al. The heart of the matter: utility of ultrasound of cardiac activity during traumatic arrest. J Trauma Acute Care Surg 2012;73:102–10.

23. Clemency BM, Tanski CT, Rosenberg M, et al. Sufficient catheter length for pneumothorax needle decompression: a meta-analysis. Prehosp Disaster Med 2015;30:249–53.

24. Mistry N, Bleetman A, Roberts KJ. Chest decompression during the resuscitation of patients in prehospital traumatic cardiac arrest. Emerg Med J 2009;26:738–40.

25. Branney SW, Moore EE, Feldhaus KM, et al. Critical analysis of two decades of experience with postinjury emergency department thoracotomy in a regional trauma center. J Trauma 1998;45:87–94 [discussion: 94–5].

26. Velmahos GC, Degiannis E, Souter I, et al. Outcome of a strict policy on emergency department thoracotomies. Arch Surg 1995;130:774–7.

27. Esposito TJ, Jurkovich GJ, Rice CL, et al. Reappraisal of emergency room thoracotomy in a changing environment. J Trauma 1991;31:881–5 [discussion: 885-7].

28. Burlew CC, Moore EE, Moore FA, et al. Western Trauma Association critical decisions in trauma: resuscitative thoracotomy. J Trauma Acute Care Surg 2012;73:1359–63.

29. Benson DM, O'Neil B, Kakish E, et al. Open-chest CPR improves survival and neurologic outcome following cardiac arrest. Resuscitation 2005;64:209–17.

30. Bradley MJ, Bonds BW, Chang L, et al. Open chest cardiac massage offers no benefit over closed chest compressions in patients with traumatic cardiac arrest. J Trauma Acute Care Surg 2016;81:849–54.

31. Levin PD, Pizov R. End-tidal carbon dioxide and outcome of out-of-hospital cardiac arrest. N Engl J Med 1997;337:1694–5.

32. Kolar M, Krizmaric M, Klemen P, et al. Partial pressure of end-tidal carbon dioxide successful predicts cardiopulmonary resuscitation in the field: a prospective observational study. Crit Care 2008;12:R115.

33. Teeter WA, Bradley MJ, Romagnoli A, et al. Treatment effect or effective treatment? Cardiac compression fraction and end-tidal carbon dioxide are higher in patients resuscitative endovascular balloon occlusion of the aorta compared with resuscitative thoracotomy and open-chest cardiac massage. Am Surg 2018;84:1691–5.

34. Teeter W, Romagnoli A, Wasicek P, et al. Resuscitative endovascular balloon occlusion of the aorta improves cardiac compression fraction versus resuscitative thoracotomy in patients in traumatic arrest. Ann Emerg Med 2018;72:354–60.

35. Bulger EM, Perina DG, Qasim Z, et al. Clinical use of resuscitative endovascular balloon occlusion of the aorta (REBOA) in civilian trauma systems in the USA, 2019: a joint statement from the American College of Surgeons Committee on Trauma, the American College of Emergency Physicians, the National

Association of Emergency Medical Services Physicians and the National Association of Emergency Medical Technicians. Trauma Surg Acute Care Open 2019;4: e000376.

36. Perron AD, Sing RF, Branas CC, et al. Predicting survival in pediatric trauma patients receiving cardiopulmonary resuscitation in the prehospital setting. Prehosp Emerg Care 2001;5:6–9.

37. Barnard EBG, Manning JE, Smith JE, et al. A comparison of selective aortic arch perfusion and resuscitative endovascular balloon occlusion of the aorta for the management of hemorrhage-induced traumatic cardiac arrest: a translational model in large swine. PLoS Med 2017;14:e1002349.

38. Wu X, Drabek T, Kochanek PM, et al. Induction of profound hypothermia for emergency preservation and resuscitation allows intact survival after cardiac arrest resulting from prolonged lethal hemorrhage and trauma in dogs. Circulation 2006; 113:1974–82.

39. Swol J, Brodie D, Napolitano L, et al. Indications and outcomes of extracorporeal life support in trauma patients. J Trauma Acute Care Surg 2018;84:831–7.

Resuscitating the Crashing Pregnant Patient

Kami M. Hu, MD[a,b,*], Aleta S. Hong, MD[b]

KEYWORDS

- Critical care • Pregnancy • Obstetrics • Maternal resuscitation • Respiratory failure
- Shock

KEY POINTS

- The physiologic changes of pregnancy can mask severe illness and early shock.
- Early specialist consultation is crucial. If needed, transfer for obstetric or pediatric specialist care should be initiated immediately or as soon as the patient is stabilized.
- The pregnant patient has an inherently difficult airway and desaturates quickly because of decreased pulmonary reserve and increased oxygen consumption.
- Most medications used in standard resuscitation can be used in pregnancy.
- Remember the 5-minute rule for perimortem cesarean section and be prepared to deliver quickly in the event of a maternal cardiac arrest.

INTRODUCTION

Critical illness in pregnancy is rare[1] and may be attributed either to an independent cause of illness that is complicated by pregnancy or to a cause associated with the pregnancy itself (**Table 1**). Caring for an unstable obstetric patient is a stressful clinical situation for the emergency physician, who must consider the welfare of two patients because the fetus is also at risk. An understanding of the physiologic changes associated with pregnancy and a solid knowledge base for treating the critically ill pregnant patient can improve care in this high-risk population.

PHYSIOLOGIC CHANGES OF PREGNANCY

Pregnancy is a dynamic state. The placenta not only connects the maternal and fetal circulation but is itself an endocrine organ, and the hormones of pregnancy set the

---

[a] Department of Emergency Medicine, University of Maryland School of Medicine, 110 South Paca Street, 6th Floor, Suite 200, Baltimore, MD 21201, USA; [b] Department of Internal Medicine, University of Maryland School of Medicine, 110 South Paca Street, 6th Floor, Suite 200, Baltimore, MD 21201, USA
* Corresponding author.
E-mail address: khu@som.umaryland.edu
Twitter: @kwhomd (K.M.H.); @hong_aleta (A.S.H.)

Emerg Med Clin N Am 38 (2020) 903–917
https://doi.org/10.1016/j.emc.2020.06.010
0733-8627/20/© 2020 Elsevier Inc. All rights reserved.
emed.theclinics.com

Table 1
Most commonly identified causes of pregnancy-related morbidity and mortality in the United States

Etiology	Percentage
Cardiovascular conditions	15.7
Sepsis/infection	12.5
Hemorrhage	11
Cardiomyopathy	11
Pulmonary embolism	9
Cerebrovascular accident	7.7
Preeclampsia/eclampsia	6.9
Amniotic fluid embolism	5.6
Other noncardiovascular causes	13.9
Unknown	6.4

Data from [CDC Pregnancy Mortality Surveillance System. Causes of pregnancy-related death in the United States: 2011-2016. 2019. Available at: https://www.cdc.gov/reproductivehealth/maternal-mortality/pregnancy-mortality-surveillancesystem.htm/www.cdc.gov/reproductivehealth/maternalinfanthealth/pregnancy-mortality-surveilance-system.htm#causes. Accessed December 1, 2019].

stage for the numerous physical changes undergone by the pregnant patient (**Table 2**). The gestational age of the fetus aids understanding of expected physiologic changes and is estimated using point-of-care ultrasound (POCUS) if unknown.

UTEROPLACENTAL PHYSIOLOGY

The two maternal uterine arteries provide approximately 700 mL/min of uteroplacental blood flow. The placental vessels have no autoregulatory capability and are maximally dilated because of circulating progesterone and nitric oxide, leaving maternal blood pressure as the primary factor in uteroplacental blood flow. Maternal hypotension, uterine contractions, alkalemia, and vasoconstricting agents (vasopressors, nicotine, cocaine) decrease uteroplacental blood flow.[8]

Transplacental gas exchange is dependent on a maternal-fetal concentration gradient; maternal respiratory alkalosis facilitates diffusion of fetal CO_2 into maternal circulation for removal. It also increases maternal hemoglobin oxygen saturation, whereas fetal hemoglobin's stronger affinity for oxygen, in comparison with maternal hemoglobin, enables oxygen transfer to the fetus.[8,9]

In the setting of acidemia the hemoglobin-oxygenation curve shifts to the right, decreasing hemoglobin-oxygen binding and decreasing oxygenation of distal tissues. In fetal hemoglobin, which already exists in a hypoxemic environment, lack of sufficient oxygen delivery quickly proceeds to anaerobic metabolism and metabolic acidosis, which in turn can lead to bradycardia and poor fetal perfusion.[9]

INITIAL STEPS
Identify Illness

Because the physiologic changes of pregnancy can mask illness and early shock, it is important to assess clinical signs of end-organ perfusion, such as mental status, capillary refill, and urine output. Physicians should notice subtle changes in vital signs and maintain a lower threshold for aggressive care, because these patients are at risk for

Table 2
Physiologic changes of pregnancy

System	Change	Clinical Relevance
Cardiovascular	↓ Systemic vascular resistance ↑ Heart rate (15–20 bpm above baseline) ↑ Cardiac output (by 30%–50%) Aortocaval compression by the uterus (≈20 wk)	↓ Blood pressure (nadirs at 24–28 wk) Supine hypotension syndrome
Respiratory	↑ Mucosal vascularity and edema Upward shift of diaphragm, decreased FRC ↑ Respiratory rate ↑ Tidal volume (caused by widening of chest wall)	Difficult airway (narrower, distorted, friable) ↓ Functional reserve and rapid desaturations Physiologic respiratory alkalosis
Renal	↑ Renin-angiotensin-aldosterone system activity ↑ Renal blood flow and glomerular filtration rate ↑ Bicarbonate secretion	↑ Total body water and circulating volume (1.5–2L) ↓ "Normal" creatinine, ↑ drug clearance Relatively normal pH
Hematologic	↑ Erythropoiesis <↑ total plasma volume ↑ White blood cell count ↑ Circulating coagulation factors ↓ Fibrinolysis	Physiologic relative anemia Hypercoagulable state
Gastrointestinal	↓ Gastric emptying/gastrointestinal motility ↓ Lower esophageal sphincter tone	Increased risk of vomiting and aspiration

FRC, functional residual capacity. *Data from* Refs.[2–7]

rapid decompensation and have narrower targets for optimal oxygenation and ventilation.

Call Consultants

As soon as severe maternal illness is recognized it is crucial to involve the obstetric team, particularly if the gestational age of the fetus has reached the age of viability, typically considered to be 24 weeks. It is similarly prudent to notify the neonatal intensive care team so that they can prepare for a precipitous delivery. In cases where the mother has comorbid chronic disease or a high-risk pregnancy, or there is fetal distress, emergent delivery may be required. These considerations are indications for urgent transfer, once the patient is stabilized, if there is no specialized obstetric or neonatal care available in-house.

Immediate Resuscitation

A sick pregnant patient with abnormal vital signs requires at least two large-bore intravenous (IV) lines. If IV access cannot be promptly achieved, intraosseous access should be pursued. Around 20 weeks of gestation and beyond, the gravid uterus can compress the inferior vena cava when the patient is lying supine, therefore IV, intraosseous, and if required, central lines, should be placed above the diaphragm to avoid a delay in fluids, blood products, and medications reaching central circulation.[10]

Similarly, supine positioning should be avoided in any patient where aortocaval compression and subsequent decrease in venous return, cardiac output, and blood pressure by an enlarged uterus is a reasonable concern. In the setting of maternal hypotension, immediately displace the uterus by moving the patient into the left lateral decubitus position or providing at least 15° of leftward tilt.[11–13] If the patient is unable to be repositioned, the uterus should be displaced leftward manually.

Any obstetric patient with hypoxia should be placed immediately on supplemental oxygen to maintain a goal oxygen saturation of greater than 95% while steps are taken to provide the patient with the additional respiratory support needed.

Specific Considerations for the Fetus

Continuous fetal heart rate and tocometry monitoring should be performed in all pregnancies beyond 24 weeks, with consideration given to continuous monitoring in pregnancy beyond 20 weeks. If cardiotocometry monitoring is unavailable, POCUS should be used for regular evaluation of fetal heart rate.

In preterm deliveries the administration of antenatal corticosteroids to the mother is strongly associated with decreased fetal morbidity and mortality.[14] The American College of Obstetricians and Gynecologists recommends administration of either dexamethasone 6 mg or betamethasone 12 mg to all pregnant women between 24 and 34 weeks of gestation who are at substantial risk of preterm delivery within the next 7 days. Administration in the previable period, between 23 and 24 weeks, can be considered.[14]

MANAGEMENT OF CRITICAL ILLNESS
Acute Respiratory Failure

The pregnant patient with respiratory illness is at risk of rapid decompensation and hypoxemia caused by increased oxygen use and decreased pulmonary reserve. Intubation of the pregnant patient presents a significant risk because of the physiologic changes of pregnancy (see **Table 2**) and should be performed in the most controlled setting possible. To this end, it is prudent to have a low threshold to intubate the pregnant patient with respiratory distress, because a crash intubation is less than ideal and even slight maternal hypoxia puts the fetus at risk.[5,9] Still, there remains a role for noninvasive ventilation in pregnant patients who may not yet require intubation. Although evidence regarding the use of noninvasive ventilation modalities in pregnancy is limited, a few case reports and data on its use in nonpregnant patients indicate that high-flow nasal cannula is a suitable option for obstetric patients with mild to moderate respiratory distress who do not require significant ventilatory support.[15–17] Although noninvasive positive pressure ventilation has been historically avoided in pregnant patients because of concerns of aspiration, there are several case reports of successful use and its initiation is reasonable in alert pregnant patients who are protecting their airway.[18] As in nonobstetric patients, it is important to monitor the patient's status because delays to intubation when needed are associated with worsened outcomes.

When preparing for intubation, ensuring appropriate patient positioning and peri-intubation oxygenation is key. To decrease the chances of desaturation, preoxygenate and provide apneic oxygenation via nasal cannula,[19,20] and keep the patient's gravid uterus off of the diaphragm by maintaining them in reverse Trendelenburg or positioned with the head of bed slightly elevated.[19,20] Limit ventilation with a bag-valve mask if possible, to prevent overdistention of the stomach and increased chance of aspiration.

The airway of a pregnant patient is more likely to be difficult, with narrowing and landmark distortion caused by edema and a high risk of bleeding caused by increased vascularity and friability.[2] The most experienced emergency clinician should intubate, use a smaller endotracheal tube to improve chances of first-pass success, and should have clear backup plans understood by the entire team to reduce the risk of complications. Nasotracheal intubation is not recommended unless absolutely necessary because of likelihood of epistaxis and secondary obscuration of the vocal cords.

Ventilator settings

As in the nonpregnant population, the maintenance of lung-protective ventilator settings including a plateau pressure less than 30 mm Hg, higher positive end-expiratory pressure strategies to maintain a driving pressure less than 15 mm Hg, and avoidance of unnecessary levels of fraction of inspired oxygen (FIO_2) remains key.[21–24]

The oxygenation goals in pregnancy are higher than in the nonpregnant population. Emergency clinicians should target a goal maternal PaO_2 of greater than 70 mm Hg, corresponding to a saturation of greater than 95%, because levels less than 60 mm Hg are associated with fetal hypoxemia.[25] As with obese patients, a slightly higher positive end-expiratory pressure may be needed to account for upward pressure on the diaphragm and increased atelectasis.

As opposed to the permissive hypercapnia widely accepted in the general population,[26] the goal in pregnancy is an average $PaCO_2$ of 30 mm Hg (**Table 3**).[4,5,20] This lower $PaCO_2$ level preserves the maternal-fetal CO_2 gradient and the appropriate level of hemoglobin-oxygen affinity.[9,20] Although lung-protective tidal volumes of 6 to 8 mL/kg of ideal body weight have become standard in ventilated patients, in pregnant patients not suffering from acute respiratory distress syndrome (ARDS), relative liberalization of tidal volumes may be reasonable as long as not at the expense of higher plateau pressures.[21] Use of sedation and even paralytics to achieve ventilator synchrony may be required in patients with severe hypoxia, hypercarbia, bronchospasm, or ARDS.[21,22]

In the intubated obstetric patient with a persistent PaO_2 less than 70 mm Hg or PaO_2:FIO_2 ratio less than 150 despite appropriate settings and therapy, early referral should be made for potential venovenous extracorporeal membrane oxygenation (ECMO).[27] Of note, proning has successfully been performed in pregnant patients with ARDS,[28] and may be worth initiating in severe refractory hypoxemia if there is a delay to intensive care unit or outside hospital transfer.

Table 3 Arterial blood gas changes in pregnancy		
Arterial Blood Gas Measurement	Nonpregnant Mean ± SD	Pregnant Mean ± SD
pH	7.43 ± 0.02	7.45 ± 0.02
PaO_2 (mm Hg)	93 ± 9	98.5 ± 10
$PaCO_2$ (mm Hg)	40 ± 2.5	32 ± 3
Serum HCO_2 (mEq/L)	25.3 ± 1.2	19.9 ± 1.3

Data from [McAuliffe F, Kametas N, Krampl E, et al. Blood gases in pregnancy at sea level and at high altitude. BJOG 2001;108:980-5].

Medications

Selecting appropriate medications for the critically ill obstetric patient is daunting because most commonly used medications cross the placenta and are not well studied in pregnancy. It is important to keep in mind that resuscitating the mother optimizes fetal status and that in the limited studies that exist, most sedatives and resuscitative medications have not been demonstrated to have long-term fetal effects.[29,30] In the event of a precipitous delivery, it is key to inform the neonatal care team of the medications administered to the mother for appropriate support of the neonate.

Use of etomidate for rapid sequence induction has been associated with transient (6 hour) decreases in neonatal cortisol levels without clinical effect[31] and therefore could be considered safe, but effects of its repeated or prolonged use has not been studied. However, the use of propofol during pregnancy is well-studied. It freely crosses the placenta but overall is considered to be safe without teratogenic effects, with caveats in relation to the side effect of lowering maternal blood pressure. In higher doses it may have short-term effects on the fetus.[29,30] Although controlled studies on the fetal effects of dexmedetomidine are lacking, multiple case series and reports have demonstrated no adverse effects in human pregnancy, it has minimal uteroplacental transfer to the fetus, and is generally considered to be safe for use.[30,32] Benzodiazepines are not ideal as first-line agents unless there is another indication, such as seizure or alcohol withdrawal syndrome, because they are known to cause respiratory depression, withdrawal symptoms, and floppy baby syndrome in the neonate.[29,30] Although ketamine was used in pregnancy before the availability of neuroaxial anesthesia, and low doses may be safe, there are conflicting data regarding potential fetal neurotoxic effects, and widespread use at this time is not recommended (**Table 4**).[33]

The commonly used paralytic agents succinylcholine, vecuronium, rocuronium, and cisatracurium are used in pregnancy. All have been noted to cross the placenta, although in small quantities that are proportional to doses given to the mother. For the purposes of rapid sequence induction, a longer-acting paralytic, such as rocuronium, may be preferred because it allows the clinician more time to manage a difficult airway. However, shorter acting neuromuscular blockade with succinylcholine may be preferred if delivery of the fetus is imminent.[30]

With respect to pain management, opioids are used as needed with the understanding that they may cause withdrawal symptoms and respiratory depression in an infant who has had prolonged exposure in utero. Nonsteroidal anti-inflammatory drugs must be avoided to prevent miscarriage, malformations, and premature closure of the fetal patent ductus arteriosus.[34]

Circulatory Shock

Despite the relative hypotension of pregnancy, hypotension should not be presumed to be normal, especially in the third trimester. If possible, a comparison of blood pressures at a patient's obstetric clinic visits and current presentation may be helpful. Management of hypotension should be tailored as soon as possible to the underlying cause. Stabilization of undifferentiated shock may be initiated with IV crystalloids, but it is crucial to limit dilutional coagulopathy in hemorrhage and overload in cardiogenic shock. Even in sepsis, the generally recommended 30 mL/kg of IV crystalloid[35] may be too much given lower colloidal pressures in pregnancy. The Society for Maternal-Fetal Medicine recommends starting with 1 to 2 L and transitioning quickly to vasopressors if the patient does not seem to be fluid responsive.[36] Hemorrhage should be managed with blood products rather than crystalloids and is specifically discussed next.

Table 4	
Commonly used medications for intubation and sedation	
Sedative Agent	Use in Pregnancy
Etomidate	RSI only
Propofol	Yes
Dexmedetomidine	Yes
Benzodiazepines	If necessary
Ketamine	Not advised

RSI, rapid sequence induction.

A mean arterial pressure greater than 65 mm Hg is a good general goal, although slightly lower mean arterial pressure may be tolerable in pregnant women if end-organ perfusion is not compromised and the fetal heart tracing is reassuring.[36] Although there is the possibility of uterine vessel vasoconstriction with the use of vasopressors or inotropes, the emergency physician should not be afraid to initiate these therapies, because without adequate maternal perfusion fetal hypoxemia and acidosis occurs.[9]

Although studies comparing norepinephrine with other vasopressors in pregnancy are limited, it has been demonstrated to be safe[37] and is recommended as the first-line vasopressor in pregnancy-associated sepsis.[36] The use of ephedrine and phenylephrine in pregnant patients is well-documented, generally in the setting of reversing hypotension because of spinal anesthesia.[38] Both are considered as adjunctive vasopressors. Phenylephrine has more recently been favored over ephedrine because of a lower risk of fetal acidosis,[38,39] but its potential effects of maternal bradycardia and lower cardiac output may limit its utility in critical illness. Finally, vasopressin is used if needed but carries the theoretic risk of stimulating contractions via its action on myometrial oxytocin and vasopressin receptors and is not recommended as a sole or first-line agent.[36,40]

There are no studies comparing inotropes in pregnancy, but cardiogenic shock should be treated with an inotropic agent, preferably dobutamine.[36,40,41] Depending on the underlying cause, the patient with profound cardiogenic shock on maximum medical therapy should be referred for potential intra-aortic balloon pump, mechanical circulatory assist device (eg, Impella, Abiomed, Danvers, MA), or venoarterial ECMO, because there are reports of pregnant patients doing well on these therapies.[42,43] A multidisciplinary team should determine the best course of action for the patient and fetus. Depending on circumstances, imminent delivery may be advisable, and for any procedural therapies it is crucial to consult the appropriate clinicians early so as to not delay care.

CRITICAL ILLNESS SPECIFIC TO PREGNANCY
Peripartum Hemorrhage

Peripartum hemorrhage is common and a major contributor to maternal mortality worldwide.[44] The causes of major hemorrhage are remembered using the "four Ts" (Table 5).

Pregnant and postpartum women are at higher risk of developing disseminated intravascular coagulation (DIC) and therefore require aggressive therapy to prevent decompensation and hemorrhage. In cases of postpartum hemorrhage, the obstetrician should be consulted immediately as the emergency physician focuses on patient

Table 5
The 4 Ts of peripartum hemorrhage and initial management

Tone	Uterine atony	Bimanual uterine massage Oxytocin infusion
Trauma	Uterine laceration or rupture Vaginal laceration Uterine inversion	Repair of lacerations Attempt manual reduction (must stop oxytocin, if running, first)
Tissue	Retained placenta Placenta accreta, increta, percreta Placenta previa	Manual removal of retained placenta Transfusion support while awaiting obstetrics arrival
Thrombin	Coagulopathy	Massive transfusion (including cryoprecipitate)

stabilization (**Fig. 1**). If an obstetrician is unavailable, the general surgeon should be consulted. The interventional radiologist should also be consulted early, because transcatheter arterial embolization can effectively manage several types of peripartum hemorrhage, potentially preserving future fertility.

Clinicians often perform poorly at estimating the volume of blood loss by visual cues,[45] and the physiologic changes to heart rate and cardiac output seen in pregnancy can hide the vital sign abnormalities typically associated with significant

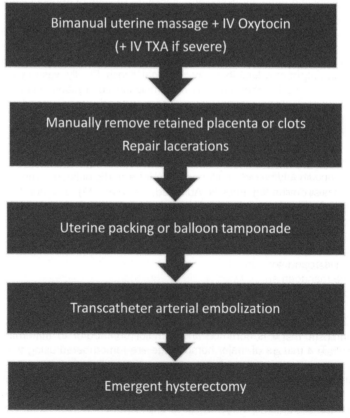

Fig. 1. Steps to control postpartum hemorrhage. IV, intravenous; TXA, tranexamic acid.

hemorrhage. More than a liter of blood may be lost before the pregnant patient becomes hypotensive.[46] Alternately, pregnant women with underlying conditions, such as anemia or preeclampsia, can experience hemorrhagic shock with smaller volumes of blood loss.[45] In general, severe peripartum hemorrhage is managed much the same way as hemorrhage from other causes, using massive transfusion, including cryoprecipitate, and avoiding actions, such as large-volume crystalloid infusion that exacerbate coagulopathy and bleeding.[47,48] Early activation of the massive transfusion protocol, with specific requisition for cryoprecipitate if not included, ensures blood products are rapidly available. If there is no time to appropriately crossmatch blood, Rhesus factor (Rh)-negative products should be used. Rh-negative individuals experiencing hemorrhage should be treated with Rhogam. Additional immediate steps to be taken include:

- Administration of tranexamic acid within the first 3 hours of life-threatening bleed, because it may decrease bleeding-related death in postpartum hemorrhage without increasing thromboembolic events.[49]
- Repair of identified uterine or vaginal lacerations and, in uterine atony, removal of any retained placenta and bimanual uterine massage in concert with oxytocin administration to promote uterine contraction. Dosing is 60 ~ 200 milliunits/min IV, titrating to appropriate uterine contraction.
- If hemorrhage persists, uterine or vaginal packing with Kerlix or gauze should be placed to provide direct pressure. Balloon tamponade with a specialized balloon catheter or even large Foley can also be attempted.[50] A Foley catheter should be inserted into the bladder before packing is placed to prevent compressive urethral obstruction and urinary retention.
- Use of thromboelastography, if available, to guide targeted management of coagulopathy, because early data have shown it to be associated with decreased bleeding and requirement of fewer transfusions.[51]

Preeclampsia with Severe Features and Eclampsia

Preeclampsia is defined as a systolic blood pressure greater than or equal to 140 mm Hg or diastolic pressure greater than or equal to 90 mm Hg, associated with proteinuria, which occurs anytime between 20 weeks of gestation and 6 weeks postpartum.[52] Occurring in approximately 4% of pregnancies, it can advance to preeclampsia with severe features (**Box 1**, or eclampsia, and must be managed aggressively to prevent poor maternal and fetal outcomes.[53] The American College of Obstetricians and Gynecologists recommends management with IV labetalol, IV hydralazine, or oral immediate-release nifedipine as the preferred agents in pregnancy.[53,54] Animal studies have found teratogenic effects with high-doses, but nifedipine has been used in the management of hypertension in pregnancy for decades without signs of fetal harm, although there are no placebo-controlled human studies investigating its use.[55]

In the setting of eclampsia, defined as the presence of seizure activity in the setting of preeclampsia, first ensure the airway is maintained. First-line treatment is IV magnesium sulfate 4 to 6 g over 15 minutes followed by a 1-2 g/h infusion, closely monitoring for signs of magnesium toxicity: vision changes, loss of reflexes, decreased mental status, difficulty breathing. If seizures remain uncontrolled, lorazepam or diazepam may also be used. Consultation with obstetrics and gynecology is essential, because if the seizures are not able to be quickly controlled imminent delivery may be indicated.

Box 1
Signs and symptoms of preeclampsia with severe features

- SBP $\geq$160 mm Hg or DBP $\geq$110 mm Hg taken twice at least 4 hours apart while resting
- Abnormal liver function tests ($\geq$2 × the upper limit of normal)
- Renal insufficiency (serum creatinine >1.1 mg/dL or 2 × baseline without other cause)
- Thrombocytopenia (platelet count <100 × 10^9/L)
- Unexplained RUQ or epigastric pain
- New-onset headache unresponsive to medication and not otherwise explained
- Visual disturbance
- Pulmonary edema

Abbreviations: DBP, diastolic blood pressure; RUQ, right upper quadrant; SBP, systolic blood pressure.

Data from [ACOG Practice Bulletin No. 202: Gestational Hypertension and Preeclampsia. Obstet Gynecol 2019;133(1):e1-25].

Amniotic Fluid Embolism

Amniotic fluid embolism (AFE) is a rare cause of maternal critical illness but has a mortality rate of 60%.[56] The underlying pathophysiology of AFE is not clear, but it is thought that amniotic fluid or other debris, such as fetal cells, enters the maternal circulation and triggers a release of inflammatory mediators, leading to cardiopulmonary dysfunction and activation of the clotting cascade, often progressing to DIC. Early recognition and aggressive resuscitative measures are key to improving survival.

The presentation of AFE is usually sudden. Initial symptoms can include shortness of breath, coughing, rigors, diaphoresis, agitation, or acute anxiety, but AFE often presents with cardiopulmonary collapse or even cardiac arrest. Although not distinguishable from high-risk pulmonary embolism, POCUS can help identify potential AFE as a cause of hemodynamic instability, because it usually demonstrates right ventricular strain with an empty left ventricle and septal bowing caused by secondary pulmonary hypertension.[56]

Management of AFE is supportive and focused on treating hypoxemia, supporting circulation, and transfusing blood products, including cryoprecipitate, if the patient is hemorrhaging with DIC.[56,57] Because there is acute right heart strain, use of IV crystalloid should be minimized to avoid further worsening right ventricular overload, and it is prudent to initiate hemodynamic resuscitation with early vasopressor or inotropic support before initiating preload-reducing positive pressure ventilation to avoid peri-intubation decompensation.[58] Norepinephrine remains the vasopressor of choice, whereas dobutamine and milrinone offer pulmonary vasodilation and are effective inotropes.[56] Pulmonary vasodilation with inhaled epoprostenol or nitric oxide, if available, should be initiated to decrease right ventricular afterload.[56] Use of circulatory assist devices and ECMO has been reported in the literature with successful outcomes and is worth serious consideration.[57]

Cardiac Arrest

Maternal cardiac arrest requires rapid action by clinicians if either the pregnant woman or fetus are to survive. The first step is to activate a maternal code, which depending on hospital resources may bring additional support from obstetrics, neonatology, anesthesia, or others.

In patients more than 20 weeks of gestation or with a uterine fundus at or above the umbilicus, the uterus should be manually displaced leftward. Of note, the most recent American Heart Association guidelines removed the recommendation for placement of a wedge or positioning the patient at a tilt, because these practices compromise the effectiveness of chest compressions.[10] Chest compressions should be performed as in the nonpregnant patient, because there are insufficient data to recommend otherwise.[10] Appropriate ventilatory support and high-quality compressions should be continued while addressing the underlying cause of arrest (See **Table 6**).

Table 6
Mnemonics for underlying causes of maternal cardiac arrest

B	Bleeding	A	Anesthetic complications
E	Embolism	B	Bleeding
A	Anesthetic complications	C	Cardiovascular
U	Uterine atony	D	Drugs
C	Cardiac disease	E	Embolism
H	Hypertension (preeclampsia/eclampsia)	F	Fever
O	Other (Hs and Ts, magnesium toxicity)	G	General nonobstetric causes
P	Placenta abruptio/previa	H	Hypertension
S	Sepsis		

Data from [Jeejeebhoy FM, Zelop CM, Lipman S, et al. Cardiac arrest in pregnancy: A scientific statement from the American Heart Association. Circulation 2015;132(18):1747-73] and [Hui D, Morrison LJ, Windrim R, et al. The American Heart Association 2019 guidelines for the management of cardiac arrest in pregnancy: consensus recommendations on implementation strategies. J Obstet Gynaecol Can 2011;33(8):858–63].

Perimortem Cesarean Section

In the event of maternal cardiac arrest, the decision to perform a perimortem cesarean section must be made immediately to obtain the appropriate supplies and deliver within 5 minutes of maternal loss of pulses. This "5-minute rule" exists because it is the time frame in which the chance of maternal and fetal survival is the highest with the most preserved neurologic function, although the mortality for both remains high.[59] It should be performed in patients presenting in cardiac arrest with a pregnancy of known gestation age greater than 24 weeks, or in a pregnancy of unknown gestational age in which the uterine fundus is above the umbilicus.

The benefit of the perimortem cesarean section is two-fold. First, after 24 weeks gestation there is a possibility of fetal survival. Second, with delivery, aortocaval compression is relieved and blood volume previously serving the uteroplacentofetal unit is shunted back to the maternal circulation, increasing cardiac output up to 80%,[3] which may increase the chance of return of spontaneous circulation.

The procedure for a perimortem cesarean section differs from the more common low transverse cesarean section because it is designed to be performed rapidly with easy visualization of structures (**Fig. 2**).[60] Using a scalpel, a vertical incision is made from the top of the uterine fundus to the pubic symphysis. Once the uterus is visualized the bladder is identified and retracted to avoid injury. The scalpel is used to quickly incise the uterus, but scissors should be used to extend the incision to avoid fetal injury, with rupture of the amniotic sac to deliver the fetus, and then clamping and cutting of the umbilical cord and delivery of the placenta. Chest compressions are held briefly while incisions are being made but should be limited to less than 10 seconds.[10,61]

PERIMORTEM C-SECTION

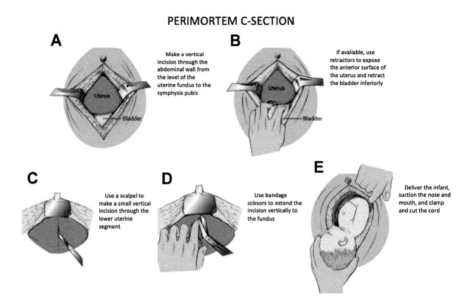

Fig. 2. Perimortem cesarean section. (*A*) Vertical incision through the abdominal wall. (*B*) Retraction of bladder inferiorly. (*C*) Incision through low uterine segment. (*D*) Extension of incision superiorly. (*E*) Delivery of fetus. (*From* Healy ME, Kozubal DE, Horn AE, et al. Care of the critically ill pregnant patient and perimortem cesarean delivery in the emergency department. J Emerg Med 2016;51(2):172-7; with permission.)

SUMMARY

Resuscitation of the critically ill obstetric patient mandates early consultation of a multidisciplinary team because two lives are at stake. Emergency clinicians should appreciate the potential difficulties in intubating the pregnant patient, target pregnancy-specific goals for oxygenation and ventilation, and aggressively support maternal blood pressure to optimize fetal oxygenation and perfusion. Although some medications may be safer in pregnancy than others, stabilizing the pregnant patient is paramount. In cardiac arrest in pregnancies beyond 24 weeks or with a fundal height above the umbilicus, a perimortem cesarean section should be performed with delivery of the fetus within 5 minutes of maternal pulselessness to maximize benefit to patient and fetus.

DISCLOSURE

The authors have nothing to disclose.

REFERENCES

1. Einav S, Leone M. Epidemiology of obstetric critical illness. Int J Obstet Anesth 2019;40:128–39.

2. Gaffney A. Critical care in pregnancy: is it different? Semin Perinatol 2014;38(6): 329–40.

3. Sanghavi M, Rutherford JD. Cardiovascular physiology of pregnancy. Circulation 2014;130(12):1003–8.

4. Yeomans ER, Gilstrap LC III. Physiologic changes in pregnancy and their impact on critical care. Crit Care Med 2005;33(10 Suppl):S256–8.
5. Hegewald MJ, Crapo RO. Respiratory physiology in pregnancy. Clin Chest Med 2011;32(1):1–13.
6. McAuliffe F, Kametas N, Krampl E, et al. Blood gases in pregnancy at sea level and at high altitude. BJOG 2001;108:980–5.
7. Guntupalli KK, Hall N, Karnad D, et al. Critical illness in pregnancy. Chest 2015; 148(4):1093–104.
8. Griffiths SK, Campbell JP. Placental structure, function and drug transfer. Contin Educ Anaesth Crit Care Pain 2015;15(2):84–9.
9. Omo-Aghoja L. Maternal and fetal acid-base chemistry: a major determinant of perinatal outcome. Ann Med Health Sci Res 2014;4(1):8–17.
10. Jeejeebhoy FM, Zelop CM, Lipman S, et al. Cardiac arrest in pregnancy: a scientific statement from the American Heart Association. Circulation 2015;132(18): 1747–73.
11. Kinsella SM. Lateral tilt for pregnant women: why 15 degrees? Anesthesia 2003; 58(9):835–6.
12. Fujita N, Higuchi H, Sakuma S, et al. Effect of right-lateral versus left-lateral tilt position on compression of the inferior vena cava in pregnant women determined by magnetic resonance imaging. Anesth Analg 2019;128(6):1217–22.
13. Higuchi H, Takagi S, Zhang K, et al. Effect of lateral tilt angle on the volume of the abdominal aorta and inferior vena cava in pregnant and nonpregnant women as determined based on magnetic resonance imaging. Anesthesiology 2015;122: 286–93.
14. Antenatal corticosteroid therapy for fetal maturation. Committee Opinion No. 713. American College of Obstetricians and Gynecologists. Obstet Gynecol 2017;130: e102–9.
15. Frat JP, Thille AW, Mercat A, et al. High-flow oxygen through nasal cannula in acute hypoxemic respiratory failure. N Engl J Med 2015;372(23):2185–96.
16. Tomohiro S, Umegaki T, Nishimoto K, et al. Use of high-flow nasal cannula oxygen therapy in a pregnant woman with dermatomyositis-related interstitial pneumonia. Case Rep Crit Care 2017;2017:4527597.
17. Stader C, Akella J. High flow oxygen in pregnancy with severe acute hypoxic respiratory failure due to community-acquired streptococcus pneumoniae. Chest 2017;152(4). Suppl.A302.
18. Allred CC, Matias Esquinas M, Caronia J, et al. Successful use of noninvasive ventilation in pregnancy. Eur Respir Rev 2014;23(131):142–4.
19. Mushambi MC, Kinsella MSM, Popat M, et al. Obstetric Anaesthetists' Association and Difficult Airway Society guidelines for the management of difficult and failed tracheal intubation in obstetrics. Anaesthesia 2015;70:1286–306.
20. Lapinsky SE. Management of acute respiratory failure in pregnancy. Semin Respir Crit Care Med 2017;38(2):201–7.
21. Duarte AG. ARDS in pregnancy. Clin Obstet Gynecol 2014;57(4):862–70.
22. Bhatia PK, Biyani G, Mohammed S, et al. Acute respiratory failure and mechanical ventilation in pregnant patient: a narrative review of literature. J Anaesthesiol Clin Pharmacol 2016;32(4):431–9.
23. Amato MBP, Meade MO, Slutsky AS, et al. Driving pressure and survival in the acute respiratory distress syndrome. N Engl J Med 2015;372:747–55.
24. Aggarwal NR, Brower RG, Hager DN, et al. Oxygen exposure resulting in arterial oxygen tensions above the protocol goal was associated with worse clinical outcomes in acute respiratory distress syndrome. Crit Care Med 2018;46(4):517–24.

25. Catanzarite VA, Willms D. Adult respiratory distress syndrome in pregnancy: report of three cases and review of the literature. Obstet Gynecol Surv 1997; 52(6):381–92.

26. O'Croinin D, Ni Chonghaile M, Higgins B, et al. Bench-to-bedside review: permissive hypercapnia. Crit Care 2005;9(1):51–9.

27. Pacheco LD, Saade GR, Hankins GDV. Extracorporeal membrane oxygenation (ECMO) during pregnancy and postpartum. Semin Perinatol 2018;42(1):21–5.

28. Ray BR, Trikha A. Prone position ventilation in pregnancy: concerns and evidence. J Obstet Anaesth Crit Care 2018;8:7–9.

29. Neuman G, Koren G. Safety of procedural sedation in pregnancy. J Obstet Gynaecol Can 2013;35(2):168–73.

30. Pacheco LD, Saade GR, Hankins GDV. Mechanical ventilation during pregnancy: sedation, analgesia, and paralysis. Clin Obstet Gynecol 2014;57(4):844–50.

31. Crozier TA, Flamm C, Speer CP, et al. Effects of etomidate on the adrenocortical and metabolic adaptation of the neonate. Br J Anaesth 1993;70(1):47–53.

32. Nair Abhijit S, Sriprakash K. Dexmedetomidine in pregnancy: review of literature and possible use. J Obstet Anaesth Crit Care 2013;3:3–6.

33. Tang Y, Liu R, Zhao P. Ketamine: an update for obstetric anesthesia. Transl Perioper Pain Med 2017;4(4):1–12.

34. Antonucci R, Zaffanello M, Puxeddu E, et al. Use of non-steroidal anti-inflammatory drugs in pregnancy: impact on the fetus and newborn. Curr Drug Metab 2012;13(4):474–90.

35. Levy MM, Evans LE, Rhodes A. The Surviving Sepsis Campaign bundle: 2018 Update. Crit Care Med 2018;46(6):997–1000.

36. Plante LA, Pacheco KD, Louis JM. SMFM Consult Series #47: sepsis during pregnancy and the puerperium. Am J Obstet Gynecol 2019;220(4):B2–10.

37. Wang X, Shen X, Liu S, et al. The efficacy and safety of norepinephrine and its feasibility as a replacement for phenylephrine to manage maternal hypotension during elective cesarean delivery under spinal anesthesia. Biomed Res Int 2018;2018:1869189.

38. Reidy J, Douglas J. Vasopressors in obstetrics. Anesthesiol Clin 2008;26(1): 75–88.

39. Practice Guidelines of Obstetric Anesthesia: An updated report by the American Society of Anesthesiologists Task Force on Obstetric Anesthesia and the Society for Obstetric Anesthesia and Perinatology. Anesthesiology 2016;124(2):270–300.

40. Thornton S, Baldwin PJ, Harris PA, et al. The role of arginine vasopressin in human labour: functional studies, fetal production and localisation of V1a receptor mRNA. BJOG 2002;109(1):57–62.

41. Fishburne JI, Meis PJ, Urban RB, et al. Vascular and uterine responses to dobutamine and dopamine in the gravid ewe. Am J Obstet Gynecol 1980;137(8): 944–52.

42. Elkayam U, Schäfer A, Chieffo A, et al. Use of Impella heart pump for management of women with peripartum cardiogenic shock. Clin Cardiol 2019;42(10): 974–81.

43. Moore SA, Dietl CA, Coleman DM. Extracorporeal life support during pregnancy. J Thorac Cardiovasc Surg 2016;151(4):1154–60.

44. Kassebaum NJ, Bertozzi-Villa A, Coggeshall MS, et al. Global, regional, and national levels and causes of maternal mortality during 1990-2013: a systematic analysis for the Global Burden of Disease Study 2013. Lancet 2014;6736(14): 1e25.

45. Pacagnella RC, Borovac-Pinheiro A. Assessing and managing hypovolemic shock in puerperal women. Best Pract Res Clin Obstet Gynaecol 2019;61: 89–105.
46. Bloomfield TH, Gordon H. Reaction to blood loss at delivery. J Obstet Gynaecol 1990;10(Suppl. 2):S13–6.
47. Pham HP, Shaz BH. Update on massive transfusion. Br J Anaesth 2013; 111(Suppl 1):i1–82.
48. Jackson DL, DeLoughery TG. Postpartum hemorrhage: management of massive transfusion. Obstet Gynecol Surv 2018;73(7):418–22.
49. WOMAN TC. Effect of early tranexamic acid administration on mortality, hysterectomy, and other morbidities in women with post-partum hemorrhage (WOMAN): an international, randomized, double-blind, placebo-controlled trial. Lancet 2017;389(10084):2105–16.
50. Bakri YN, Amri A, Abdul Jabbar F. Tamponade-balloon for obstetrical bleeding. Int J Gynaecol Obstet 2001;74(2):139–42.
51. McNamara H, Kenyon C, Smith R, et al. Four years' experience of a ROTEM-guided algorithm for treatment of coagulopathy in obstetric hemorrhage. Anaesthesia 2019;74(8):984–91.
52. Sibai BM. Evaluation and management of severe preeclampsia before 34 weeks' gestation. Am J Obstet Gynecol 2011;205(3):191–8.
53. El-Sayed YY, Borders AE. The ACOG Committee on Obstetric Practice. ACOG committee opinion no. 767: Emergent therapy for acute-onset, severe hypertension during pregnancy and the postpartum period. Obstet Gynecol 2019;133(2): 174–80.
54. Espinoza J, Vidaeff A, Pettker CM, Simhan H. ACOG Committee on Practice Bulletins-Obstetrics. ACOG Practice Bulletin No. 222: Gestational hypertension and preeclampsia. Obstet Gynecol 2019;135(6):e237–60.
55. Smith P, Anthony J, Johanson R. Nifedipine in pregnancy. BJOG 2000;107: 299–307.
56. Pacheco LD, Clark SL, Klassen M, et al. Amniotic fluid embolism: principles of early clinical management. Am J Obstet Gynecol 2020;222(1):48–52.
57. Kaur K, Bhardwaj M, Kumar P, et al. Amniotic fluid embolism. J Anaesthesiol Clin Pharmacol 2016;32(2):153–9.
58. Dalabih M, Rischard F, Mosier JM. What's new: the management of acute right ventricular decompensation of chronic pulmonary hypertension. Intensive Care Med 2014;40:1930–3.
59. Katz VL, Dotters DJ, Droegemueller W. Perimortem cesarean delivery. Obstet Gynecol 1986;68:571–6.
60. Healy ME, Kozubal DE, Horn AE, et al. Care of the critically ill pregnant patient and perimortem cesarean delivery in the emergency department. J Emerg Med 2016;51(2):172–7.
61. Sato Y, Weil MH, Sun S, et al. Adverse effects of interrupting precordial compression during cardiopulmonary resuscitation. Crit Care Med 1997;25(5):733–6.

Pearls and Pitfalls in the Crashing Geriatric Patient

David P. Yamane, MD[a,b,]*

KEYWORDS

- Geriatric • Emergency clinician • Critical care • Intensive care

KEY POINTS

- The geriatric population is growing and is the largest utilizer of emergency and critical care services; the emergency clinician should be comfortable in the management of the acutely ill geriatric patient.
- There are important physiologic changes in geriatric patients, which alters their clinical presentation and management.
- Age alone should not determine the prognosis for elderly patients. Premorbid functional status, frailty, and severity of illness should be considered carefully for the geriatric population.
- Emergency clinicians should have honest conversations about goals of care based not only a patient's clinical presentation but also the patient's values.

INTRODUCTION

The definition of "old" varies greatly. The most common definition of the geriatric patient, including that of the World Health Organization, is an adult greater than or equal to age 65 years.[1] Within the United States, this population increased 1000%, from 3.1 million (1 in every 25 persons) in 1900 to more than 35 million people (1 in every 8 persons) in 2000. The geriatric population is the largest growing age group, accounting for more than 13% of the population, with an expected increase to 70 million, or 16% to 25% of the population, by 2050. The oldest-old group ($\geq$85 years) is the fastest growing, with an expected climb from 1% to 5% of the population (1 in 20 Americans) by 2050.[2,3]

One in 4 older adults visits the emergency department (ED) each year, and ED care is one of the highest utilized health resources by this population. Geriatric patients account for approximately 15% of ED visits and utilize ambulances 38% more than any other age group. These patients have higher disease acuity and higher probability of needing hospital admission.[4] This growing population is also increasingly utilizing critical care services. Over the past 20 years, admissions to the intensive care unit (ICU)

[a] Emergency Medicine, George Washington University, Washington, DC, USA;
[b] Anesthesiology and Critical Care Medicine, George Washington University, Washington, DC, USA
* 2120 L street NW, suite 400, Washington DC 20037, USA
E-mail address: dyamane@email.gwu.edu
Twitter: @donth8intubate (D.P.Y.)

Emerg Med Clin N Am 38 (2020) 919–930
https://doi.org/10.1016/j.emc.2020.06.011
0733-8627/20/© 2020 Elsevier Inc. All rights reserved.

have increased for the geriatric population, with those for the greater than 80-year-old cohort increasing at the fastest rate. Geriatric ICU admission accounts for 25% to 50% of all ICU admissions and the geriatric population stays longer in the ICU, accounting for 60% of total ICU days.[1,3,5–7] This growing population requiring critical care resources is projected to lead to a severe shortage of ICU beds. This shortage will require emergency physicians to care for critically ill geriatric patients for longer periods and be ready to respond to their specific needs if they deteriorate.

GERIATRIC PATIENTS ARE NOT JUST OLD ADULTS: PHYSIOLOGIC CHANGES IN THE GERIATRIC POPULATION

The geriatric population has a loss of physiologic reserve due to the aging process, making them vulnerable to stressors, such as infection and injury.[2] The exact mechanism of the aging process is not well understood, involving an interplay of genetic, oxidative free radical, and cellular-level changes.[7] The geriatric patient has specific physiologic changes that the emergency clinician must be attuned to (**Table 1**).

Neurologic Changes

The aging brain decreases in size, with a decrease in functional neurons resulting in loss of cognitive function, motor function, hearing vision, and memory. The decrease in size with the adherence of the dura to the skull bases places the strain on the bridging vessels, increasing the risk for subdural hematomas in response to even minor traumas. The geriatric brain also has baseline decreased cerebral perfusion; declines in perfusion pressure from critical illnesses (eg septic shock) may result in concomitant neurologic insults.[8] The geriatric patient also is less sensitive to pain, which may result in later-stage presentations of illness.[9] The clinician should be attuned that the lack of pain cannot rule out serious illness.

Cardiovascular Changes

The geriatric patient population is at increased risk for cardiovascular ischemia. More than 40% of deaths in the geriatric population stem from cardiovascular disease, and silent myocardial infarctions occur in over 40% of patients older than 75 years.[7,10,11] In addition the geriatric population is at increased risk to arrhythmias, including sick sinus syndrome, atrial arrhythmias, ventricular arrhythmias, and bundle branch blocks, as a result of connective tissue and fat replacing the autonomic tissues. Atrial fibrillation is common in the elderly, with a prevalence of 10% in patients over 80 years old.[2,7,10,12]

Both systolic and diastolic heart failure are common in the elderly population, and several effects of aging contribute to the high prevalence.[13] With age, the cardiac myocytes are replaced by fibrous tissue, reducing the ejection fraction and overall cardiac output. In addition, the decrease in elasticity of the aorta increases cardiac afterload and hypertension. In response to the increased cardiac afterload, there is left ventricular hypertrophy decreasing the cardiac compliance placing these patients at risk for diastolic dysfunction. The geriatric heart responds to demands of increased cardiac output by increasing ventricular filling and stroke volume. The geriatric patient is in a preload dependent state, very susceptible to even minor changes in volume status.[2]

At rest, cardiac output can be maintained; however, the aging heart has a blunted response to sympathetic stimulation (hyposympathetic state) and is unable to respond to increased demands by increasing the heart rate. Geriatric patients suffering from hypovolemia may not mount the tachycardic response clinicians expect. Similarly,

Table 1
Summary of physiologic and functional changes in the geriatric population

Physiologic Changes	Functional Changes
Neurologic	
Decreased brain size	Decline in cognitive function
Decreased cerebral perfusion	Increased risk for additional neurologic insult
Cardiovascular	
Increased fibrosis of the myocardium and autonomic tissue	Increased arrhythmia risk
	Decreased cardiac output
Increase aortic wall thickness and decreased elasticity	Increased afterload
Pulmonary	
Decreased chest wall compliance	Decreased maximal inspiratory and expiratory force, forced expiratory volume in the first second of expiration
Decreased alveolar surface area, surfactant, ciliary clearance	
Increased residual volume	Decreased cough, increased pneumonia risk
	Increased ventilation/perfusion mismatch
Gastrointestinal	
Decreased motility and delayed gastric emptying	Increased aspiration risk
	Increased malnutrition risk
Decreased in nutritional absorption	Increased risk of gastrointestinal bleeds and bacterial translocation
Decreased gastric acid secretion and mucous production	
Renal	
Decrease renal size	Decreased GFR
Decrease renal blood flow	Increased risk of acute renal failure
Increase sclerosis of nephrons	
Musculoskeletal	
Decrease in lean muscle mass	Increased risk of falls and injury
Integumentary	
Decrease subcutaneous adipose	Increased risk of infection
Decreased epidermal skin layer	Increased risk of decubitus ulcers
Decease dermal vasculature	Poor wound healing

normotensive geriatric patients may be masking inadequate perfusion, and these changes make shock insidious in the geriatric patient. Emergency clinicians must be vigilant for changes in mental status, oliguria, and clammy skin as evidence of shock. During resuscitation, the clinician must carefully balance the need to maintain adequate preload with the increased risks of pulmonary edema from heart failure.

Airway Changes

Airway management and intubation in the elderly population can be challenging. Bag-valve masking a patient can be a challenge with the loss of muscular facial and pharyngeal support, and edentulousness can make a mask seal challenging. Mouth opening, mandibular protrusion, thyromental distance, neck mobility, and submandibular compliance decrease with age, while the Mallampati score increases. The emergency clinician, therefore, should be prepared for a potentially difficult airway when intubating a geriatric patient.[14]

Pulmonary Changes

The geriatric patient has many changes in the pulmonary system. Structural changes, such as kyphosis, vertebral compression fractures, increased chest wall stiffness, and increased anteroposterior diameter, result in decreases in chest wall compliance. The chest wall compliance decreases by 10% after age 50,[15] and lungs have a loss of elastic recoil. Along with a 25% decline in respiratory muscle strength, these changes lead to a decrease of the maximal inspiratory and expiratory forces of up to 50%.[3,16]

Geriatric patients have a reduction in total lung capacity, vital capacity, and forced expiratory volume in the first second of expiration, with increases in functional residual capacity and residual volume.[3] Alveolar surface area decreases from 70 m^2 at age 20 to approximately 60 m^2 at age 70, for a reduced gas exchange area leading to a decline in Pao_2 of 0.3 mm Hg/y after age 30.[17] There are no changes in the $Paco_2$ with age, however.[18]

The physiologic response to hypoxia decreases by 50% and hypercapnia by 40%, making the geriatric patient less able to respond to changes.[7] With the decrement in elastic recoil, there is subsequent airway narrowing and collapse, which may lead to ventilation-perfusion mismatch. These physiologic changes result in higher rates of mechanical ventilation and longer ventilation needs in the geriatric patient population.[3] Additionally, they are at risk for higher rates of ventilator-associated pneumonia and failure to wean from the ventilator. Noninvasive ventilation should be considered to avoid intubation when possible.

Renal Changes

The kidneys decrease in size up to 30% and blood flow up to 50% by age 80. By age 85%, 40% of the nephrons become sclerotic, while the remaining nephrons hypertrophy to compensate. This loss of physiologic reserve places geriatric patients at high risk of acute renal failure from even minor perfusion changes. Diminished renal function leads to an inability to concentrate urine, conserve sodium, and excrete hydrogen, making the geriatric patient susceptible to dehydration and sodium and acid-base imbalances. Clinicians should be cautious because a loss of up to 50% of a functioning glomerular filtration rate (GFR) may not be reflected in the creatinine because patients' lean body mass also decreases over this time period.[6,7,12]

AGE IS JUST A NUMBER: BEYOND CHRONOLOGIC AGE

The common adage, "age is just a number," often is incorporated into documentation when it is stated that a patient "appears younger (or older) than stated age." There are more scientific approaches to classifying geriatric patients, however. As with pediatrics, there are phases in geriatrics, including the young-old, middle-old, and oldest-old. The young-old typically represents patients 65 to 75 years old, the middle-old 75 to 85 years old, and the oldest-old greater than or equal to 85 years old.[8,19] Geriatric patients often progress from being healthy independent individuals in the first category to progressive dependence on others for performing their instrumental activities of daily living (IADLs), which include operating a phone, shopping, food preparation, housekeeping, and laundry, and for help with activities of daily living (ADLs), including bathing, dressing, toileting, transfers, and feeding. Although these stages help frame thinking of the geriatric patients, not all patients age at the same rate. Physiologic changes vary between individuals due to genetics, lifestyle, and environment, and a patient's physiologic age may not align with chronologic age.[7,8]

Although the mortality of the geriatric patient is higher than that of the younger population, age alone does not predict mortality from critical illness.[3,4,20] Severity of presenting illness, admission from a chronic care facility, comorbid illness, prior health, and functional status have shown to correlate more strongly with mortality. Patients 65 to 84 years old have on average 2.6 ± 2.2 comorbid conditions, and those greater than 85 years old have 3.6 ± 2.3 comorbid conditions.[1] Comorbid conditions associated with worse outcomes include degenerative brain disease, cerebrovascular disease, congestive heart failure, chronic pulmonary disease, diabetes mellitus, and malnutrition.[20] Mechanical ventilation and longer ICU stays also are associated with higher mortality in the geriatric patient.[4,21] In cases of out-of-hospital cardiac arrest, time to cardiopulmonary resuscitation and clinical characteristics, including a shockable rhythm, a lactate less than 5 mg/dL, and a lower cumulative dose of epinephrine, correlate with mortality and neurologic outcomes better than age does.[9]

Frailty

More important than chronologic age is the concept of frailty, a syndrome of reduced physical, physiologic, and cognitive reserve. Frailty is characterized by decreased mobility, muscle mass, weakness, poor nutritional status, and diminished cognitive function, making individuals more susceptible to extrinsic stressors. Frailty and comorbid conditions are more common in the geriatric population, but advanced age is not synonymous with either frailty or comorbidity. Frail geriatric patients account for 25% of the population over the age of 65% and 50% over the age of 85.[22–24] Frailty has been linked to increases in both in-hospital and long-term mortality. More meaningful to the geriatric population, however, is that frailty has been linked to a reduced chance of returning home, functional disability, and decreased quality of life.[25–27] There are multiple validated screening tools to quantify frailty; however, many are cumbersome and too complex to complete in ED setting, with up to 30 to 70 items assessed.[25,26,28] One well-studied, simple tool is the Clinical Frailty Scale, which is a 9-level assessment, with levels 1 to 4 being nonfrail, 5 to 6 mildly to moderately frail, and greater than or equal to 7 severely frail (**Table 2**).[24,29,30] This scale has been proved to be reliably performed by emergency clinicians.[31] Increases in the Clinical Frailty Scale are associated with higher mortality.[1,24] The identification of frailty and its impact may help guide emergency clinicians in management decisions or discussions of goals of care in the critically ill.

DANGER DRUGS: CRITICAL CARE PHARMACOLOGY IN THE GERIATRIC PATIENT

The critically ill geriatric patient is at an increased risk of adverse drug reactions,[32,33] due to changes in physiology, metabolism, and polypharmacy. Diminished first-pass effect and decreased gastric motility may increase the availability in the systemic circulation, but this may be offset some by the decreased absorption of the geriatric gastrointestinal system. The geriatric patient has an increased proportion of body fat content of 15% to 30% and decreases in total body water of 12% to 15%, affecting volume of distribution.[34] For lipophilic drugs, there is an increased volume of distribution with a prolonged half-life, whereas water-soluble drugs have a decreased volume of distribution. Protein bound drugs, like warfarin, phenytoin, and digoxin, may have a reduced binding capacity in elderly patients with higher concentration of unbound (active) drug[2] (**Table 3**).

Drug excretion also is altered in the geriatric patient. Due to the physiologic decline in GFR in the geriatric population, there is a decrease in renal excretion of drugs. The hepatic clearance of drugs is slowed but the clinical significance in the geriatric population is unknown.[3]

Table 2
Clinical Frailty Scale

Level	Description
1. Very fit	Robust, active, energetic, well-motivated, fit; exercise regularly; fittest for their age
2. Well	No active disease symptoms, less fit than group 1; active occasionally (eg seasonally)
3. Managing well	Medical problems are well controlled; no regular activity beyond routine walking
4. Apparently vulnerable	Not frankly dependent, disease symptoms limit activity; commonly complain of feeling "slow" or being tired during the day
5. Mildly frail	More evident slowing; limited dependence on high-order IADLs (finances, transportation, heavy housework, and medications)
6. Moderately frail	Need help in in both IADLs and ADLs, such as all outside activities and keeping house; often have problems with stairs and need help with bathing
7. Severely frail	Completely dependent on others for ADLs; stable and not at risk of dying (<6 mo)
8. Very severely frail	Completely dependent; approaching end of life; could not recover from minor illness
9. Terminally ill	Life expectancy <6 mo who otherwise are not evidently frail

Data from Rockwood K, Song X, Macknight C, et al. A global clinical measure of fitness and frailty in elderly people. CMAJ. 2005;173(5):489-95 and Juma S, Taabazuing MM, Montero-odasso M. Clinical Frailty Scale in an Acute Medicine Unit: a Simple Tool That Predicts Length of Stay. Can Geriatr J. 2016;19(2):34-9.

Polypharmacy is associated with adverse outcomes and should be avoided. In the critical care setting, this may be impossible, but efforts should be made to minimize the number of medications a geriatric patient receives.[7]

Drugs and Delirium: A Doubly Dangerous Combination

Delirium is an acute-onset disorder characterized by fluctuations of attention and global cognitive function.[35] Delirium is nearly ubiquitous in the geriatric critical care population, with rates greater than or equal to 70%,[36,37] and serious consequences.

Table 3
Commonly prescribed drugs in the critical care setting[3]

Drug	Route of Elimination	Volume of Distribution	Half-Life	Dose Adjustment
Midazolam	Hepatic (CYP3a)	Unchanged	Increased	Decrease
Lorazepam	Hepatic	Decreased	Unchanged	Decrease
Diazepam	Hepatic (CYP3a)	Increased	Increased	Decrease
Digoxin	Renal	Decreased	Increased	Decrease
Furosemide	Hepatic, Renal	Decreased	Increased	Decrease
Propofol	Renal	Decreased	Increased	Decrease
Morphine	Renal	Decreased	Increased	Decrease

Delirium may result in inadvertent removal of life-support devices, requirement of physical restraints, and prolonged mechanical ventilation. Delirium has been linked to increased morbidity, mortality, ICU length of stay, and hospital length of stay, and, specific to the geriatric population, loss of cognitive function, nursing home placement, and loss of independence.[4,35,38,39]

Drugs associated with delirium are digoxin, antihistamines, opiates, antiparkinsonian medications, antipsychotics, antidepressants, and sedative or analgesic medications, especially benzodiazepines.[7,9,40] To treat the symptoms of delirium, pharmacologic agents like antipsychotics, such as haloperidol or olanzapine, can be considered.[7] Because antipsychotics treat only the symptoms of delirium and not delirium itself, their use should be limited and discontinued as soon as possible. Antipsychotics have been linked to long-term mortality and are discouraged by the American Geriatrics Society.[1,9] Benzodiazepines should be avoided in the geriatric patient population at all costs, because their use has been associated with increased delirium.[1,9]

DO NOT RESUSCITATE/DO NOT INTUBATE DOES NOT MEAN DO NOT PROVIDE CRITICAL CARE: ESTABLISHING GOALS OF CARE AND TRIAGING CRITICAL CARE INTERVENTIONS

Many geriatric patients have set limits to their care. These limits may have clear definitions like "do not resuscitate" whereas others may be more nebulous and individualized. Even though patients may have limitations to their treatment plans, that does not exclude them the benefit of critical care interventions.

In all geriatric patients presenting with critical illness, clearly establishing goals of care is important. This often can be a challenge while resuscitating an acutely ill geriatric patient because time and information are limited. Often geriatric patients have advanced directives in place, which can guide the emergency clinician; these wishes should be confirmed with the patient or surrogate. if possible. When no advanced directives are available, patients should be asked directly about their wishes. When patients are unable to speak for themselves, a surrogate must be sought. This may require a phone call to a patient's home, facility, or next of kin. When none of these is available, the emergency clinician should default to resuscitation.[14]

There is a great degree of uncertainty with critical care, even more so with the geriatric patient. Often, it is uncertain if a patient would benefit from critical care interventions, and patients may be unsure about their goals of care or the options for critical care support. For those who cannot express their wishes, surrogates may not truly understand a patient's preferences or may not be able to consider how acute changes in clinical prognosis would alter the patient's beliefs.

With so much uncertainty around prognosis, clinicians are challenged with triaging who would benefit from critical care. In 1 series, only 30% to 50% of all geriatric patients with definitive need for ICU admission (abnormal vital signs or high-intensity condition or diagnoses) were admitted to the ICU.[3] There often is a high refusal rate of admission to the ICU for the elderly, up to 73% for patients greater than or equal to 80 years old, critical care providers citing either being too well (28%) or too sick (44%) to benefit from ICU admission.[41] The population of "too sick" patients, however, had a mortality less than 100%, and those "too well" patients a mortality greater than 0%, representing a potential underutilization of critical care admission.[41] Life-sustaining therapies often are denied to the geriatric population, with less likelihood of having renal replacement, vasopressors, tube feeding, major surgical interventions, and mechanical interventions.[21]

Although geriatric patients are more likely to place limitations on care, poor physician-patient communications often underestimate the geriatric patient's desire for aggressiveness of care and pursuit of life-sustaining interventions.[1,27,42] Chronologic age should not be used to discriminate against patients who potentially may benefit from critical interventions. Factors shown to better predict outcomes, including frailty, physiologic reserve, comorbid illnesses, severity of illness, and premorbid functional status, should be considered, along with the patient's goals of care and treatment limitations.[7,21] Decisions to withhold critical care interventions should be based on a patient's values and the those predictors, not based on age alone.

For geriatric patients with an unclear benefit of resuscitation or an unsure surrogate, a "trial of ICU" may be offered. A trial of ICU is a time-limited trial with pursuit of specified ICU interventions and a specified goal of recovery. If a patient deteriorates over this time period, the patient should be transitioned to comfort measures, and, if the patient improves, directed therapy should continue. If uncertainty remains after the trial of ICU, another trial may be initiated. This trial must have a predefined period of care, after which clinicians and the family re-evaluate the clinical situation. There are no strict guidelines on how long this time period should be, but many recommend at least 24 hours to 72 hours, up to 10 days to 12 days for patients with lower rates of organ failure. Worsening clinical status within 3 days to 5 days of initiating a trial of ICU, however, can serve as a reliable endpoint. The directed therapies and limitations of care should be agreed on. The clinician care team should guide the recommendations to ensure they are internally consistent with the stated goals.[27,43]

FATE FAR WORSE THAN DEATH: NAVIGATING END-OF-LIFE AND GOALS-OF-CARE DISCUSSIONS

The mortality of the critically ill geriatric patient is high; 30% of older adults are admitted to the ICU in the last 30 days of their life,[27] and 14% of patients greater than 85 years old die during the ICU admission.[21] Many patients are admitted to the ICU in the terminal portion of their illness, and more than 40% of these patients die in the ICU, accounting for 25% of Medicare expenditures.[7]

Although many studies focus on mortality outcomes, most geriatric patients have an understanding of the inevitability of death, and mortality may not be the most important outcome for them. Many focus on the quality of life remaining, valuing maintaining function and returning to their previous functional state.[44,45] Many geriatric patients rate conditions like ventilator dependence and bowel or bladder incontinence worse than death. The geriatric patient may be uninterested in care if the result is an unacceptable quality of life.[27]

Geriatric survivors of sepsis have a 50% risk of developing a new or worsening disability and only 25% of patients greater than 80 years old ever return to their pre-functional status after ICU admission.[27] Hospitalized geriatric patients who required mechanical ventilation had worse disability scores compared with those who were not hospitalized, with a greater decline in functioning in the year after hospitalization. ICU admission in the elderly is associated with 2.3 times the risk of developing dementia. At 12 months after a critical illness, 25% of geriatric patients had cognitive impairment similar to Alzheimer disease and a third were impaired to the level of a moderate traumatic brain injury.[46] Although patients may survive their acute critical illness, they may go on to develop chronic critical illness, with prolonged organ failures and mechanical ventilation dependence.[4] In patients with acute respiratory failure, age is associated with longer duration of mechanical ventilation and ICU length of stay. Patients greater than or equal to 80 years old are more likely to be discharged to a long-term care facility than are younger cohorts, and those discharged to a long-term facility had a higher long-term mortality[7,21]; 20% of all patients admitted to a longer-term care facility require readmission to the hospital within 30 days, decreasing their chances of ever returning home.[27] To a geriatric patient who values independence and quality of life, chronic dependence on mechanical support without hope of return to previous function can be a fate worse than death.

Clinicians should have frank conversations with geriatric patients and their families about their goals of care and prognosis. Discussions should occur with every geriatric patient, ideally before a patient needs resuscitation, to ensure provision of care respectful of the patient's values and goals. These conversations should consider the patient's premorbid functional status, frailty, severity of illness, and expected prognosis. It is crucial to inform patients and their loved ones of poor expected outcomes so they may make informed decisions about their goals of care.

PHONE A FRIEND: ROLES OF GERIATRICS AND PALLIATIVE CARE CONSULTATION

Both geriatrics and palliative care medicine have important roles in the care of the critically ill geriatric patients. Clinicians may specialize in either or both specialties.

Geriatricians provide a specialized approach to geriatric patients and their unique challenges, focusing on prevention of functional decline and restoration of independent functioning in acutely ill patients. They provide a complete approach to the geriatric patient's care, integrating social work, dietitians, and physical and occupational therapists. They address issues, such as polypharmacy, delirium, dementia, failure to thrive, elder abuse/neglect, malnutrition, and depression.[4] Geriatricians have been shown improve outcomes, including delirium treatment and discharge to home.[47]

Palliative care medicine follows the principles of improving quality of life for patients with serious illness through pain and symptom management, providing psychosocial support and facilitating conversation about patients' preferences and complex medical decision making. Despite these benefits, palliative care consults are underutilized and often initiated late in the clinical course. This likely is due to the misconception that consulting palliative care is inconsistent with continued medical care or is the same as hospice care. Palliative care consultation has shown improvements with increased advanced directives, decreases in nonbeneficial ICU treatments, and reductions in ICU length of stay and ICU readmissions.[4]

SUMMARY

The geriatric population is the largest growing age group, accounting for more than 13% of the population, with an expected increase to 70 million, or 16% to 25% of the population, by 2050. The oldest-old group ($\geq$85 years) is the fastest growing, with an expected climb from 1% to 5% of the population by 2050 (1 in 20 Americans). The geriatric population has a loss of physiologic reserve due to the aging process, making them vulnerable to stressors, such as infection and injury. All organ systems undergo significant changes in the aging process, and understanding these changes is imperative for emergency clinicians who are resuscitating geriatric patients. Although age correlates with frailty and comorbidities, frailty is a more important marker of outcomes than age alone. Clinicians should discuss goals of care with all geriatric patients but should not assume that patients will not benefit from critical care interventions. When the goals are in flux, a clearly defined trial of critical care may be in order. Both geriatricians and palliative care clinicians can be invaluable in assisting in the care of older patients.

REFERENCES

1. Guidet B, Vallet H, Boddaert J, et al. Caring for the critically ill patients over 80: a narrative review. Ann Intensive Care 2018;8(1):114.
2. Pisani MA. Considerations in caring for the critically ill older patient. J Intensive Care Med 2009;24(2):83–95.
3. Nagappan R, Parkin G. Geriatric critical care. Crit Care Clin 2003;19(2):253–70.
4. Hazzard WR. Principles of geriatric medicine and gerontology. New York: McGraw-Hill; 2003.
5. Angus DC, Kelley MA, Schmitz RJ, et al. Caring for the critically ill patient. Current and projected workforce requirements for care of the critically ill and patients with pulmonary disease: can we meet the requirements of an aging population? JAMA 2000;284:2762–70.
6. Menaker J, Scalea TM. Geriatric care in the surgical intensive care unit. Crit Care Med 2010;28(9):S452–9.
7. Marik PE. Management of the critically ill geriatric patient. Crit Care Med 2006; 34(9):s176–82.
8. Walker M, Spivak M, Sebastian M. The impact of aging physiology in critical care. Crit Care Nurs Clin North Am 2014;26(1):7–14.
9. Joyce MF, Reich JA. Critical care issues of the geriatric patient. Anesthesiol Clin 2015;33(3):551–61.
10. The GUSTO investigators. An international randomized trial comparing four thrombolytic strategies for acute myocardial infarction. N Engl J Med 1993;329: 673–82.
11. The International Study Group. In-hospital mortality and clinical course of 20 891 patients with suspected acute myocardial infarction Older ICU Patients/randomised between alteplase and streptokinase with or without heparin. Lancet 1990;336:71–5.
12. Boss GR, Seegmiller JE. Age-related physiological changes and their clinical significance. West J Med 1981;135(6):434–40.
13. Crispell KA. Common cardiovascular issues encountered in geriatric critical care. Crit Care Clin 2003;19:677–91.
14. Perera T, Cortijo-brown A. Geriatric Resuscitation. Emerg Med Clin North Am 2016;34(3):453–67.
15. Anthonisen NR. Tests of mechanical function. Bethesda (MD): American Physiologic Society; 1986.
16. Chen HI, Kuo CS. Relationship between respiratory muscle function and age, sex, and other factors. J Appl Physiol (1985) 1989;66:943–8.
17. Brandstetter RD, Kazemi H. Aging and the respiratory system. Med Clin North Am 1983;67:419–31.
18. Sorbini CA, Grassi V, Solinas E, et al. Arterial oxygen tension in relation to age in healthy subjects. Respiration 1968;25:3–13.
19. Aronson L. Elderhood, redefining aging, transforming medicine, reimagining life. New York: Bloomsbury Publishing; 2019.
20. Chelluri L, Pinsky MR, Donahoe MP, et al. Long-term outcome of critically ill elderly patients requiring intensive care. JAMA 1993;269(24):3119–23.
21. Bagshaw SM, Webb SA, Delaney A, et al. Very old patients admitted to intensive care in Australia and New Zealand: a multi-centre cohort analysis. Crit Care 2009; 13(2):R45.
22. Clegg A, Young J, Iliffe S, Rikkert MO, Rockwood K. Frailty in elderly people. Lancet 2013;381(9868):752–62.

23. Hoover M, Rotermann M, Sanmartin C, et al. Validation of an index to estimate the prevalence of frailty among community-dwelling seniors. Health Rep 2013; 24(9):10–7.
24. Rockwood K, Song X, Macknight C, et al. A global clinical measure of fitness and frailty in elderly people. CMAJ 2005;173(5):489–95.
25. Darvall JN, Gregorevic KJ, Story DA, et al. Frailty indexes in perioperative and critical care: A systematic review. Arch Gerontol Geriatr 2018;79:88–96.
26. Muscedere J, Waters B, Varambally A, et al. The impact of frailty on intensive care unit outcomes: a systematic review and meta-analysis. Intensive Care Med 2017; 43(8):1105–22.
27. Mittel A, Hua M. Supporting the geriatric critical care patient: decision making, understanding outcomes, and the role of palliative care. Anesthesiol Clin 2019; 37(3):537–46.
28. De vries NM, Staal JB, Van ravensberg CD, et al. Outcome instruments to measure frailty: a systematic review. Ageing Res Rev 2011;10(1):104–14.
29. Juma S, Taabazuing MM, Montero-odasso M. Clinical frailty scale in an acute medicine unit: a simple tool that predicts length of stay. Can Geriatr J 2016; 19(2):34–9.
30. Islam A, Muir-Hunter S, Speechley M, et al. Facilitating frailty identification: comparison of two methods among community-dwelling older adults. J Frailty Aging 2014;3(4):216–21.
31. Ringer T, Thompson C, Mcleod S, et al. Inter-rater agreement between self-rated and staff-rated clinical frailty scale scores in older emergency department patients: a prospective observational study. Acad Emerg Med 2019;27(5):419–22.
32. Lazarou J, Pomeranz BH, Corey PN. Incidence of adverse drug reactions in hospitalized patients: a meta-analysis of prospective studies. JAMA 1998;279: 1200–5.
33. Onder G, Pedone C, Landi F, et al. Adverse drug reactions as cause of hospital admissions: results from the Italian Group of Pharmacoepidemiology in the Elderly (GIFA). J Am Geriatr Soc 2002;50:1962–8.
34. Shock NW, Watkin DM, Yiengst MJ, et al. Age differences in the water content of the body as related to basal oxygen consumption in males. J Gerontol 1963; 18:1–8.
35. Inouye SK. Delirium in older persons. N Engl J Med 2006;354:1157–65.
36. McNicoll L, Pisani MA, Zhang Y, et al. Delirium in the intensive care unit: occurrence and clinical course in older patients. J Am Geriatr Soc 2003;51:591–8.
37. Pisani MA, Murphy TE, Van Ness PH, et al. Characteristics associated with delirium in older patients in a medical intensive care unit. Arch Intern Med 2007;167:1629–34.
38. Ely EW, Gautam S, Margolin R, et al. The impact of delirium in the intensive care unit on hospital length of stay. Intensive Care Med 2001;27:1892–900.
39. Milbrandt EB, Deppen S, Harrison PL, et al. Costs associated with delirium in mechanically ventilated patients. Crit Care Med 2004;32:955–62.
40. Dubois MJ, Bergeron N, Dumont M, et al. Delirium in an intensive care unit: a study of risk factors. Intensive Care Med 2001;27:1297–304.
41. Garrouste-orgeas M, Timsit JF, Montuclard L, et al. Decision-making process, outcome, and 1-year quality of life of octogenarians referred for intensive care unit admission. Intensive Care Med 2006;32(7):1045–51.
42. Fowler RA, Sabur N, Li P, et al. Sex-and age-based differences in the delivery and outcomes of critical care. CMAJ 2007;177(12):1513–9.

43. Vink EE, Azoulay E, Caplan A, et al. Time-limited trial of intensive care treatment: an overview of current literature. Intensive Care Med 2018;44(9):1369–77.
44. Cosgriff JA, Pisani M, Bradley EH, et al. The association between treatment preferences and trajectories of care at the end-of-life. J Gen Intern Med 2007;22: 1566–71.
45. Fried TR, Bradley EH, Towle VR, et al. Understanding the treatment preferences of seriously ill patients. N Engl J Med 2002;346:1061–6.
46. Pandharipande PP, Girard TD, Jackson JC, et al. Long-term cognitive impairment after critical illness. N Engl J Med 2013;369:1306–16.
47. Brooks SE, Peetz AB. Evidence-based care of geriatric trauma patients. Surg Clin North Am 2017;97(5):1157–74.

Current Controversies in Caring for the Critically Ill Pulmonary Embolism Patient

Samuel Francis, MD[a],*, Christopher Kabrhel, MD, MPH[b]

KEYWORDS

- Pulmonary embolism • Thrombolysis • Deep venous thrombosis
- Venous thromboembolism

KEY POINTS

- Appropriate classification of the patient with pulmonary embolism (PE) into high-risk, intermediate-risk, or low-risk allows physicians to start proper resuscitative strategies.
- Due to the pathophysiology of PE, intravenous (IV) fluids and positive pressure ventilation can lead to deterioration of hemodynamic status, and physicians need to recognize if and when that occurs.
- Timely thrombolytic administration in the correct cohort of patients saves lives and can improve hemodynamic status of those with high-risk PE.

INTRODUCTION

Five percent of patients with pulmonary embolism (PE) present with hemodynamic instability, and death from PE usually occurs within the first hour.[1–4] Typical approaches to resuscitation, however, can be detrimental to patients with acute right ventricular (RV) overload due to PE. Emergency resuscitation, therefore, must be targeted to the unique pathophysiology of PE.

PULMONARY EMBOLISM PATHOPHYSIOLOGY

Acute pulmonary thromboembolism increases pulmonary vascular resistance and RV pressure, which leads to increased RV distention, septal bowing, and decreased left ventricular (LV) preload. Because RV distention asymmetrically compresses the intraventricular septum, LV volume can be compromised in the setting of severe RV

a Division of Emergency Medicine, Department of Surgery, Duke University Hospital, DUH Box 3096, 2301 Erwin Road, Durham, NC 27710, USA; b Department of Emergency Medicine, Center for Vascular Emergencies, Massachusetts General Hospital, Zero Emerson Place, Suite 3B, Boston, MA 02114, USA
* Corresponding author.
E-mail address: Samuel.francis@duke.edu
Twitter: @edmullet (S.F.); @chriskabrhel (C.K.)

Emerg Med Clin N Am 38 (2020) 931–944
https://doi.org/10.1016/j.emc.2020.06.012
0733-8627/20/© 2020 Elsevier Inc. All rights reserved.

overload, decreasing cardiac output (**Fig. 1**).[5] Individuals with preexisting heart disease or congestive heart failure are particularly prone to shock from PE.[6]

PE also can cause ventilation/perfusion (V/Q) mismatch, increased alveolar dead space, and a low mixed venous O_2 level.[5,7,8] Although hypoxia from V/Q mismatch usually is reversible with supplemental oxygen, hypoxic pulmonary vasoconstriction can worsen pulmonary hypertension, and myocardial ischemia can decrease cardiac output.

PULMONARY EMBOLISM CLASSIFICATION

Current terminology classifies PE as (1) high-risk, or massive; (2) intermediate-risk, or submassive; or (3) low-risk[1] (**Table 1**). Treatment, management, and disposition of patients depend on risk class, although the classification of PE can change over the course of a patient's care as new data become available or circumstances change[9]; 5% to 8% of patients clinically deteriorate or die from their PE after hospital admission.[10,11]

High-Risk or Massive Pulmonary Embolism

Patients with massive PE present with hypotension or shock. These patients are critically ill, so prompt recognition and resuscitation are required. Patients qualify as high-risk PE with either (1) systemic hypotension with systolic arterial pressure less than 90 mm Hg or a drop in systolic arterial pressure of at least 40 mm Hg for 15 minutes, not caused by a dysrhythmia or other etiology, or (2) shock manifested by tissue hypoperfusion or hypoxia. Shock can include altered level of consciousness, oliguria, or cool clammy extremities.[2,12] PE patients with arterial hypotension have greater than 25% mortality. PE is a common cause of cardiac arrest. One decision instrument found that greater than 50% of individuals less than 65 years old with pulseless electrical activity (PEA) as the initial rhythm had PE as the cause of cardiac arrest.[13] Patients with PE who present in cardiac arrest have mortality of greater than 90%.[5]

Intermediate-Risk or Submassive Pulmonary Embolism

Normotensive patients with RV dysfunction do not qualify as high-risk PE but have a higher all-cause mortality, 4% to 21%, compared with patients with normal RV function.[1,2,14,15] **Box 1** outlines criteria that define an intermediate-risk PE.[16] Approximately 35% to 40% of PE patients manifest at least 1 of these findings.[1,17] The 2019 European Society of Cardiology guidelines incorporate the Pulmonary Embolism Severity Index (**Table 2**) or its simplified version (**Table 3**)[18,19] and further delineate

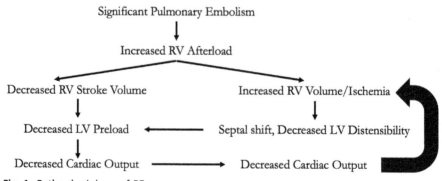

Fig. 1. Pathophysiology of PE.

Table 1
Pulmonary embolism classification

Type	Percentage of Total Pulmonary Embolism	Mortality at 3 Months
High-risk/massive	5%	58%
Systolic blood pressure <90		
Systolic blood pressure drop >90 mm Hg for $\geq$15 min		
Shock with tissue hypoperfusion or hypoxia		
Intermediate-risk/submassive	40%	21%
RV dilation on echocardiogram or CTPA		
Elevation of BNP or NT-proBNP		
Elevation of troponin		
ECG changes		
Low-risk	55%	<1%

Data from Kasper W, Konstantinides S, Geibel A, et al. Management strategies and determinants of outcome in acute major pulmonary embolism: results of a multicenter registry. J Am Coll Cardiol. 1997;30(5):1165-1171.

intermediate-risk PE into intermediate-high and intermediate-low categories based on positive biomarkers. Intermediate-high patients have both RV dysfunction on transthoracic echocardiogram or computed tomography pulmonary angiography (CTPA) and elevated cardiac troponin levels. Intermediate-low patients can have 1 of RV dysfunction or elevated troponin, or neither.[12]

Low-Risk Pulmonary Embolism

Hemodynamically stable patients without RV dysfunction are considered low risk.

Box 1
Criteria for intermediate-risk pulmonary embolism

1. RV dilation by RV diameter/LV diameter >0.9 or RV systolic dysfunction as noted on echocardiography

2. RV dilation by RV diameter/LV diameter greater than 0.9 on CTPA

3. Elevation of BNP (>90 pg/mL)

4. Elevation of NT-proBNP (>500 pg/mL)

5. ECG changes (new incomplete or complete right bundle branch block, anteroseptal ST segment changes, or anteroseptal T-wave inversion)

6. Myocardial necrosis by troponin testing (troponin I >0.4 ng/mL; troponin T >0.1 ng/mL)

Data from Jaff MR, McMurtry MS, Archer SL, et al. Management of massive and submassive pulmonary embolism, iliofemoral deep vein thrombosis, and chronic thromboembolic pulmonary hypertension: a scientific statement from the American Heart Association. Circulation. 2011;123(16):1788-1830.

Table 2
The Pulmonary Embolism Severity Index score

Age	___ years	
Sex	Female, 0 points	Male, +10 points
History of cancer	No, 0 points	Yes, +30 points
History of heart failure	No, 0 points	Yes, +10 points
History of chronic lung disease	No, 0 points	Yes, +10 points
Heart rate ≥110 beats per minute	No, 0 points	Yes, +20 points
Systolic BP <100 mm Hg	No, 0 points	Yes, +30 points
Respiratory rate ≥ 30/minute	No, 0 points	Yes, +20 points
Temperature <36C°	No, 0 points	Yes, +20 points
Altered mental status	No, 0 points	Yes, +60 points
O_2 saturation <90%	No, 0 points	Yes, +20 points

Total Score	Risk Category	30-day Mortality
0–65	I: very low	0%–1.6%
66–85	II: low	1.7%–3.5%
86–105	III: intermediate	3.2%–7.1%
106–125	IV: high	4%–11.4%
>125	V: very high	10%–24.5%

Data from Drahomir Aujesky, D. Scott Obrosky, Roslyn A. Stone, Derivation and Validation of a Prognostic Model for Pulmonary Embolism. Am J Respir Crit Care Med. 2005 Oct 15; 172(8): 1041–1046. Published online 2005 Jul 14. https://doi.org/10.1164/rccm.200506-862OC.

INITIAL EVALUATION AND TESTING

Bedside tests cannot confirm a diagnosis of PE but can increase suspicion and help risk-stratify patients.

Point-of-care echocardiography

In the critically ill patient too unstable to obtain confirmatory chest imaging (eg, CTPA), point-of-care echocardiography showing new RV dilatation (a ratio of the RV to LV internal diameter in diastole [RV:LV ratio] >1:1 [**Fig. 2**]) should increase physician suspicion of PE.[20] RV dilatation also can risk-stratify a patient with confirmed PE to the intermediate-risk category.[21] Visualization of a thrombus in the right-sided chambers of the heart, clot-in-transit, is associated with higher mortality (21% vs 11%) and can be an indication for surgical thromboembolectomy or thrombolysis.[22]

Electrocardiogram

Electrocardiogram (ECG) findings in PE typically are associated with new-onset RV dysfunction. Studies have demonstrated that patients with isolated T-wave inversions in either the precordial or inferior leads (**Fig. 3**) are more likely to have PE than acute coronary syndrome.[23,24] PE can be associated ST segment elevation in aVR with diffuse ST depression, a finding that can be confused with primary cardiac etiologies.[25,26] The ECG findings most predictive of cardiovascular collapse in patients with PE were new precordial T-wave inversions, new heart block, and atrial fibrillation.[27]

Table 3
The simplified Pulmonary Embolism Severity Index score

Age in years	≤80, 0 points	>80, +1 point
History of cancer	No, 0 points	Yes, +1 point
History of heart or lung disease	No, 0 points	Yes, +1 point
Heart rate ≥110 beats per minute	No, 0 points	Yes, +1 point
Systolic blood pressure <100 mm Hg	No, 0 points	Yes, +1 point
O_2 saturation <90%	No, 0 points	Yes, +1 point

Total Score	Risk Category	30-day Mortality
0	Low	1.1%
≥1	High	8.9%

Data from Jiménez D, Aujesky D, Moores L, et al. Simplification of the pulmonary embolism severity index for prognostication in patients with acute symptomatic pulmonary embolism. Arch Intern Med. 2010;170(15):1383-1389. https://doi.org/10.1001/archinternmed.2010.199.

Troponin

Elevated troponin in a PE patient indicates myocardial injury from a type II non–ST-elevation myocardial infarction. An elevated troponin is associated with higher mortality after PE and is one of the criteria for intermediate-risk PE.[28] The degree of troponin elevation predicts the degree of RV strain and mortality from PE.[29] The appropriate use of high sensitivity troponin assays are yet to be determined for PE.

B-type natriuretic peptide and N-terminal pro–B-type natriuretic peptide

B-type natriuretic peptide (BNP) and N-terminal pro–B-type BNP are released from cardiac myocytes in the setting of elevated RV pressure. Patients with PE and high BNP/NT-proBNP levels are at increased risk of a complicated in-hospital course and 30-day mortality.[30,31]

Lactate

Normotensive patients with PE and a plasma lactate greater than or equal to 2 mmol/L have higher mortality and are more likely to develop of shock or hypotension and require intubation or CPR.[32]

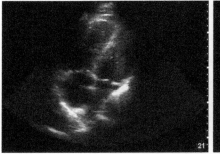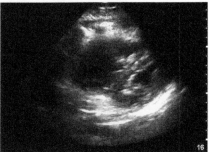

Fig. 2. Echocardiogram demonstrating apical 4 chamber (*left*) and parasternal long (*right*) view of RV dilatation in intermediate-risk PE. (Credit to Drs. Breslin & Gurysh.)

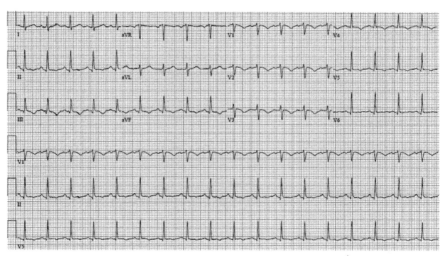

Fig. 3. ECG demonstrating anterior Y-wave inversions (V1–V4) seen in a patient with PE.

ADVANCED IMAGING IN THE PATIENT WITH PULMONARY EMBOLISM
Computed Tomography Pulmonary Angiogram

CTPA (**Fig. 4**) is the most common imaging modality used to confirm a diagnosis of PE. PE clot burden is readily apparent on CTPA. Some studies have shown that clot burden is useful in risk-stratifying patients with acute PE,[33,34] whereas other studies have not.[35] Compared with a gold standard of echocardiography, RV:LV ratio on CT has a lower positive predictive value.[36] Thus, the presence of RV dysfunction on CT should be confirmed with echocardiography. Unless there are data to suggest otherwise, lack of RV dysfunction seen on CTPA likely is correct owing to a sensitivity of 88% for this finding.

Ventilation/Perfusion Imaging

V/Q scan results are indeterminate in up to 70% of studies,[37,38] but V/Q imaging can be a useful study for patients with elevated creatinine or iodine dye allergy, those unable to lie flat for a CTPA, or those unable to fit in a CT scanner.[39]

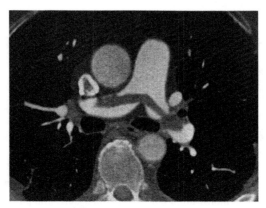

Fig. 4. CTPA demonstrating a saddle embolus.

INITIAL RESUSCITATION
Respiratory Support

Supplemental oxygenation
Hypoxemia from PE, which mostly is due to V/Q mismatch, typically responds to noninvasive supplemental oxygen. To minimize hypoxic pulmonary vasoconstriction and pulmonary hypertension, the emergency physician should aim to maintain oxygenation at or above 90% utilizing nasal cannula, high-flow nasal cannula, or nonrebreather masks.

Noninvasive positive pressure ventilation
Evidence for noninvasive positive pressure ventilation (eg, bilevel positive airway pressure) in patients with PE is limited.[40,41] Noninvasive PPV can open atelectatic lung, overcome pulmonary vascular shunting, and allow time for the physician to begin resuscitation.[42] Positive pressure also has the potential to impair RV function and decrease preload, worsening hemodynamic instability. Because noninvasive positive pressure ventilation can be removed easily in the case of hypotension, it is reasonable to trial for patients who cannot oxygenate or ventilate with supplemental oxygen.

Endotracheal intubation and mechanical ventilation
In patients with impending respiratory failure, intubation sometimes is necessary. Physicians must recognize, however, that intubation of a patient with PE can decrease preload and compress an already compressed LV. In high-risk PE patients who are intubated, 19% have cardiac arrest on induction and another 17% have cardiac arrest shortly afterward.[43,44] Therefore, intubation should be avoided if at all possible. If intubation is necessary, the authors recommend induction with a medication that minimizes hypotension (eg, ketamine) and having a vasopressor (eg, norepinephrine) ready.

Extracorporeal membranous oxygenation
In patients with refractory hypoxia or hypotension, venoarterial extracorporeal membrane oxygenation can provide a bridge to definitive PE therapy like systemic thrombolysis, catheter-directed lysis, or surgical embolectomy. Literature on this subject is limited to case reports and series, but selected patients appear to have good long-term outcomes.[45,46]

Circulatory Support

Intravenous fluids
Intravenous (IV) fluids can be helpful in PE by increasing preload.[47] Excessive IV fluids, however, can increase RV pressures, exacerbate septal bowing, lead to collapse of the LV during systole, and worsen hypotension in patients with severe PE. Expert recommendations recommend careful, not aggressive, fluids in acute PE.[12] A reasonable approach is an IV fluid bolus of 500 mL, if the patient has a history, examination findings, or laboratory findings that suggest hypovolemia, and re-evaluation after the initial bolus. If a patient develops worsening hypotension after IV fluid administration, fluids should be discontinued and vasopressor support started.

Vasopressors
Vasopressor support should be considered early in the resuscitation of patients with hypotension due to PE. Peripheral administration of vasopressors appears safe for the first 24 hours[48] and reduces the risk of large vessel injury that can lead to bleeding when thrombolytics are used. Norepinephrine, titrated to systolic blood pressure greater than 90 mm Hg,[49] is recommended as first-line vasopressor for patients

with PE. Epinephrine and dopamine increase chronotropy, which can exacerbate hypotension.[50–52] Dobutamine can increase cardiac index and decrease vascular resistance in patients with PE,[53] but it also is associated with systemic vasodilation, which can worsen hypotension. The authors recommend adding dobutamine if additional inotropic support is required in addition to norepinephrine.

Nitric oxide

Inhaled nitric oxide's ability to decrease pulmonary vascular resistance without affecting systemic blood pressure makes it a tantalizing potential therapy in patients with PE.[54] A clinical trial examining inhaled nitric oxide in patients with intermediate-risk PE, however, showed improvement in RV hypokinesis and dilation but no benefit in the primary study outcome.[55]

ANTICOAGULATION, THROMBOLYSIS, AND THROMBOEMBOLECTOMY

Anticoagulation

All patients without absolute contraindications should receive prompt anticoagulation after a diagnosis of PE. In patients with a high probability of PE, empiric treatment with anticoagulation is recommended, especially if diagnosis is expected to be delayed. For patients in whom an advanced intervention (thrombolysis or thromboembolectomy) is being considered, intravenous unfractionated heparin commonly is recommended because it can be discontinued easily. Direct-acting oral anticoagulants (DOACs), such as apixaban or rivaroxaban, and low-molecular-weight heparin (LMWH), all are reasonable first-line treatments for most stable patients with PE. For pregnant patients with confirmed PE, both the American College of Chest Physicians and American College of Obstetricians and Gynecologists recommend LMWH or heparin for the treatment of PE.[56,57] In pregnant patients with stable PE, LMWH is preferred over heparin. DOACs have not been widely studied in pregnant women.

Systemic Thrombolysis

Systemic thrombolysis can be lifesaving but also is associated with an increased risk of major intracranial and fatal hemorrhages. Thrombolysis is indicated for high-risk, hemodynamically unstable PE and may be considered for some intermediate-risk PE. Thrombolysis is not indicated for low-risk PE (**Table 4**).

Table 4	
Contraindications to thrombolysis administration in pulmonary embolism	
Absolute Contraindications	**Relative Contraindications**
Prior intracranial hemorrhage	Age >75 y
Known intracranial vascular malformation	Currently on anticoagulation
	Pregnancy
Known intracranial malignancy	>10 min of cardiopulmonary resuscitation
Recent significant facial or closed head injury	Noncompressible vascular punctures
	Internal bleeding within the past month
Recent spinal or intracranial surgery	History of uncontrolled or severe hypertension
Active bleeding or bleeding diathesis	Hypertension >180 mm Hg systolic or >110 mm Hg diastolic on presentation
Aortic dissection suspected	
Ischemic stroke within 3 mo	Dementia
	Ischemic stroke >3 mo old
	Major surgery within 3 wk

Absent contraindications, patients with high-risk PE should be treated with thrombolytics. When thrombolytics are indicated, delay in administration is associated with increased mortality.[58,59] The typical dose is 100 mg of tissue plasminogen activator (tPA) over 2 hours.[60] Weight-based tenecteplase also can be used. Compared with anticoagulation alone, meta-analyses demonstrate a 55% reduction in death or recurrent PE in high-risk PE patients treated with systemic thrombolytics,[61] with intracranial hemorrhage occurring in up to 2% and major extracranial bleeding occurring in 6% of patients.[11] For patients who present in cardiac arrest, societal guidelines suggest thrombolysis when a physician suspects PE.[16,56,62] Empiric thrombolysis in undifferentiated cardiac arrest, however, does not improve mortality benefit.[63]

For pregnant women in developed countries, PE causes 11% to 20% of maternal deaths.[64,65] As with nonpregnant patients, the mortality of high-risk PE in pregnant women is high, and delayed treatment increases mortality.[58,66] Thrombolysis should not be withheld in a pregnant woman with high-risk PE.[67,68] Neither tPA nor streptokinase crosses the placenta.[69] A recent systematic review of 127 pregnant high-risk PE patients treated with systemic thrombolysis found 6% maternal mortality and 12% fetal mortality. This same review found major bleeding complications of 18% and 58%, respectively, in the prepartum and postpartum periods.[70]

Thrombolytics therapy for patients with intermediate-risk PE is controversial. Full-dose thrombolysis appears to decrease the rate of hemodynamic compensation but does not reduce mortality, long-term morbidity, or chronic thromboembolic pulmonary hypertension.[61,71,72] Thrombolysis is associated with an increased risk of intracranial hemorrhage and major bleeding, particularly in patients over 65 years old.[73] Half-dose (ie, 50 mg) thrombolysis has been suggested as an approach to reduce major bleeding.[74,75] Similarly, this approach has been associated with improvement in RV function but not mortality.

Catheter-Directed Interventions

Catheter-directed intervention techniques include catheter-directed thrombolysis, clot maceration, and rheolytic and suction thrombectomy. In patients with high-risk or intermediate-risk PE, catheter-directed intervention may be beneficial, although data are sparse. To date, only 1 randomized controlled trial has compared catheter-directed thrombolysis to anticoagulation alone. This study, and several registries, have demonstrated short-term improvement in RV function, but no difference in mortality.[76]

Surgical Thromboembolectomy

Surgical thromboembolectomy should be considered in patients with high-risk PE in whom there are contraindications to systemic thrombolytic administration or after thrombolysis has failed.[77] Early patient identification and appropriate patient selection are associated with better mortality. Case series have demonstrated immediate improvement in RV function and high 1-month survival after successful embolectomy.[78,79]

Pulmonary Embolism Response Teams

PE response teams (PERTs) comprise multidisciplinary specialists who provide clinical expertise and expedite the care and disposition of patients with life-threatening PE. These teams are now in place across the United States and in many other countries. PERTs have been shown to improve disposition times, access to advanced therapies, and improve overall care.[80,81]

SUMMARY

Emergency physicians must be prepared to diagnose and resuscitate patients with PE rapidly. Certain aspects of PE resuscitation, however, run counter to typical approaches to resuscitation, so specific understanding of the pathophysiology of PE is required to guide resuscitation and avoid cardiovascular collapse. Once PE is diagnosed, treatment is guided by a patient's risk class. Although anticoagulation remains the mainstay of PE treatment, emergency physicians also must understand the indications and contraindications for thrombolysis and also should be aware of new therapies and models of care that may improve outcomes.

DISCLOSURE

Dr C. Kabrhel has received grant funding, paid to his institution, from Diagnostica Stago, Janssen, and Siemens Healthcare Diagnostics. He has consulted for Boston Scientific and EKOS Corporation.

REFERENCES

1. Goldhaber SZ, Visani L, De Rosa M. Acute pulmonary embolism: clinical outcomes in the International Cooperative Pulmonary Embolism Registry (ICOPER). Lancet 1999;353(9162):1386–9.
2. Kasper W, Konstantinides S, Geibel A, et al. Management strategies and determinants of outcome in acute major pulmonary embolism: results of a multicenter registry. J Am Coll Cardiol 1997;30(5):1165–71.
3. Goldhaber SZ, Hennekens CH, Evans DA, et al. Factors associated with correct antemortem diagnosis of major pulmonary embolism. Am J Med 1982;73(6): 822–6.
4. Laporte S, Mismetti P, Decousus H, et al. Clinical predictors for fatal pulmonary embolism in 15,520 patients with venous thromboembolism: findings from the Registro Informatizado de la Enfermedad TromboEmbolica venosa (RIETE) Registry. Circulation 2008;117(13):1711–6.
5. Wood KE. Major pulmonary embolism: review of a pathophysiologic approach to the golden hour of hemodynamically significant pulmonary embolism. Chest 2002;121(3):877–905.
6. Monreal M, Munoz-Torrero JF, Naraine VS, et al. Pulmonary embolism in patients with chronic obstructive pulmonary disease or congestive heart failure. Am J Med 2006;119(10):851–8.
7. D'Alonzo GE, Dantzker DR. Gas exchange alterations following pulmonary thromboembolism. Clin Chest Med 1984;5(3):411–9.
8. Manier G, Castaing Y, Guenard H. Determinants of hypoxemia during the acute phase of pulmonary embolism in humans. Am Rev Respir Dis 1985;132(2):332–8.
9. Konstantinides S, Geibel A, Olschewski M, et al. Association between thrombolytic treatment and the prognosis of hemodynamically stable patients with major pulmonary embolism: results of a multicenter registry. Circulation 1997;96(3): 882–8.
10. Casazza F, Becattini C, Bongarzoni A, et al. Clinical features and short term outcomes of patients with acute pulmonary embolism. The Italian Pulmonary Embolism Registry (IPER). Thromb Res 2012;130(6):847–52.
11. Meyer G, Vicaut E, Konstantinides SV. Fibrinolysis for intermediate-risk pulmonary embolism. N Engl J Med 2014;371(6):581–2.

12. Konstantinides SV, Meyer G, Becattini C, et al, The Task Force for the diagnosis and management of acute pulmonary embolism of the European Society of Cardiology (ESC). 2019 ESC Guidelines for the diagnosis and management of acute pulmonary embolism developed in collaboration with the European Respiratory Society (ERS): The Task Force for the diagnosis and management of acute pulmonary embolism of the European Society of Cardiology (ESC). Eur Respir J 2019;54(3):1901647.

13. Courtney DM, Kline JA. Prospective use of a clinical decision rule to identify pulmonary embolism as likely cause of outpatient cardiac arrest. Resuscitation 2005; 65(1):57–64.

14. Grifoni S, Olivotto I, Cecchini P, et al. Short-term clinical outcome of patients with acute pulmonary embolism, normal blood pressure, and echocardiographic right ventricular dysfunction. Circulation 2000;101(24):2817–22.

15. Ribeiro A, Lindmarker P, Juhlin-Dannfelt A, et al. Echocardiography Doppler in pulmonary embolism: right ventricular dysfunction as a predictor of mortality rate. Am Heart J 1997;134(3):479–87.

16. Jaff MR, McMurtry MS, Archer SL, et al. Management of massive and submassive pulmonary embolism, iliofemoral deep vein thrombosis, and chronic thromboembolic pulmonary hypertension: a scientific statement from the American Heart Association. Circulation 2011;123(16):1788–830.

17. Pollack CV, Schreiber D, Goldhaber SZ, et al. Clinical characteristics, management, and outcomes of patients diagnosed with acute pulmonary embolism in the emergency department: initial report of EMPEROR (Multicenter Emergency Medicine Pulmonary Embolism in the Real World Registry). J Am Coll Cardiol 2011;57(6):700–6.

18. Jimenez D, Aujesky D, Moores L, et al. Simplification of the pulmonary embolism severity index for prognostication in patients with acute symptomatic pulmonary embolism. Arch Intern Med 2010;170(15):1383–9.

19. Aujesky D, Obrosky DS, Stone RA, et al. Derivation and validation of a prognostic model for pulmonary embolism. Am J Respir Crit Care Med 2005;172(8):1041–6.

20. Dresden S, Mitchell P, Rahimi L, et al. Right ventricular dilatation on bedside echocardiography performed by emergency physicians aids in the diagnosis of pulmonary embolism. Ann Emerg Med 2014;63(1):16–24.

21. Dahhan T, Siddiqui I, Tapson VF, et al. Clinical and echocardiographic predictors of mortality in acute pulmonary embolism. Cardiovasc Ultrasound 2016;14(1):44.

22. Torbicki A, Galie N, Covezzoli A, et al. Right heart thrombi in pulmonary embolism: results from the International Cooperative Pulmonary Embolism Registry. J Am Coll Cardiol 2003;41(12):2245–51.

23. Sinha N, Yalamanchili K, Sukhija R, et al. Role of the 12-lead electrocardiogram in diagnosing pulmonary embolism. Cardiol Rev 2005;13(1):46–9.

24. Sukhija R, Aronow WS, Ahn C, et al. Electrocardiographic abnormalities in patients with right ventricular dilation due to acute pulmonary embolism. Cardiology 2006;105(1):57–60.

25. Harhash AA, Huang JJ, Reddy S, et al. aVR ST segment elevation: Acute STEMI or Not? Incidence of an acute coronary occlusion. Am J Med 2019;132(5): 622–30.

26. Brenes-Salazar JA. ST-segment elevation in lead aVR: a visual reminder of potential catastrophe. JAMA Intern Med 2018;178(6):847–8.

27. Shopp JD, Stewart LK, Emmett TW, et al. Findings from 12-lead electrocardiography that predict circulatory shock from pulmonary embolism: systematic review and meta-analysis. Acad Emerg Med 2015;22(10):1127–37.

28. Becattini C, Vedovati MC, Agnelli G. Prognostic value of troponins in acute pulmonary embolism: a meta-analysis. Circulation 2007;116(4):427–33.
29. Andrews J, MacNee W, Murchison J. Measurement of cardiac troponin identifies patients with moderate to large pulmonary emboli and right ventricular strain. Eur Respir J 2014;44(Suppl 58):P2407.
30. Klok FA, Mos IC, Huisman MV. Brain-type natriuretic peptide levels in the prediction of adverse outcome in patients with pulmonary embolism: a systematic review and meta-analysis. Am J Respir Crit Care Med 2008;178(4):425–30.
31. Lega JC, Lacasse Y, Lakhal L, et al. Natriuretic peptides and troponins in pulmonary embolism: a meta-analysis. Thorax 2009;64(10):869–75.
32. Vanni S, Jimenez D, Nazerian P, et al. Short-term clinical outcome of normotensive patients with acute PE and high plasma lactate. Thorax 2015;70(4):333–8.
33. Patel A, Kassar K, Veer M, et al. Clot burden serves as an effective predictor of 30 day mortality in patients with acute pulmonary embolism. J Am Coll Cardiol 2018;71(11 Supplement):A1933.
34. Hariharan P, Dudzinski DM, Rosovsky R, et al. Relation among clot burden, right-sided heart strain, and adverse events after acute pulmonary embolism. Am J Cardiol 2016;118(10):1568–73.
35. Vedovati MC, Becattini C, Agnelli G, et al. Multidetector CT scan for acute pulmonary embolism: embolic burden and clinical outcome. Chest 2012;142(6): 1417–24.
36. Dudzinski DM, Hariharan P, Parry BA, et al. Assessment of right ventricular strain by computed tomography versus echocardiography in acute pulmonary embolism. Acad Emerg Med 2017;24(3):337–43.
37. Fennerty T. The diagnosis of pulmonary embolism. BMJ 1997;314(7078):425–9.
38. Investigators P. Value of the ventilation/perfusion scan in acute pulmonary embolism. Results of the prospective investigation of pulmonary embolism diagnosis (PIOPED). JAMA 1990;263(20):2753–9.
39. Moore AJE, Wachsmann J, Chamarthy MR, et al. Imaging of acute pulmonary embolism: an update. Cardiovasc Diagn Ther 2018;8(3):225–43.
40. Noble WH, Kay JC. Effect of continuous positive-pressure ventilation on oxygenation after pulmonary microemboli in dogs. Crit Care Med 1985;13(5):412–6.
41. Antonelli M, Conti G, Moro ML, et al. Predictors of failure of noninvasive positive pressure ventilation in patients with acute hypoxemic respiratory failure: a multicenter study. Intensive Care Med 2001;27(11):1718–28.
42. Green RS, Fergusson DA, Turgeon AF, et al. Resuscitation Prior to Emergency Endotracheal Intubation: Results of a National Survey. West J Emerg Med 2016;17(5):542–8.
43. Rosenberger P, Shernan SK, Shekar PS, et al. Acute hemodynamic collapse after induction of general anesthesia for emergent pulmonary embolectomy. Anesth Analg 2006;102(5):1311–5.
44. Bennett JM, Pretorius M, Ahmad RM, et al. Hemodynamic instability in patients undergoing pulmonary embolectomy: institutional experience. J Clin Anesth 2015;27(3):207–13.
45. Al-Bawardy R, Rosenfield K, Borges J, et al. Extracorporeal membrane oxygenation in acute massive pulmonary embolism: a case series and review of the literature. Perfusion 2019;34(1):22–8.
46. Kjaergaard B, Kristensen JH, Sindby JE, et al. Extracorporeal membrane oxygenation in life-threatening massive pulmonary embolism. Perfusion 2019;34(6): 467–74.

47. Mercat A, Diehl JL, Meyer G, et al. Hemodynamic effects of fluid loading in acute massive pulmonary embolism. Crit Care Med 1999;27(3):540–4.

48. Cardenas-Garcia J, Schaub KF, Belchikov YG, et al. Safety of peripheral intravenous administration of vasoactive medication. J Hosp Med 2015;10(9):581–5.

49. Ventetuolo CE, Klinger JR. Management of acute right ventricular failure in the intensive care unit. Ann Am Thorac Soc 2014;11(5):811–22.

50. Ghignone M, Girling L, Prewitt RM. Effect of increased pulmonary vascular resistance on right ventricular systolic performance in dogs. Am J Physiol 1984;246(3 Pt 2):H339–43.

51. Vasu MA, O'Keefe DD, Kapellakis GZ, et al. Myocardial oxygen consumption: effects of epinephrine, isoproterenol, dopamine, norepinephrine, and dobutamine. Am J Physiol 1978;235(2):H237–41.

52. Boulain T, Lanotte R, Legras A, et al. Efficacy of epinephrine therapy in shock complicating pulmonary embolism. Chest 1993;104(1):300–2.

53. Jardin F, Genevray B, Brun-Ney D, et al. Dobutamine: a hemodynamic evaluation in pulmonary embolism shock. Crit Care Med 1985;13(12):1009–12.

54. Capellier G, Jacques T, Balvay P, et al. Inhaled nitric oxide in patients with pulmonary embolism. Intensive Care Med 1997;23(10):1089–92.

55. Kline JA, Puskarich MA, Jones AE, et al. Inhaled nitric oxide to treat intermediate risk pulmonary embolism: A multicenter randomized controlled trial. Nitric Oxide 2019;84:60–8.

56. Kearon C, Akl EA, Comerota AJ, et al. Antithrombotic therapy for VTE disease: Antithrombotic Therapy and Prevention of Thrombosis, 9th ed: American College of Chest Physicians Evidence-Based Clinical Practice Guidelines. Chest 2012; 141(2 Suppl):e419S–96S.

57. ACOG Practice Bulletin No. 196: Thromboembolism in Pregnancy. Obstet Gynecol 2018;132(1):e1–17.

58. Beydilli I, Yilmaz F, Sonmez BM, et al. Thrombolytic therapy delay is independent predictor of mortality in acute pulmonary embolism at emergency service. Kaohsiung J Med Sci 2016;32(11):572–8.

59. Wang Y, Yang Y, Wang C, et al. Delay in thrombolysis of massive and submassive pulmonary embolism. Clin Appl Thromb Hemost 2011;17(4):381–6.

60. Weinberg I, Jaff MR. Treating large pulmonary emboli: do the guidelines guide us? Curr Opin Pulm Med 2013;19(5):413–21.

61. Wan S, Quinlan DJ, Agnelli G, et al. Thrombolysis compared with heparin for the initial treatment of pulmonary embolism: a meta-analysis of the randomized controlled trials. Circulation 2004;110(6):744–9.

62. Monsieurs KG, Nolan JP, Bossaert LL, et al. European resuscitation council guidelines for resuscitation 2015: Section 1. Executive summary. Resuscitation 2015;95:1–80.

63. Bottiger BW, Arntz HR, Chamberlain DA, et al. Thrombolysis during resuscitation for out-of-hospital cardiac arrest. N Engl J Med 2008;359(25):2651–62.

64. Benhamou D, Chassard D, Mercier FJ, et al. [The seventh report of the confidential enquiries into maternal deaths in the United Kingdom: comparison with French data]. Ann Fr Anesth Reanim 2009;28(1):38–43.

65. Clark SL, Belfort MA, Dildy GA, et al. Maternal death in the 21st century: causes, prevention, and relationship to cesarean delivery. Am J Obstet Gynecol 2008; 199(1):36.e1-5 [discussion: 91–2.e7-11].

66. Kucher N, Rossi E, De Rosa M, et al. Massive pulmonary embolism. Circulation 2006;113(4):577–82.

67. Lindquist A, Kurinczuk JJ, Redshaw M, et al. Experiences, utilisation and outcomes of maternity care in England among women from different socio-economic groups: findings from the 2010 National Maternity Survey. BJOG 2015;122(12):1610–7.

68. Holden EL, Ranu H, Sheth A, et al. Thrombolysis for massive pulmonary embolism in pregnancy–a report of three cases and follow up over a two year period. Thromb Res 2011;127(1):58–9.

69. te Raa GD, Ribbert LS, Snijder RJ, et al. Treatment options in massive pulmonary embolism during pregnancy; a case-report and review of literature. Thromb Res 2009;124(1):1–5.

70. Martillotti G, Boehlen F, Robert-Ebadi H, et al. Treatment options for severe pulmonary embolism during pregnancy and the postpartum period: a systematic review. J Thromb Haemost 2017;15(10):1942–50.

71. Kline JA, Nordenholz KE, Courtney DM, et al. Treatment of submassive pulmonary embolism with tenecteplase or placebo: cardiopulmonary outcomes at 3 months: multicenter double-blind, placebo-controlled randomized trial. J Thromb Haemost 2014;12(4):459–68.

72. Konstantinides SV, Vicaut E, Danays T, et al. Impact of Thrombolytic Therapy on the Long-Term Outcome of Intermediate-Risk Pulmonary Embolism. J Am Coll Cardiol 2017;69(12):1536–44.

73. Chatterjee S, Chakraborty A, Weinberg I, et al. Thrombolysis for pulmonary embolism and risk of all-cause mortality, major bleeding, and intracranial hemorrhage: a meta-analysis. JAMA 2014;311(23):2414–21.

74. Levine M, Hirsh J, Weitz J, et al. A randomized trial of a single bolus dosage regimen of recombinant tissue plasminogen activator in patients with acute pulmonary embolism. Chest 1990;98(6):1473–9.

75. Sharifi M, Bay C, Skrocki L, et al. Moderate pulmonary embolism treated with thrombolysis (from the "MOPETT" Trial). Am J Cardiol 2013;111(2):273–7.

76. Kucher N, Boekstegers P, Muller OJ, et al. Randomized, controlled trial of ultrasound-assisted catheter-directed thrombolysis for acute intermediate-risk pulmonary embolism. Circulation 2014;129(4):479–86.

77. Fukuda I, Daitoku K. Surgical embolectomy for acute pulmonary thromboembolism. Ann Vasc Dis 2017;10(2):107–14.

78. Stein PD, Alnas M, Beemath A, et al. Outcome of pulmonary embolectomy. Am J Cardiol 2007;99(3):421–3.

79. Keeling WB, Sundt T, Leacche M, et al. Outcomes after surgical pulmonary embolectomy for acute pulmonary embolus: a multi-institutional study. Ann Thorac Surg 2016;102(5):1498–502.

80. Kabrhel C, Rosovsky R, Channick R, et al. A multidisciplinary pulmonary embolism response team: initial 30-month experience with a novel approach to delivery of care to patients with submassive and massive pulmonary embolism. Chest 2016;150(2):384–93.

81. Chaudhury P, Gadre S, Schneider E, et al. Impact of multidisciplinary pulmonary embolism response team availability on management and outcomes. Am J Cardiol 2019;124(9):1465–9.

Extracorporeal Membrane Oxygenation in the Emergency Department

Jenelle H. Badulak, MD[a],*, Zachary Shinar, MD[b]

KEYWORDS

- Extracorporeal membrane oxygenation • ECMO • Extracorporeal life support
- ECLS • Extracorporeal cardiopulmonary resuscitation • ECPR • VA ECMO

KEY POINTS

- Venovenous extracorporeal membrane oxygenation (ECMO) provides pulmonary bypass for severe respiratory failure, and venoarterial ECMO provides cardiac and pulmonary bypass for severe cardiac failure including cardiac arrest.
- Inclusion criteria for extracorporeal cardiopulmonary resuscitation (ECPR): reversible cause of arrest, witnessed arrest with bystander CPR, total chest compression time of less than 60 minutes, no known preexisting chronic terminal illnesses.
- The initiation of ECMO is divided into 3 stages: (1) vascular access, (2) insertion of ECMO cannulas and connection to the circuit once the patient is determined to be an ECMO candidate, (3) pump initiation.
- Post-circuit initiation critical care for ECPR includes establishing an arterial line and managing vasopressors, defibrillation if needed, checking an arterial blood gas on right upper extremity, therapeutic hypothermia, adding an inotrope for left ventricular distention, placing a distal perfusion catheter, and treating the underlying cause of arrest.

 Video content accompanies this article at http://www.emed.theclinics.com.

INTRODUCTION

Extracorporeal membrane oxygenation (ECMO) is an invasive form of artificial life support used for severe cardiac and/or pulmonary failure. The worldwide use of ECMO is rapidly growing and indications for its application are expanding. In the past decade, use of venoarterial (VA) ECMO to restore perfusion in patients with refractory cardiac

[a] Division of Pulmonary, Critical Care and Sleep Medicine, Department of Emergency Medicine, University of Washington, Harborview Medical Center, Box 359702, 325 Ninth Avenue, Seattle, WA 98104-2499, USA; [b] Department of Emergency Medicine, Sharp Memorial Hospital, 7901 Frost Street, San Diego, CA 92130, USA
* Corresponding author.
E-mail address: badulakj@uw.edu
Twitter: @JenelleBadulak (J.H.B.); @ZackShinar (Z.S.)

Emerg Med Clin N Am 38 (2020) 945–959
https://doi.org/10.1016/j.emc.2020.06.015
0733-8627/20/© 2020 Elsevier Inc. All rights reserved.
emed.theclinics.com

arrest, called extracorporeal cardiopulmonary resuscitation (ECPR), has increased in emergency departments and in the prehospital setting.[1-6] This article highlights circuit configurations and physiology of ECMO, guidance for running an ECPR code, description of the cannulation procedure, postcircuit initiation critical care, patient selection, and the evidence for use of ECMO.

EXTRACORPOREAL MEMBRANE OXYGENATION MODES AND CIRCUIT CONFIGURATION

In VA ECMO, blood is drained from the central venous system, pumped through a membrane lung (ML), and returned to the central arterial system providing cardiopulmonary bypass. VA ECMO provides hemodynamic support. In venovenous (VV) ECMO, blood is drained from the central venous system, pumped through a ML and returned to the central venous system providing pulmonary bypass. VV ECMO provides no hemodynamic support, as the return blood is isolated to the venous system.

VA ECMO is used for severe cardiogenic or obstructive shock requiring mechanical circulatory support and for cardiac arrest refractory to advanced cardiac life support (ACLS). In peripheral VA ECMO, a venous drainage cannula is placed in the femoral vein draining blood from the right atrium and vena cava and blood is returned via a cannula in the femoral artery (**Fig. 1**).

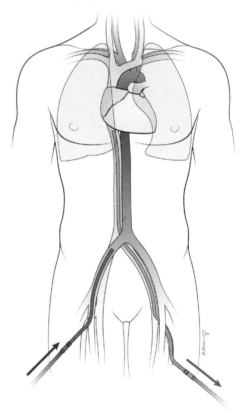

Fig. 1. Venous drainage cannula in the right femoral vein and return cannula in the femoral artery. (Image used with permission from CollectedMed.)

VV ECMO is used for hypoxemia and/or hypercarbia refractory to conventional therapies. In the most common configuration for VV ECMO, a venous drainage cannula is placed in the femoral vein draining blood from the inferior vena cava and blood is returned via a cannula in the right internal jugular vein with blood flow directed across the tricuspid valve (**Fig. 2**).

The basic ECMO circuit is composed of a venous drainage cannula, a centrifugal pump that pushes blood through an ML, and a return cannula. All of these components are connected with tubing. A flow probe is attached to the tubing and measures the rate of blood flow through the circuit. Sweep gas is composed of oxygen or a blend of oxygen and air that is supplied to the ML where blood is oxygenated and carbon dioxide (CO_2) is removed. A heat exchanger is connected to the ML and regulates temperature of the blood in the circuit. Some circuits have additional capabilities to monitor pressures throughout the system, detect air bubbles, and monitor hemoglobin and oxygen saturation (**Fig. 3**).

General Extracorporeal Membrane Oxygenation Physiology

Most adult ECMO circuits use a centrifugal pump; therefore, speed, in revolutions per minute (RPMs), is the independent variable set by the clinician, which controls blood flow. As blood flow increases, inlet pressures will become more negative and return pressures more positive.

Centrifugal pumps are preload dependent and afterload sensitive. Therefore, impediments to venous drainage (preload) including hypovolemia, a small, kinked, or

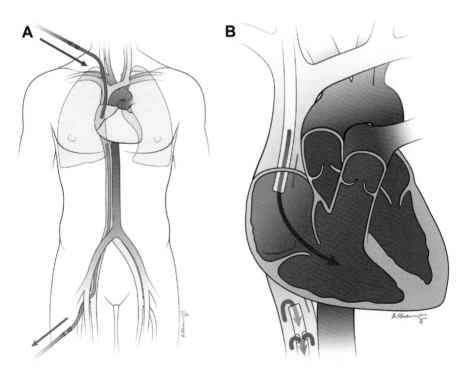

Fig. 2. (*A*) Venous drainage cannula in the right femoral vein and return cannula in the right internal jugular vein. (*B*) Blood is drained from the IVC and returned across the tricuspid valve into the right heart. (Image used with permission from CollectedMed.)

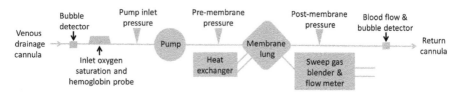

Fig. 3. Schematic of an example ECMO circuit.

clotted drainage cannula, tamponade, tension pneumothorax/hemothorax, or abdominal compartment syndrome will result in lower blood flow at a given speed. Causes of high afterload including a small, kinked, or clotted return cannula, clotted ML, or high systemic vascular resistance (only in VA ECMO) will also result in lower blood flow.

Sweep gas runs through the lumens of small tubules bathed in blood within the ML (**Fig. 4**). The rate at which the sweep gas is pushed through the ML is called the sweep gas flow rate, which determines the partial pressure of carbon dioxide (P_{CO_2}) exiting the ML. As the sweep flow is increased, P_{CO_2} decreases. A blender can be used to change the percentage of oxygen in the sweep gas, called fraction of delivered oxygen (FdO_2). As long as the ML is functioning and the sweep gas is >0.5 L/min, blood leaving the ML will be 100% saturated with O_2.

Venoarterial Extracorporeal Membrane Oxygenation Physiology

Total blood flow in the arterial system (Q) during VA ECMO is the combination of native cardiac output and ECMO blood flow. ECMO blood flow is titrated to target ~80% of estimated resting cardiac output based on the patient's body surface area. In addition, echocardiography is used to guide ECMO blood flow titration. As ECMO flow is increased, more venous blood is drained leading to decreased native heart preload and ventricular decompression. At the same time, native heart afterload is increased due to retrograde ECMO flow up the aorta, which will eventually lead to left ventricular dilation. The goal is to find the ECMO blood flow that (1) achieves a perfusing mean arterial pressure (MAP), and (2) maximally decompresses the right ventricle without leading to left ventricular dilation. Although Q has a significant impact on MAP, additional increases in MAP can be achieved using vasopressors to increase systemic vascular resistance (SVR) as well as volume administration to address central venous pressure (CVP).

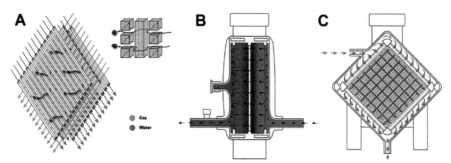

Fig. 4. (A) Red blood cells travel in-between tubules containing sweep gas in the lumen. (B) Deoxygenated blood enters the ML and oxygenated blood exits after interacting with the ML tubules. (C) Sweep gas enters the ML, travels through the lumen of the tubules and is exhausted out of the bottom of the ML. (Image used with permission from CollectedMed.)

$$MAP = (SVR \times Q) + CVP$$

The degree of cardiac failure determines where the mixing point is in the aorta between blood from the native heart and retrograde flow from the ECMO pump (**Fig. 5**). This concept is important because the O_2 and CO_2 content of the blood will depend on whether it is coming from the native lungs or the ML. If the native lungs are functioning poorly in the setting of native heart recovery, poorly oxygenated blood will be ejected from the native heart leading to upper body hypoxemia. This is termed differential oxygenation or north-south syndrome. Thus oxygenation via pulse oximeter or arterial blood gas is monitored on the right upper extremity for early detection of this pathologic state.

Venovenous Extracorporeal Membrane Oxygenation Physiology

When using VV ECMO, blood flow is circulated entirely within the venous system, therefore VV ECMO has no direct effect on hemodynamics. Blood is oxygenated and CO_2 is removed in the ML. The blood is then returned to the patient's right atrium where it moves through the native heart and lungs, thus obviating the requirement of the native lungs to contribute to gas exchange. When ECMO blood

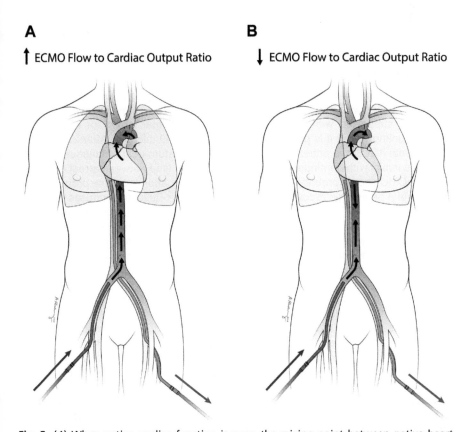

A ↑ ECMO Flow to Cardiac Output Ratio

B ↓ ECMO Flow to Cardiac Output Ratio

Fig. 5. (*A*) When native cardiac function is poor, the mixing point between native heart blood flow and ECMO blood flow is in the proximal aorta. (*B*) When native cardiac function improves, the mixing point moves further down the aorta. (Image used with permission from CollectedMed.)

flow is increased, the fraction of oxygenated blood entrained into the heart increases, raising the mixed venous oxygen saturation and subsequently raising the arterial oxygen saturation.

PATIENT SELECTION

In general, ECMO can be used for severe cardiac and/or pulmonary failure refractory to conventional therapies.[7] ECMO is a form of life support and is thus not a treatment but a bridge to native heart/lung recovery or durable organ replacement. Therefore, a patient should ideally only be placed on ECMO with a predetermined exit strategy. General contraindications for ECMO include multiorgan failure with a high risk of death despite use of ECMO, severe neurologic disease with poor neurologic prognosis or other preexisting terminal illness such as metastatic malignancy, end-stage organ dysfunction (lung, heart, liver, kidney) without possibility of transplant, severe coagulopathy, advanced age with poor functional status, and inadequate vascular access for implantation of cannulas. Although the bleeding patient was traditionally excluded from ECMO implementation, growing experience has shown that systemic anticoagulation is probably able to be safely held for periods of time, especially given the widespread use of heparin-bonded circuits.[8] Additional contraindications for VA ECMO include untreated aortic dissection and aortic valve insufficiency. For VV ECMO, prolonged high-intensity mechanical ventilation >7 to 10 days is associated with poor outcomes and is thus a relative contraindication.[9–12]

Extracorporeal Cardiopulmonary Resuscitation

For ECPR, the goal is to select previously high-functioning patients without known terminal illnesses who had a witnessed cardiac arrest from a reversible cause who have been supported with high-quality CPR. The optimal timing for initiation of ECMO is unknown but it is probably between 25 and 60 minutes. After 25 minutes of traditional ACLS, the patient is unlikely to achieve return of spontaneous circulation and survival with continued ACLS is dismal.[13] The time between arrest and initiation of ECMO should probably not exceed 60 minutes, after which the probability of a meaningful neurologic recovery steeply declines.[14,15] Reversible causes of arrest may include myocardial infarction treated with revascularization, massive pulmonary embolism treated with anticoagulation, thrombolytics, and/or thrombectomy, cardiotoxic drug overdose that resolves after drug metabolism or decontamination, and accidental hypothermia, which is easily corrected with rewarming on the ECMO circuit. Many centers have developed their own ECPR criteria that follow these general principles.[1–6,16]

The evidence for ECPR involves case series, registry data, and propensity analyses.[1–3,16–19] No randomized trials have been published to date. SAVE-J was a prospective observational study that compared out-of-hospital cardiac arrest survival between patients sent to ECPR centers versus hospitals without ECPR capability. Patients sent to ECPR centers had a statistically significant fourfold increased survival.[2] The most impressive ECPR case series have come from Minneapolis where out-of-hospital cardiac arrests are taken directly to the cardiac catheterization laboratory. Neurologically intact survivorship has been greater than 40% from that institution.[6,20] An emergency department in San Diego using emergency physician-initiated ECPR showed statistically significant improved survivorship for ECPR patients compared with ECPR-eligible patients who did not receive ECPR. In addition, this study showed that most of those who died did so early in their hospitalization. Prolonged hospitalizations among nonsurvivors were few.[5]

Venoarterial Extracorporeal Membrane Oxygenation for Shock

VA ECMO is most often used for patients with cardiogenic shock and obstructive shock due to massive pulmonary embolism.[21] For cardiogenic shock, VA ECMO can be rapidly deployed at the bedside to rescue an undersupported patient failing medical therapy or other temporary mechanical circulatory support (MCS) devices by providing full biventricular support. Ethical concerns regarding lack of equipoise between offering or withholding MCS for patients with critical cardiogenic shock make randomized controlled trials unlikely. However, multiple observational studies show improved survival when VA ECMO is used.[22–24] Medical causes of cardiogenic shock likely to be encountered in the emergency department include acute myocardial infarction,[25] myocarditis,[26] acute decompensated heart failure,[27] and cardiotoxic drug overdose.[28] Some centers consider use of VA ECMO for refractory septic shock with mixed results.[29–31] Expeditious transfer of the patient in cardiogenic shock to cardiogenic shock centers equipped with temporary MCS and other durable organ replacement options should be considered.[32]

Venovenous Extracorporeal Membrane Oxygenation for Respiratory Failure

VV ECMO can be used for patients with severe respiratory failure refractory to conventional support. Disease states include severe hypoxemia secondary to acute respiratory distress syndrome (ARDS) despite conventional therapies. Other examples include severe asthma exacerbations,[33] traumatic airway injuries, or bronchopleural fistulas, which all pose significant ventilatory challenges. VV ECMO can also be used when unable to establish a definitive airway via intubation or surgical airway.

Initial studies for use of VV ECMO for ARDS showed tentatively optimistic data but varied significantly as to when VV ECMO was initiated.[34–37] The question remained whether VV ECMO should be used early in respiratory failure or after all other therapies had failed. Recently, the large EOLIA trial was stopped early secondary to futility,[38] with much controversy surrounding the interpretation of the outcome.

RUNNING AN EXTRACORPOREAL CARDIOPULMONARY RESUSCITATION CODE

One key concept in not only ECPR but any new resuscitative technology is to ensure the resuscitation leading up to that intervention is optimized. Before jumping to advanced technologies, it is important to assess for simpler, rapidly correctable causes of cardiac arrest. A witnessed ventricular fibrillation arrest requires defibrillation, not ECMO. A patient in pseudo-pulseless electrical activity needs vasopressors and evaluation for rapidly correctable causes before ECMO initiation. Using your resources to efficiently optimize your traditional resuscitation efforts in concert with the added complexities of an ECMO initiation is key.

The first component in running the ECMO code is to set up a prearranged place for each medical device and health care provider in the room. Each institution will need to decide the optimal strategy and design of this room, but keeping uniformity within this design is ideal. Common medical devices used during ECMO codes include ultrasounds for cardiac imaging as well as vascular access, code cart with defibrillator, computer on wheels for charting and organization, mechanical chest compression device, airway equipment, and a stool for manual chest compressions. In addition to this standard equipment, 2 small procedural tables, covered with a large sterile drape at the end of the patient gurney extend the working space for ECMO-related equipment. This equipment includes cannulas for both femoral vein and artery, ECMO circuit, dilators, stiff and floppy guidewires, and clamps. Toomey syringes are needed with a crystalloid basin for the underwater seal necessary for circuit connection.

The second component involves limiting the number of people in the room to those directly involved in the resuscitation. Each person should have a dedicated place to stand and no other personnel should be allowed in the room.

The final component is defining the roles of each of the providers in the room. The most critical role is the code team leader. There are many advantages to assigning a nurse to this role. Their job is to be the sole voice in the room. They control the room and oversee the quality of chest compressions, dosing of medications, chest compression free times, and defibrillation. The second is the physician team leader. The job of this physician is to secure an airway and then determine the patient's inclusion/exclusion for ECMO. They will gather the patient's medical history and decide if deviations from the standard resuscitation are necessary. They need to resist, if possible, participating in the cannulation procedure. The third role is the physician cannulator who performs the cannulation procedure. The fourth role that is underappreciated, but imperative, is a wire assistant. This provider assists the cannulator in guidewire insertion and dilation particularly during the difficult task of femoral arterial cannulation (**Fig. 6**).

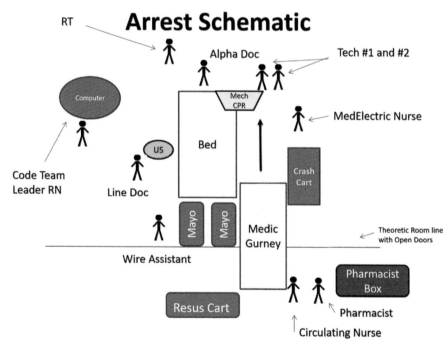

Fig. 6. ECPR provider roles. RT: respiratory therapist operating ventilator, Alpha Doc: doctor team leader who establishes airway and gathers patient's medical history to determine ECMO candidacy of patient, Tech #1 and #2 run mechanical CPR device (Mech CPR), MedElectric nurse: uses Crash Cart administering medications and electricity for defibrillation, Pharmacist: prepares medications, Circulating Nurse: primes and operates ECMO pump, Medic Gurney: location for paramedic's gurney, Mayo: additional small tables to extend working surface of emergency department bed, Resus Cart: location of ECMO supplies and equipment, Wire Assistant: assists Line Doc with cannulation, Line Doc: performs cannulation procedure using ultrasound, Code Team Leader RN: nurse who directs standard ACLS and records with computer.

Each provider should understand the basic metrics of minimizing interruptions in chest compressions, optimizing defibrillation, providing high-quality chest compressions, and troubleshooting medical equipment. This allows for the code to run quietly and standard resuscitation to be optimized. Frequent feedback about the initial phases of the resuscitation in addition to the ECMO specific components should be discussed during code debriefing and simulated training sessions. ECPR simulation at regular intervals is imperative to maintain personnel skillsets.

EXTRACORPOREAL CARDIOPULMONARY RESUSCITATION CANNULATION PROCEDURE

Although cannulation can be performed with 1 cannulator and 1 wire assistant, it is best done with 2 cannulators and 2 wire assistants. Ultrasound guidance is critical for minimizing vessel trauma and confirming that the correct vessel has been accessed. Sometimes, when ideal circumstances occur (right-handed cannulator on right femoral vessels with optimal ultrasound imagery), 1 cannulator can complete cannulation of both vessels before the opposite groin is accessed.

Cannulation starts with typical Seldinger insertion of a guidewire into the femoral vein and artery. Placeholder lines in the form of a 5-Fr arterial and 9-Fr venous sheath are used for blood pressure monitoring and medication administration while the decision to initiate ECMO is in question. Once the decision to initiate ECMO has been confirmed, the longer (150 cm) guidewires are inserted through the placeholder sheaths. Some long guidewires are floppy and some are stiff. There is some advantage to the stiff wires as they resist kinking; however, overly aggressive line/dilator/cannula insertion must be avoided. The mantra of "slow is smooth, smooth is fast" should be repeated frequently.

During cardiac arrest, differentiation of arterial from venous blood is difficult, and with chest compressions, ultrasound images can be misinterpreted. This makes confirmation of wires in the correct vessels difficult but still paramount. Fluoroscopy is ideal but not usually accessible. Ultrasound of the femoral vessels, inferior vena cava (IVC) and aorta or an abdominal radiograph after long wire insertion can be helpful. Once wires are in place and before insertion of the cannulas, a heparin bolus is administered.

Over the long guidewires, serial dilation is necessary to enlarge the venotomy and arteriotomy to the appropriate cannula size. For adult ECPR, arterial cannulas are typically between 15 and 19 Fr and venous are between 19 and 25 Fr. After dilation, the cannulas are inserted. Ideally the tip of the venous cannula sits at the IVC/right atrial junction and the arterial cannula will sit in the common iliac or distal aorta (Video 1).

Once cannulas are inserted, clamps are placed after removal of the internal obturator and guidewire. The cannulas are then connected to the circuit using the underwater seal technique in which continuous crystalloid is poured over the top to ensure no air bubbles are in the circuit (Video 2).

Before circuit initiation, the circuit is inspected to ensure it is air free and the sweep gas is set at a 1:1 ratio with the targeted blood flow (~4 L/min). Initiation occurs with removal of the clamp on the venous tubing of the circuit, increasing the RPMs to ensure no backflow, and removal of the arterial clamp on the circuit tubing (Video 3). RPMs should be increased to achieve a flow of 3 to 4 L/min.

On ECPR initiation, "chatter" is commonly encountered where the tubing shakes or jolts (Video 4). This is caused by inadequate pump preload manifest by a cyclic "suck down" of the drainage cannula onto the endothelium of the vena cava generating excessively negative suction pressures, followed by release once central venous blood pools. This should be treated by decreasing the RPMs and administering volume, for example, crystalloid or blood, as the cause is commonly hypovolemia. Tension pneumothorax, tamponade, and abdominal compartment syndrome can also cause chatter and should be ruled out if it persists.

POST EXTRACORPOREAL MEMBRANE OXYGENATION INITIATION MANAGEMENT IN THE EMERGENCY DEPARTMENT

Once ECMO has been initiated for ECPR, the provider should first visualize the circuit. The venous drainage blood should be dark and arterial return blood should be bright. If not, troubleshooting may involve confirming correct vessel cannulation and double-checking sweep gas settings and connections (**Fig. 7**).

Second, the provider should reassess the patient's rhythm. If the patient is in ventricular fibrillation, repeat defibrillation after a few minutes with a perfusing MAP. It is important to have an ejecting left ventricle (LV) on ECMO to prevent LV distention.

Third, a right radial arterial line should be inserted. This allows accurate measurement of the MAP, especially if the patient has nonpulsatile blood flow. Commonly, vasopressors, transfusion of blood, and/or crystalloid infusion are necessary. As with all patients on MCS, the MAP goal for an ECMO patient is typically 60 to 80 mm Hg. The MAP must be high enough to perfuse organs and low enough to avoid excessive afterload for the native heart and ECMO centrifugal pump. An arterial blood gas (ABG) from the right radial arterial line should be sent to determine if native circulation is sending poorly oxygenated blood to the coronaries and brain, that is, differential oxygenation or north-south syndrome. In this case, hypoxemia should be corrected with the ventilator. The ABG is also used to adjust the sweep gas flow rate.

Fourth, most patients should be started on an inotrope to prevent LV distention. This is especially important if the pulse pressure is narrow, that is, less than 10 mm Hg, or an echocardiogram reveals that the LV is distended and the aortic valve is not opening. If the distended LV does not eject, this will lead to myocardial ischemia and pulmonary edema, as well as stasis of blood, which leads to intracardiac clot.[39,40] If LV distention is not improved with an inotrope, an LV vent, such as an Impella (Abiomed, Danvers, MA), intra-aortic balloon pump, or atrial septostomy may be needed.[41]

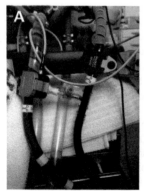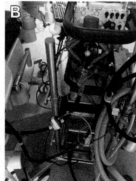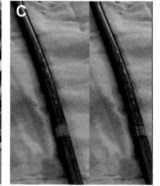

Fig. 7. (*A*) In a correctly functioning circuit, the drainage tubing is dark red and the return tubing is bright red. (*B*) If the ML is not functioning, most commonly due to a sweep gas disconnection, both drainage and return tubing are dark red. (*C*) If both drainage and return tubing are bright red, they may both be located in arteries or veins.

Important next steps in the process include the initiation of targeted temperature management and placement of a distal perfusion catheter in an artery in the leg with the arterial return cannula to prevent leg ischemia.[42] Clinicians should also evaluate for the etiology of the arrest and initiate appropriate treatment, such as transfer to the cardiac catheterization laboratory for acute coronary syndrome.[43,44]

SUMMARY

Indications
- ECMO, also called extracorporeal life support (ECLS), is a form of mechanical life support for the lungs and/or heart
  - VV ECMO provides pulmonary bypass for respiratory failure
  - VA ECMO provides cardiac and pulmonary bypass for cardiac failure with or without respiratory failure
  - ECPR uses VA ECMO for patients in cardiac arrest
    - Patients in cardiac arrest are potential candidates for ECPR if they have the following:
      - Reversible cause of arrest
      - Witnessed arrest
      - Bystander cardiopulmonary resuscitation (CPR)
      - Total chest compression time of less than 60 minutes
      - No known preexisting terminal illness
  - When running an ECPR code, care must be taken to continue high-quality traditional CPR in addition to ECMO initiation

Procedure
- Initiation of ECMO is divided into 3 stages:
  - Stage I: femoral and arterial sheaths are inserted into the femoral vessels and used for medication administration and hemodynamic monitoring while ECMO candidacy is determined
  - Stage II: if the patient is determined to be an ECMO candidate, the arterial and vascular sheaths are replaced with larger ECMO cannulas and connected to the primed ECMO circuit
  - Stage III: ECMO pump flow initiation

Postprocedure
- Post pump initiation considerations include the following:
  - Early right radial ABG and pressure monitoring
  - Defibrillate persistent ventricular fibrillation
  - Manage vasopressors and volume expanders based on arterial pressure tracings
  - Use the heat exchanger for therapeutic hypothermia
  - Start an inotrope to prevent LV distention
  - Early coronary revascularization in the cardiac catheterization laboratory for suspected acute coronary syndrome
  - Plan for distal perfusion catheter insertion

ECMO provides heart and/or lung bypass for the patient with severe cardiopulmonary failure. ECPR uses VA ECMO to restore perfusion in the patient with refractory cardiac arrest and can be deployed in the emergency department. Successful ECPR requires a well-rehearsed protocol with clear team-member roles to facilitate high-quality cardiac arrest resuscitation and a staged approach to vascular access, cannula insertion, and circuit initiation. Patient selection criteria for ECMO should be clear and predetermined and usually includes a witnessed arrest, bystander

CPR, a reasonable down time, and no known preexisting terminal illnesses. Post-ECMO circuit initiation critical care is crucial to ensure adequate perfusion pressure, gas exchange, perfusing rhythm, LV unloading, distal leg perfusion, therapeutic hypothermia, and steps to treat the underlying cause of arrest. Current evidence suggests a substantial benefit to ECPR compared with traditional ACLS for patients with refractory cardiac arrest; however, data are limited given lack of randomized trials.

DISCLOSURE

The authors have nothing to disclose.

SUPPLEMENTARY DATA

Supplementary data related to this article can be found online at https://doi.org/10.1016/j.emc.2020.06.015.

REFERENCES

1. Stub D, Bernard S, Pellegrino V, et al. Refractory cardiac arrest treated with mechanical CPR, hypothermia, ECMO and early reperfusion (the CHEER trial). Resuscitation 2015;86:88–94.
2. Sakamoto T, Morimura N, Nagao K, et al. Extracorporeal cardiopulmonary resuscitation versus conventional cardiopulmonary resuscitation in adults with out-of-hospital cardiac arrest: a prospective observational study. Resuscitation 2014;85(6):762–8.
3. Lamhaut L, Hutin A, Puymirat E, et al. A pre-hospital extracorporeal cardio pulmonary resuscitation (ECPR) strategy for treatment of refractory out hospital cardiac arrest: an observational study and propensity analysis. Resuscitation 2017;117:109–17.
4. Johnson NJ, Acker M, Hsu CH, et al. Extracorporeal life support as rescue strategy for out-of-hospital and emergency department cardiac arrest. Resuscitation 2014;85(11):1527–32.
5. Shinar Z, Plantmason L, Reynolds J, et al. Emergency physician-initiated resuscitative extracorporeal membrane oxygenation. J Emerg Med 2019;56(6):666–73.
6. Yannopoulos D, Bartos JA, Martin C, et al. Minnesota Resuscitation Consortium's advanced perfusion and reperfusion cardiac life support strategy for out-of-hospital refractory ventricular fibrillation. J Am Heart Assoc 2016;5(6):1–11.
7. Extracorporeal Life Support Organization - ECMO and ECLS > Resources > Guidelines. Available at: https://www.elso.org/Resources/Guidelines.aspx. Accessed December 27, 2019.
8. Krueger K, Schmutz A, Zieger B, et al. Venovenous extracorporeal membrane oxygenation with prophylactic subcutaneous anticoagulation only: an observational study in more than 60 patients. Artif Organs 2017;41(2):186–92.
9. Brogan TV, Thiagarajan RR, Rycus PT, et al. Extracorporeal membrane oxygenation in adults with severe respiratory failure: a multi-center database. Intensive Care Med 2009;35(12):2105–14.
10. Pranikoff T, Hirschl RB, Steimle CN, et al. Mortality is directly related to the duration of mechanical ventilation before the initiation of extracorporeal life support for severe respiratory failure. Crit Care Med 1997;25(1):28–32.
11. Schmidt M, Zogheib E, Rozé H, et al. The PRESERVE mortality risk score and analysis of long-term outcomes after extracorporeal membrane oxygenation for

severe acute respiratory distress syndrome. Intensive Care Med 2013;39(10): 1704–13.

12. Schmidt M, Bailey M, Sheldrake J, et al. Predicting survival after extracorporeal membrane oxygenation for severe acute respiratory failure: The Respiratory Extracorporeal Membrane Oxygenation Survival Prediction (RESP) score. Am J Respir Crit Care Med 2014;189(11):1374–82.

13. Grunau B, Reynolds J, Scheuermeyer F, et al. Relationship between Time-to-ROSC and survival in out-of-hospital cardiac arrest ECPR candidates: when is the best time to consider transport to hospital? Prehosp Emerg Care 2016; 20(5):615–22.

14. Otani T, Sawano H, Natsukawa T, et al. Low-flow time is associated with a favorable neurological outcome in out-of-hospital cardiac arrest patients resuscitated with extracorporeal cardiopulmonary resuscitation. J Crit Care 2018;48: 15–20.

15. Reynolds JC, Grunau BE, Elmer J, et al. Prevalence, natural history, and time-dependent outcomes of a multi-center North American cohort of out-of-hospital cardiac arrest extracorporeal CPR candidates. Resuscitation 2017; 117(–):24–31.

16. Chen YS, Lin JW, Yu HY, et al. Cardiopulmonary resuscitation with assisted extracorporeal life-support versus conventional cardiopulmonary resuscitation in adults with in-hospital cardiac arrest: an observational study and propensity analysis. Lancet 2008;372(9638):554–61.

17. Haas NL, Coute RA, Hsu CH, et al. Descriptive analysis of extracorporeal cardiopulmonary resuscitation following out-of-hospital cardiac arrest-An ELSO registry study. Resuscitation 2017;119:56–62.

18. Matsuoka Y, Ikenoue T, Hata N, et al. Hospitals' extracorporeal cardiopulmonary resuscitation capabilities and outcomes in out-of-hospital cardiac arrest: a population-based study. Resuscitation 2019;136:85–92.

19. Patricio D, Peluso L, Brasseur A, et al. Comparison of extracorporeal and conventional cardiopulmonary resuscitation: a retrospective propensity score matched study. Crit Care 2019;23(1). https://doi.org/10.1186/s13054-019-2320-1.

20. Bartos JA, Carlson K, Carlson C, et al. Surviving refractory out-of-hospital ventricular fibrillation cardiac arrest: Critical care and extracorporeal membrane oxygenation management. Resuscitation 2018;132:47–55.

21. Meneveau N, Guillon B, Planquette B, et al. Outcomes after extracorporeal membrane oxygenation for the treatment of high-risk pulmonary embolism: a multicentre series of 52 cases. Eur Heart J 2018;39(47):4196–204.

22. Ouweneel DM, Schotborgh JV, Limpens J, et al. Extracorporeal life support during cardiac arrest and cardiogenic shock: a systematic review and meta-analysis. Intensive Care Med 2016;42(12):1922–34.

23. Hryniewicz K, Sandoval Y, Samara M, et al. Percutaneous venoarterial extracorporeal membrane oxygenation for refractory cardiogenic shock is associated with improved short- and long-term survival. ASAIO J 2016;62(4):397–402.

24. Sun T, Guy A, Sidhu A, et al. Veno-arterial extracorporeal membrane oxygenation (VA-ECMO) for emergency cardiac support. J Crit Care 2018;44:31–8.

25. Muller G, Flecher E, Lebreton G, et al. The ENCOURAGE mortality risk score and analysis of long-term outcomes after VA-ECMO for acute myocardial infarction with cardiogenic shock. Intensive Care Med 2016;42(3):370–8.

26. Lorusso R, Centofanti P, Gelsomino S, et al. Venoarterial extracorporeal membrane oxygenation for acute fulminant myocarditis in adult patients: a 5-year multi-institutional experience. Ann Thorac Surg 2016;101(3):919–26.

27. Aso S, Matsui H, Fushimi K, et al. In-hospital mortality and successful weaning from venoarterial extracorporeal membrane oxygenation: analysis of 5,263 patients using a national inpatient database in Japan. Crit Care 2016;20(1):1–7.

28. Chenoweth JA, Colby DK, Sutter ME, et al. Massive diltiazem and metoprolol overdose rescued with extracorporeal life support. Am J Emerg Med 2017; 35(10):1581.e3-5.

29. Park TK, Yang JH, Jeon K, et al. Extracorporeal membrane oxygenation for refractory septic shock in adults. Eur J Cardiothorac Surg 2014;47(2):e68–74.

30. Falk L, Hultman J, Broman LM. Extracorporeal membrane oxygenation for septic shock. Crit Care Med 2019;47(8):1097–105.

31. Park TK, Yang JH, Jeon K, et al. Extracorporeal life support for adults with refractory septic shock. Crit Care Med 2018;47(8):1097–105.

32. Rab T, Ratanapo S, Kern KB, et al. Cardiac shock care centers: JACC review topic of the week. J Am Coll Cardiol 2018;72(16):1972–80.

33. Yeo HJ, Kim D, Jeon D, et al. Extracorporeal membrane oxygenation for life-threatening asthma refractory to mechanical ventilation: analysis of the Extracorporeal Life Support Organization registry. Crit Care 2017;21(1):297.

34. Peek GJ, Mugford M, Tiruvoipati R, et al. Efficacy and economic assessment of conventional ventilatory support versus extracorporeal membrane oxygenation for severe adult respiratory failure (CESAR): a multicentre randomised controlled trial. Lancet 2009;374(9698):1351–63.

35. Pham T, Combes A, Roze H, et al. Extracorporeal membrane oxygenation for pandemic influenza a(h1n1)-induced acute respiratory distress syndrome a cohort study and propensity-matched analysis. Am J Respir Crit Care Med 2013;187(3):276–82.

36. Noah MA, Peek GJ, Finney SJ, et al. Referral to an extracorporeal membrane oxygenation center and mortality among patients with severe 2009 influenza A(H1N1). JAMA 2011;306(15):1659–68.

37. The Australia and New Zealand Extracorporeal Membrane Oxygenation (ANZ ECMO) Influenza Investigators. ECMO with H1N1. JAMA 2011;302(17): 1888–95.

38. Goligher EC, Tomlinson G, Hajage D, et al. Extracorporeal membrane oxygenation for severe acute respiratory distress syndrome and posterior probability of mortality benefit in a post hoc bayesian analysis of a randomized clinical trial. JAMA 2018;320(21):2251–9.

39. Truby LK, Takeda K, Mauro C, et al. Incidence and implications of left ventricular distention during venoarterial extracorporeal membrane oxygenation support. ASAIO J 2017;63(3):257–65.

40. Williams B, Bernstein W. Review of venoarterial extracorporeal membrane oxygenation and development of intracardiac thrombosis in adult cardiothoracic patients. J Extra Corpor Technol 2016;48(4):162–7.

41. Russo JJ, Aleksova N, Pitcher I, et al. Left ventricular unloading during extracorporeal membrane oxygenation in patients with cardiogenic shock. J Am Coll Cardiol 2019;73(6):654–62.

42. Kaufeld T, Beckmann E, Ius F, et al. Risk factors for critical limb ischemia in patients undergoing femoral cannulation for venoarterial extracorporeal membrane oxygenation: Is distal limb perfusion a mandatory approach? Perfusion 2019; 34(6):453–9.

43. Lamhaut L, Tea V, Raphalen JH, et al. Coronary lesions in refractory out of hospital cardiac arrest (OHCA) treated by extra corporeal pulmonary resuscitation (ECPR). Resuscitation 2018;126:154–9.
44. Yannopoulos D, Bartos JA, Raveendran G, et al. Coronary artery disease in patients with out-of-hospital refractory ventricular fibrillation cardiac arrest. J Am Coll Cardiol 2017;70(9):1109–17.

UNITED STATES POSTAL SERVICE ®
Statement of Ownership, Management, and Circulation
(All Periodicals Publications Except Requester Publications)

1. Publication Title	2. Publication Number	3. Filing Date
EMERGENCY MEDICINE CLINICS OF NORTH AMERICA	000 – 714	9/18/2020

4. Issue Frequency	5. Number of Issues Published Annually	6. Annual Subscription Price
FEB, MAY, AUG, NOV	4	$352.00

7. Complete Mailing Address of Known Office of Publication (Not printer) (Street, city, county, state, and ZIP+4®)

ELSEVIER INC.
230 Park Avenue, Suite 800
New York, NY 10169

Contact Person
Malathi Samayan

Telephone (Include area code)
91-44-4299-4507

8. Complete Mailing Address of Headquarters or General Business Office of Publisher (Not printer)

ELSEVIER INC.
230 Park Avenue, Suite 800
New York, NY 10169

9. Full Names and Complete Mailing Addresses of Publisher, Editor, and Managing Editor (Do not leave blank)

Publisher (Name and complete mailing address)

Dolores Meloni, ELSEVIER INC.
1600 JOHN F KENNEDY BLVD. SUITE 1800
PHILADELPHIA, PA 19103-2899

Editor (Name and complete mailing address)

Colleen Dietzler, ELSEVIER INC.
1600 JOHN F KENNEDY BLVD. SUITE 1800
PHILADELPHIA, PA 19103-2899

Managing Editor (Name and complete mailing address)

PATRICK MANLEY, ELSEVIER INC.
1600 JOHN F KENNEDY BLVD. SUITE 1800
PHILADELPHIA, PA 19103-2899

10. Owner (Do not leave blank. If the publication is owned by a corporation, give the name and address of the corporation immediately followed by the names and addresses of all stockholders owning or holding 1 percent or more of the total amount of stock. If not owned by a corporation, give the names and addresses of the individual owners. If owned by a partnership or other unincorporated firm, give its name and address as well as those of each individual owner. If the publication is published by a nonprofit organization, give its name and address.)

Full Name	Complete Mailing Address
WHOLLY OWNED SUBSIDIARY OF REED/ELSEVIER US HOLDINGS	1600 JOHN F KENNEDY BLVD. SUITE 1800 PHILADELPHIA, PA 19103-2899

11. Known Bondholders, Mortgagees, and Other Security Holders Owning or Holding 1 Percent or More of Total Amount of Bonds, Mortgages, or Other Securities. If none, check box ▶ ☐ None

Full Name	Complete Mailing Address
N/A	

12. Tax Status (For completion by nonprofit organizations authorized to mail at nonprofit rates) (Check one)
The purpose, function, and nonprofit status of this organization and the exempt status for federal income tax purposes:

☒ Has Not Changed During Preceding 12 Months
☐ Has Changed During Preceding 12 Months (Publisher must submit explanation of change with this statement)

PS Form 3526, July 2014 [Page 1 of 4 (see instructions page 4)] PSN: 7530-01-000-9931   PRIVACY NOTICE: See our privacy policy on www.usps.com.

---

13. Publication Title	14. Issue Date for Circulation Data Below
EMERGENCY MEDICINE CLINICS OF NORTH AMERICA	MAY 2020

15. Extent and Nature of Circulation			Average No. Copies Each Issue During Preceding 12 Months	No. Copies of Single Issue Published Nearest to Filing Date
a. Total Number of Copies (Net press run)			250	219
b. Paid Circulation (By Mail and Outside the Mail)	(1)	Mailed Outside-County Paid Subscriptions Stated on PS Form 3541 (Include paid distribution above nominal rate, advertiser's proof copies, and exchange copies)	136	84
	(2)	Mailed In-County Paid Subscriptions Stated on PS Form 3541 (Include paid distribution above nominal rate, advertiser's proof copies, and exchange copies)	0	0
	(3)	Paid Distribution Outside the Mails Including Sales Through Dealers and Carriers, Street Vendors, Counter Sales, and Other Paid Distribution Outside USPS®	58	53
	(4)	Paid Distribution by Other Classes of Mail Through the USPS (e.g., First-Class Mail®)	0	0
c. Total Paid Distribution (Sum of 15b (1), (2), (3), and (4))		▶	194	137
d. Free or Nominal Rate Distribution (By Mail and Outside the Mail)	(1)	Free or Nominal Rate Outside-County Copies included on PS Form 3541	39	65
	(2)	Free or Nominal Rate In-County Copies included on PS Form 3541	0	0
	(3)	Free or Nominal Rate Copies Mailed at Other Classes Through the USPS (e.g., First-Class Mail)	0	0
	(4)	Free or Nominal Rate Distribution Outside the Mail (Carriers or other means)	0	0
e. Total Free or Nominal Rate Distribution (Sum of 15d (1), (2), (3) and (4))		▶	39	65
f. Total Distribution (Sum of 15c and 15e)		▶	233	202
g. Copies not Distributed (See Instructions to Publishers #4 (page #3))		▶	17	17
h. Total (Sum of 15f and g)		▶	250	219
i. Percent Paid (15c divided by 15f times 100)		▶	83.26%	67.82%

* If you are claiming electronic copies, go to line 16 on page 3. If you are not claiming electronic copies, skip to line 17 on page 3.

16. Electronic Copy Circulation	Average No. Copies Each Issue During Preceding 12 Months	No. Copies of Single Issue Published Nearest to Filing Date
a. Paid Electronic Copies ▶		
b. Total Paid Print Copies (Line 15c) + Paid Electronic Copies (Line 16a) ▶		
c. Total Print Distribution (Line 15f) + Paid Electronic Copies (Line 16a) ▶		
d. Percent Paid (Both Print & Electronic Copies) (16b divided by 16c × 100) ▶		

☒ I certify that 50% of all my distributed copies (electronic and print) are paid above a nominal price.

17. Publication of Statement of Ownership

☒ If the publication is a general publication, publication of this statement is required. Will be printed in the NOVEMBER 2020 issue of this publication.   ☐ Publication not required.

18. Signature and Title of Editor, Publisher, Business Manager, or Owner	Date
Malathi Samayan - Distribution Controller *Malathi Samayan*	9/18/2020

I certify that all information furnished on this form is true and complete. I understand that anyone who furnishes false or misleading information on this form or who omits material or information requested on the form may be subject to criminal sanctions (including fines and imprisonment) and/or civil sanctions (including civil penalties).

PS Form 3526, July 2014 (Page 2 of 4)   PRIVACY NOTICE: See our privacy policy on www.usps.com

Moving?

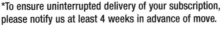

Make sure your subscription moves with you!

To notify us of your new address, find your **Clinics Account Number** (located on your mailing label above your name), and contact customer service at:

Email: journalscustomerservice-usa@elsevier.com

800-654-2452 (subscribers in the U.S. & Canada)
314-447-8871 (subscribers outside of the U.S. & Canada)

Fax number: 314-447-8029

Elsevier Health Sciences Division
Subscription Customer Service
3251 Riverport Lane
Maryland Heights, MO 63043

*To ensure uninterrupted delivery of your subscription, please notify us at least 4 weeks in advance of move.